Asylum Doctor

For Layton McCurdy,
Friend, colleague,
and scholar,
With appreciation
and warm regards,
Charles S. Bryan

July 1, 2014

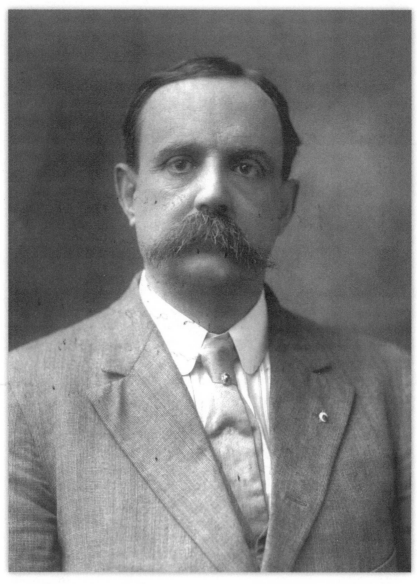

James Woods Babcock (April 11, 1856–March 3, 1922).
Courtesy: Arthur St. J. Simons II.

Asylum
Doctor

*James Woods Babcock
and the Red Plague of Pellagra*

CHARLES S. BRYAN

The University of South Carolina Press

© 2014 University of South Carolina

Published by the University of South Carolina Press
Columbia, South Carolina 29208

www.sc.edu/uscpress

Manufactured in the United States of America

23 22 21 20 19 18 17 16 15 14   10 9 8 7 6 5 4 3 2 1

Library of Congress Cataloging-in-Publication Data can be found
at http://catalog.loc.gov/.

This book was printed on a recycled paper with 30 percent
postconsumer waste content.

For Shane Mull, Arthur Simons, and Robert Walkup

In many ways, the Old South disappeared along with pellagra.

—*Arturo Warman, 2003*

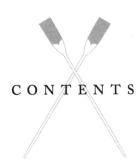

CONTENTS

ILLUSTRATIONS

Tables

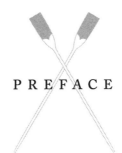

PREFACE

THIS BOOK TRACES BACK TO 1944–1946 when I was a toddler living with relatives in Anderson, South Carolina, where my uncle ran a textile mill. A silver bowl of tan-colored tablets sat on the mahogany dining table. I snitched them by the handful. I loved the taste—brewer's yeast.

When my father came back from the war we returned to Columbia, where he resumed his dermatology practice at 1515 Bull Street. The older boys in the neighborhood teased us incessantly: "Bull Street . . . Bull Street!" When I went off to grammar school I kept it a secret that Dad's office was on Bull Street.

During the summer of 1961 my best friend was Arthur Simons. I never went to his house without admiring a pair of crossed racing oars. The inscriptions marked races won and Arthur said they'd been his grandfather's.

Unwittingly, I followed a path blazed by the oarsman.

I went north, rowed on the Charles River as an undergraduate (albeit in a wherry, not a racing shell), studied medicine, and, after missing out on my era's racial excitement (the dismantling of Jim Crow), returned home to spend my career within a three-mile radius of where the oarsman spent his— the old asylum on Bull Street and, later, the Waverley Sanitarium. I learned more about the oarsman through articles by my late friends William S. Hall ("Psychiatrist, Humanitarian, and Scholar: James Woods Babcock, M.D.") and S. Hope Sandifer ("Pellagra in South Carolina"). Like the oarsman I found myself, because of my chosen medical specialty, in the vanguard against a mysterious, highly-lethal, new disease (HIV/AIDS) that affected nearly every organ system and caused among the general public great concern, sometimes bordering on hysteria. Like him I started a task force, taught my colleagues and the public, arranged for care of the disadvantaged in central South Carolina (through a federal grant), and became concerned especially for African American women, who suffered disproportionately. Also like him I rose to a senior administrative position for which I was unprepared, knew the frustrations of titular authority without real power over other doctors, proved more adept at tracing the history of institutional problems than at solving them, and sublimated by turning to history and biography.

In 1998 Shane Mull, then a first-year medical student and now Doctor Mull, approached me about a summer project on Babcock, the oarsman. Could Babcock claim priority for recognizing epidemic pellagra in the United States? Babcock said no. Whenever someone gave him such credit, as the governor of South Carolina once did before a large audience, he immediately deferred to others. And he would tell us that recognizing a full-blown case of pellagra does not count for much—it's an easy call if you've read a description of the disease.

We next examined whether Babcock understood the dietary-deficiency hypothesis before 1914, when the U.S. Public Health Service turned its pellagra effort over to Joseph Goldberger, the story's eventual hero. Babcock reminded us that for nearly two centuries, beginning with the Spaniard Gaspar Casál, nearly all students of pellagra advocated better diet. And Babcock never speculated about causation except for a general sympathy with the "Zeists" (those who thought corn had a lot to do with it). He had little if any training in research and was a busy asylum superintendent. I eventually learned, however, that he was among the first to see the analogy between pellagra and two other vitamin-deficiency diseases, beriberi and scurvy.

Shane Mull did an outstanding job during the summer of 1999 and a subsequent elective rotation but graduated from medical school, finished a residency, started a family, and now practices emergency medicine and serves as a lieutenant colonel in the National Guard. Dr. Charles N. Still, the third member of our band, dropped out for other pursuits. I was left staring at the prospect of a full-length biography involving extensive primary and secondary sources. Was the project worthwhile?

I ultimately said yes for several reasons.

First, three distinguished historians—Edward Beardsley of the University of South Carolina, Peter McCandless of the College of Charleston, and Todd Savitt of East Carolina University—all felt Babcock deserved a biography. He was South Carolina's first trained psychiatrist or "alienist," an asylum superintendent during a difficult time in the history of asylums, a conspicuous public figure, and, shortly after his death, one of two South Carolina physicians listed in the *Dictionary of American Biography*.

Second, Babcock's leadership in the American response to pellagra is well known. All contemporaries credited him for starting and maintaining a National Association for the Study of Pellagra. Its three triennial meetings at a most unlikely venue, Babcock's woefully underfunded South Carolina State Hospital for the Insane, became milestones in the conquest of pellagra: a call-to-arms (1909), the introduction of the vitamin-deficiency hypothesis on American soil (1912), and the announcement of Joseph Goldberger's breakthrough (1915). As opposition arose to Goldberger's inconvenient truth that the root cause was southern poverty, Babcock tried but failed to preserve the cooperation and goodwill that had theretofore characterized the American pellagra effort. The consequences were tragic for thousands of Americans.

Finally, no previous book has dealt exclusively with the pre-Goldberger era of pellagra in the United States (that is, between 1907 and 1914). This era, I suggest, constitutes a significant chapter in the coming-of-age of American medical science. Americans felt deep inferiority to Europeans. English was not yet the *lingua franca* for scientific discourse. The extent to which a patchwork coalition of practicing physicians, asylum superintendents, and local health officials established an American competence in a newly recognized disease and chased its cause had no precedent. Social historians have written extensively about reactions to Goldberger's inconvenient truth, but less attention has been paid to what happened before February 1914, when Goldberger boarded a southbound train.

A story-within-the-story concerns the charismatic European Louis Sambon who, committed to his creative idea that flies of the genus *Simulium* transmitted pellagra, led Americans down a primrose path. My principal thesis holds that Sambon's obsession led to the Thompson-McFadden Commission, which gave health officials, politicians, and others a "scientific" counterpoint to the dietary-deficiency hypothesis. Goldberger's need to refute the Thompson-McFadden Commission's conclusions probably delayed his ultimate discovery: the preventative and curative power of brewer's yeast. Thousands died as a result.

As with any project of this scope there were many helpers. I am indebted especially to Peter McCandless, who read and criticized early drafts, and to Ed Beardsley, who criticized the penultimate draft. I am indebted to Allen Stokes, Henry Fulmer, and their staff at the South Caroliniana Library at the University of South Carolina, Columbia, and to Susan Hoffius and her

staff at the Waring Historical Library at the Medical University of South
Carolina, Charleston. Audrey Graft, an honors student at the University of
South Carolina, helped catalog the Babcock Papers at the South Caroliniana
Library. (The Babcock materials at the Waring Historical library have now
been catalogued by Susan Hoffius and her staff.) A second honors student,
Alina Arbuthnot, did research at the National Library of Medicine, and a
third, Taylor Turnbull, helped clean up loose ends. I owe numerous favors
to the staffs of the South Carolina Department of Archives and History,
the South Carolina State Library, and the National Archives and Records
Administration in College Park, Maryland. I am indebted to librarians,
archivists, and staff at Clemson University (Special Collections, University Libraries), the University of North Carolina, Chapel Hill (Southern
Historical Collection, Wilson Library), New York-Presbyterian/Weill
Cornell Medical College, New York (Medical Center Archives), the Uni-
versity of Virginia (Claude Moore Health Sciences Library), the Harvard
Medical Library in the Francis A. Countway Library of Medicine, Boston,
the Sheppard Pratt Health System, Baltimore (Robert W. and Diane E.
Gibson Museum), Phillips Exeter Academy in Exeter, New Hampshire,
the London School of Hygiene and Tropical Medicine, the Boston Public
Library, the New York Academy of Medicine, the National Library of
Medicine, the Lillian & Clarence de la Chapelle Medical Archives of the
New York University Health Sciences Libraries, and the archives of Harvard
University and the University of Illinois. For insights into specific persons
I thank Arthur St. J. Simons II and the late James B. Meriwether (James
Woods Babcock, their grandfather), Edouard L. Desrochers (Babcock's
years at Phillips Exeter Academy), B. Walter Taylor Jr. and Edmund Taylor
(Benjamin Walter Taylor and Julius Heyward Taylor), Anne Christensen
Pollitzer (Neils Christensen Jr.), Eddie Williams Sr. (Frederick Williams),
Joan Echtenkamp Klein (Claude Lavinder), John M. Bryan (Robert Mills),
Uta Anderson (Eleanora Bennette Saunders), Harry M. Bayne (Henry
Bellaman), Gordon Cook (Sir Patrick Manson), Matthew Chipping (Louis
Sambon), Arlene Parr (George Zeller), Charles R. Roberts (Stewart R.
Roberts), and Michael Flannery (Carl Grote). I thank Paul R. Housley for
reviewing my account of the biochemistry and pharmacology of niacin and
Walter Edgar for insights into South Carolina history through the years.
Rebecca Wilson helped with the illustrations. I also thank as readers, in
addition to Peter McCandless and Ed Beardsley, E. A. Driggers, Elizabeth
Etheridge, Michael Jones, Woodrow Harris, and Shane Mull. I am deeply
indebted to Alexander Moore of the University of South Carolina Press for
encouragement and suggestions. I thank the South Carolina Department

of Mental Health for permission to explore the old asylum buildings. I thank the Waring Library Society for a generous subvention allowing the book to be offered at a reasonable price with more illustrations and fuller documentation than would otherwise be the case. Finally, I thank my wife, Donna, who has patiently endured this fifteen-year obsession with the old asylum on Bull Street, pellagra, and James Woods Babcock.

Brewer's yeast ... Bull Street ... a pair of racing oars—the South of today is a far cry from the South of my childhood just as the South of my childhood was a far cry from the South of the story that follows.

Charles S. Bryan
Columbia, South Carolina
November 2013

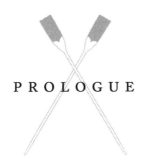

PROLOGUE

IN THE FALL OF 1908 Mildred Corley began to act strangely. She seemed distant. She neglected her children. She dressed poorly. She stared into space, heard voices, and talked to people who weren't there. Her family doctor sent her to the State Hospital for the Insane in Columbia. When relatives visited the next summer she barely recognized them, and vice versa. Her behavior had become even stranger. They commented on a sunburn-like rash on her neck and the backs of her hands. That winter she did not know them at all. She lay expressionless in bed and rarely spoke. She had frequent diarrhea and was getting bedsores. She died a few months later. The death certificate read, "Pellagra."

Pellagra. "Pel-LAY-gra," "pel-LAG-ra," and "pel-LAH-gra" are all acceptable pronunciations. Most Americans are dimly aware of it, if they've heard of it at all. Medical students memorize it as "the disease of 4Ds"—dermatitis, diarrhea, dementia, and death—caused by deficiency of niacin (vitamin B_3). They learn it as one of the classic vitamin-deficiency diseases, the others being scurvy, beriberi, rickets, and vitamin A deficiency.[1] By one estimate pellagra affected 250,000 Americans at its peak and caused about 7,000 deaths each year in the fifteen southern states.[2] Between 1907 and 1915, the period covered here, pellagra was a huge story in South Carolina and beyond. In 1910 Dr. Robert Wilson Jr., chairman of the State Board of Health, wrote that "no disease in the history of the State has ever aroused so much interest among the members of the medical profession and the laity"; in 1911 he called it "so prevalent that it forms a topic of conversation in the churches, in the streets, in the clubs and in the homes"; and in 1912 he added that it "menaces the industrial prosperity of South Carolina" by its toll on textile workers.[3] Mildred Corley was one of untold thousands of Americans who died of pellagra before 1937, when investigators at the University of Wisconsin identified the deficient vitamin, leading to its addition to foodstuffs.

The conquest of pellagra is commonly associated with a single name: Joseph Goldberger. In February 1914 Surgeon General Rupert Blue of the U.S. Public Health Service made Goldberger his chief pellagra investigator. Goldberger concluded within four months that the cause was inadequate, monotonous diet, not infection as many people thought.[4] By the fall of 1915 Goldberger had both prevented and caused pellagra by dietary manipulation alone. Public health officials, politicians, and others rejected the dietary explanation, especially since it indicted southern poverty. Goldberger devoted the rest of his life to pellagra and, before his death from cancer, found an inexpensive way to prevent and treat the disease: brewer's yeast. After Goldberger's ashes were scattered into the Potomac River on January 18, 1929, Surgeon General Hugh Cumming wrote that "the disease which baffled the best medical talent of Europe for two centuries had yielded well within a decade to the researches of one American scientist."[5]

The story is not so simple. In 1963 medical historian Owsei Temkin told the present author's class of first-year medical students: "Great discoveries are seldom the work of one person. There is usually something 'in the air,' so to speak." That same year historian of science Thomas Kuhn coined the term "paradigm shift" for his thesis that new theories arise when older theories make us insecure by failing to account for all the facts.[6] More recently Steven Johnson reviews what scholars call "the multiple"—a scientist goes public with a new idea only to find that others independently came up with the same idea—adding: "Good ideas are not conjured out of thin air; they are built out of a collection of existing parts."[7] Innovation springs "not from geniuses acting alone but from accumulated knowledge, constructive errors, and the 'information spillover' that emerges from collaborative settings."[8] However, the present author's goal is to burnish, not blemish, Goldberger's iconic image. Goldberger never told the story in quite the way it's been told to later generations. Goldberger, a great man and apparently a nice man as well, gave ample credit to others on both sides of the Atlantic.

When Goldberger went south in February 1914 the idea that faulty diet caused pellagra was very much "in the air," although it was not the most popular explanation at that time. The idea that pellagra was an infectious disease was relatively new. For nearly two centuries Europeans associated pellagra with monotonous, corn-based diets. In 1810 an Italian named

Marzari proposed that corn might *lack* something essential to good health. Goldberger's timing could not have been more propitious. In 1912, just two years before Goldberger became involved, Casimir Funk, a Polish-born chemist working in London, coined the term "vitamine" and suggested that pellagra, beriberi, and scurvy might all be vitamine-deficiency diseases. Funk's hypothesis did not go unnoticed.

This book focuses on the period between 1907 and 1914, or what might be called the pre-Goldberger era of pellagra in the United States. Before 1907 little had been written about pellagra in English and nothing in the United States aside from occasional case reports. William Osler, the most famous physician in the English-speaking world, stated flatly in his best-selling textbook that pellagra "has not been observed in the United States." According to Osler, pellagra occurred mainly in parts of Italy, Spain, and southern France, and was thought due "in some way with the use of maize [corn] which . . . is fermented or diseased."[9] By 1914 Americans had established a competence in the disease, sifted through an enormous body of contradictory facts and theories, and largely rejected the "spoiled corn" hypothesis. When Goldberger entered the fray the hypothesis *du jour* was that of a charismatic European doctor, Louis Sambon, who claimed pellagra was an infectious disease (perhaps caused by a protozoan parasite) transmitted by an insect (perhaps flies of the genus *Simulium*). Sadly, two relatively-well-funded groups of American researchers claimed their studies pointed away from faulty diet and toward an infectious cause. Less well-known is that some Americans, beginning in 1912, saw the analogy between pellagra and two better-known deficiency diseases—scurvy and beriberi—and aired Funk's new "vitamine" hypothesis as a plausible explanation.

At the center of the American response to pellagra was an unlikely doctor in an unlikely place: James Woods Babcock, superintendent of the South Carolina State Hospital for the Insane. In 1913 a Maine physician, for example, wrote: "Dr. Babcock of Columbia, S.C., who has drawn attention to the disease in this country more than any other man, tersely sums up the situation as follows: 'I think the deeper one gets into the pellagra problem, the less inclined he is to dogmatize about it.'"[10] Working with limited resources and spending his own money, Babcock became a national authority. Shy, self-effacing, and exquisitely sensitive to criticism, he never sought the limelight. Indeed, he was quick to focus it on others.

In brief, Babcock (1) verified that pellagra in South Carolina was the same disease that occurred in Italy; (2) helped sound the alarm that the United States had a major public health problem on its hands; (3) sponsored the first American conference on the disease, indeed the first conference in an

English-speaking country; (4) produced the first monograph on pellagra in English; (5) organized what became the National Association for the Study of Pellagra; and (6) coordinated that organization's triennial conferences. Those conferences, held in 1909, 1912, and 1915, all took place at the South Carolina State Hospital for the Insane in Columbia, where conditions were deplorable even by that era's standards.[11]

Each of the triennial conferences in Columbia became a turning point. The 1909 conference called attention to pellagra as a national problem, not just a southern problem, stimulated physicians throughout the United States, and resulted in Babcock obtaining assistance from the U.S. Public Health and Marine Hospital Service. The 1912 conference included the suggestion by Dr. Fleming Sandwith of London that pellagra might result from deficiency of an as-yet-undiscovered "vitamine." Comments by Blue, Babcock, and others confirm that the dietary-deficiency hypothesis was very much "in the air." By 1914 the tide of opinion ebbed away from the spoiled-corn hypothesis, but commitment to the infection hypothesis was far from universal. The 1915 conference featured Goldberger's breakthrough announcement. Tragically, the cooperation and goodwill that characterized the pre-Goldberger era vaporized as many people, especially southerners, refused to blame such a terrible disease on poverty and backwardness. It is perhaps unfortunate that Babcock, under pressure from South Carolina's Governor Coleman L. Blease, left public life in 1914 just as Goldberger began his heroic odyssey. Contact between the two men was limited, although they obviously liked and respected each other. There was little overlap between what might be called the "Babcock era" and the Goldberger era in the study of pellagra.

Babcock would almost certainly object to a book based on his work on pellagra. With characteristic modesty he downplayed his own contributions. Moreover, the years between 1907 and 1914 encompass but a brief period of a useful and varied life. He would want us to remember him, if at all, as an "asylum doctor," a superintendent during a difficult time and at a difficult place. After Babcock's resignation in 1914, a fellow superintendent wrote: "In South Carolina, its one state hospital, through legislative and public indifference and neglect, has become a disgrace to the commonwealth. . . . The recent state administration . . . made matters still worse by removing Dr. Babcock" who had worked "amid most disheartening conditions, appealing without success for better financial support, reciting over and over the needs of the institution, to the apparently deaf ears of a legislature which in 1910 ignored the report of its own committee."[12]

To what extent, if any, should Babcock be held accountable for deplorable conditions at the South Carolina State Hospital for the Insane at the turn of the twentieth century? Readers will want to draw their own conclusions.

Let us begin these parallel stories: James Woods Babcock as an asylum doctor and James Woods Babcock as an early figure in the eventual conquest of pellagra. We can be reasonably certain that Mildred Corley and thousands like her would want to know more.

CHAPTER I

Jimmie

"To Fit Ourselves for Future Usefulness"

CHESTER, SOUTH CAROLINA, LATE EVENING OF FEBRUARY 16, 1865. A Confederate army surgeon holds up his eight-year-old son and points to a lit-up spot on the horizon. "Jimmie," the man says grimly, "that's Columbia burning."

The boy would transcend the mediocre primary and secondary schools of post-Civil War South Carolina by going north for 17 years. There he received the finest education to be had for his eventual career choice: Phillips Exeter Academy, Harvard College, Harvard Medical School, and the nation's premier private psychiatric facility, McLean Asylum. He would make his mark on that lit-up spot only to endure fireworks of a different nature.

A Chester Boyhood

Babcocks came to America from the south of England during the seventeenth century. They prospered especially in Rhode Island and Connecticut, the men often attending Yale College and becoming printers in Hartford or New Haven, Connecticut. During the War of 1812, one of them, William Rogers Babcock, left Yale and enlisted in the Navy.[1]

William Rogers Babcock jumped ship when chased by a British privateer and took refuge in Charleston, South Carolina, with an uncle who had gone there to establish a branch of the family printing business. The uncle returned to New Haven after the war, leaving William in charge. The business prospered and expanded, and by 1830 the firm of S. Babcock & Co., at Franklin's Head, King Street, besides printing, publishing, and bookselling offered for sale "Elegant Fancy Boxes, Harmonicas, Splendid Card Racks and Fire Screens, Battledoors and Shuttlecocks, Waterloo Rockets,

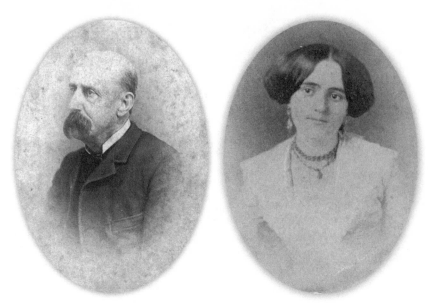

Sydney Eugene Babcock (1829–1892) and Margaret Woods Babcock (1834–1864).
Courtesy: Arthur St. J. Simons II.

Embroidery Boxes, Miniature Trunks, Youth's Walking Sticks, Elegant Snuff Boxes, Medals, Premiums, Ever Pointed Pencils, Albums, Souvenirs and Forget-Me-Nots for old and young, beautiful new Engravings, very suitable for presents, elegantly bound Miniature Bibles, Work and Dressing Boxes, Mantle Ornaments, Fancy Baskets, Busts of Napoleon, a great variety of new and suitable Books for the occasion, and other pretty things."[2] Following an attack of malaria, William sought recovery in the backcountry where he met and later married Elizabeth Jane Chisholm of Chester, South Carolina. They had three sons and two daughters. The second son, Sydney Eugene Babcock, studied medicine in New York City and then Paris, where he received his degree. He set up practice in Chester and married a Chester native, Margaret Faucette Woods. They had two sons, James Woods Babcock, who concerns us here, and William Frederick Babcock, known in the family as "Brooks."

The Civil War disrupted the Babcocks as it did nearly all Southern families. Sydney Babcock was among the 1,941 men of Chester who enlisted in the Confederate Army. He began as a private in the Sixth Regiment of South Carolina Volunteers and was in Charleston on April 11, 1861, when the first shots were fired at Fort Sumter. He spent most of 1862 and 1863 attending Confederate sick and wounded as an assistant surgeon in various hospitals in Richmond and Petersburg. In 1864 he transferred to the hospitals of Columbia, South Carolina, possibly because his wife had contracted tuberculosis, allegedly from caring for diseased soldiers. She died in September of that year. On April 1, 1865, the Confederacy in death throes, he was sent to Chester, where a railroad depot received carnage from battlefields throughout the South. He converted a large carriage factory into an infirmary, every cot of which was soon occupied. Survivors were sent back to their homes across the countryside. When the hospital closed in August 1865, Sydney Babcock returned to his medical practice and raising the boys as a single parent.[3]

The town of Chester arose between the Catawba and Broad Rivers in what had been a hilly no man's land between the Catawba Indians and the mighty Cherokee Nation. Chester prospered after the 1852 completion of the Charlotte and South Carolina Railroad and sustained only moderate damage during William Tecumseh Sherman's march through the Carolinas. However Southern whites were socially, politically, and economically devastated by the war.

Few details of Jimmie's boyhood survive except a story about his coming into a large supply of gunpowder. Shortly after the war a train broke down in Chester and for some reason two cars were left behind after a new locomotive

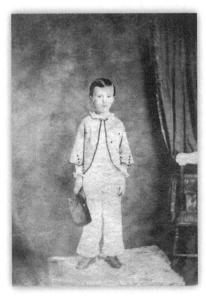
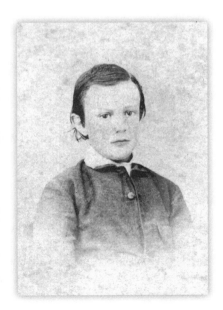

James Woods Babcock as a boy.
Courtesy: Arthur St. J. Simons II.

had been secured. Jimmie and his younger brother Brooks bored a hole into the floor of one of the cars and found it filled with gunpowder, which entertained them for months. A favorite trick was to place and then light a trail of gunpowder leading to the tail of a certain cat. (Tradition holds the animal was unharmed.) Leftover gunpowder from the Civil War suggests a metaphor for the Chester County of Jimmie's boyhood, as whites resisted Republican rule, federal laws, and the Freedmen's Bureau by every means at their disposal, including violence. In March 1870, a month before Jimmie's fourteenth birthday, a skirmish between hundreds of armed and mounted whites and more than a hundred armed blacks near Chester left at least five blacks and one white dead.[4]

Jimmie collected stamps and Native-American artifacts but found school unchallenging. Regional poverty, teacher shortages, and social unrest contributed to the sorry shape of public education, which had been spotty even before the war. He received his primary and secondary educations at the Chester Male Academy except for one year at a school near Brevard, North Carolina. Records at Chester Male Academy indicate good behavior and near-perfect attendance, and he invariably stood first in his class. He wrote essays on "Rice" and "Robinson Crusoe." He later lamented: "Most of my life has been spent in Chester, and I may say that with the exception of a year spent in the mountains of North Carolina my whole life up to my 18th year was wasted under the wretched school system of that town."[5]

Phillips Exeter Academy

To Jimmie Babcock's intellectual rescue came Edward Henry Strobel, a former childhood playmate whose Charleston family had sought refuge in Chester during the war. Strobel, who later became a professor of international law at Harvard and legal adviser to the King of Siam, suggested during a visit to Chester that Jimmie go north to Phillips Exeter Academy in Exeter, New Hampshire.

Despite or perhaps because of his meager education to that point, Babcock applied himself at Exeter and finished the academic year 1874–75 at the top of his class of forty-nine pupils. The next year he won the academy's highest honor, the Bancroft Scholarship with its $140 annual stipend. He stayed at Exeter four years, taking the prescribed curriculum heavily weighted toward Latin, Greek, history, and mathematics. He fit in well with fellow students. The only other southerner in his class, Thomas P. Ivy of Alabama, later wrote: "Jim Babcock was deservedly popular with everyone. His looks, his manners, his lovely black eyes, his soft, gentle voice, almost feminine, all gave to him an attraction that one could not escape."[6] Years later the academy's *Bulletin* described him as "a strikingly handsome man of exceptional charm, but modest and gentle," adding "no student was more popular."[7]

Babcock's nonconfrontational personality explains in part his popularity at Exeter and in later life. He avoided conflict and did not like loud, obstreperous, or aggressive behavior. A classmate later reminded him of his "bashful spirit."[8] He was nevertheless active in the Golden Branch, a debating society that met twice monthly for readings, declamations, and formal debates. Between 1875 and 1876 he debated on the negative "that the Eastern and Southern States do not offer as good an opening for a young man as the Western States," "that of the learned professions that of a physician is preferable," and "that the Lake Shore and Michigan Southern Railroad Company did take necessary precautions against incident at the time of the Ashtabula disaster." He debated on the affirmative "that dancing at public places has a bad effect on society" and "that immigration ought to be encouraged." The Golden Branch established the first library on the Phillips Exeter campus to which members contributed books. Jim Babcock later became an avid book collector, a bibliophile bordering on bibliomania.

In June 1877 Babcock was elected president of the Golden Branch for the next term. His inaugural address in September 1877 featured a sober reflection on education as preparation for a life of service: "We have all now had one or more years experience in the Academy and the longer this experience has been, the more will be expected of us; this each of us realizes, and so we have made resolutions to work more faithfully than before to fit ourselves for future usefulness." He continued: "From the schools we derive our literary culture, from our intercourse with each other we choose our friends and form the happy associations which are to last us through life; and here in the Golden Branch we take our first lessons in the practical part of our education. The school work is in the hands of experienced gentlemen, and we have only to do well what they see fit to give us, and that part will be accomplished. The rest of our culture is, in a great measure, in our hands, and with each of us individually rests the responsibility for making the best of it."

"Can not some, if not all of us," he concluded, "'be true to the dreams of our youth?'"[9] These sentiments evince Ralph Waldo Emerson's essay on "Self-Reliance," and in June 1878 Babcock had the honor of introducing Emerson, who addressed the Golden Branch on "Education."[10]

Although he had debated against the proposition "that of the learned professions, that of a physician is most preferable," Babcock decided at Exeter to go to medical school. Being by then 22 years of age, he was willing to go

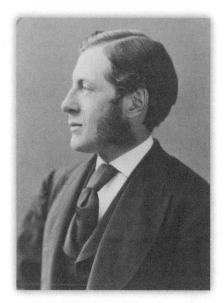

Charles William Eliot (1834–1926) became president of Harvard in 1869 and transformed the undergraduate curriculum and also Harvard Medical School. *Courtesy:* Harvard University Archives, HUP Eliot, Charles W. (22a).

directly from the preparatory school and could have done so given that era's lax pre-medical requirements. His father urged him to go to college first. In the fall of 1878 Babcock entered Harvard College.

Harvard College—and the Race of His Life

The 1870s and 1880s were an exciting time at Harvard largely because of the vision and energy of Charles William Eliot, who substantially improved higher education during America's Gilded Age (the period between roughly 1870 and the turn of the twentieth century). In 1863 Eliot, after being denied the Harvard professorship he sought, went to Europe and studied educational methods both in the universities and in everyday life. Returning to the United States, he published in February and March of 1869 a two-part article in the *Atlantic Monthly* on "The New Education: Its Organization." Americans, he wrote, were "fighting the wilderness, physical and moral," and "for this fight we must be trained and armed." Members of the Harvard Corporation took notice and in May 1869 elected the 35-year-old Eliot president. During his forty-year presidency Eliot transformed the small provincial college with its run-of-the-mill graduate schools into a world-class research university. He held the ultimate aims of a liberal education to be character and the ability to make wise choices. To that end he replaced the inflexible, one-size-fits-all undergraduate curriculum with its emphasis on the classics to a system that allowed students to choose many of their courses, and from an expanded range of options.

Babcock concentrated in natural history with strong interests in German and English. He twice applied for and received scholarships. He probably earned money by serving as a chapel monitor all four years, during which his attendance was perfect. He lived on the Yard, the first two years in College House and the last two in Hollis. During the latter part of his senior year he roomed with his friend Edward Henry Strobel, then a tutor at Harvard. Although he later wrote that he "never had a regular chum" in college,[11] he was again well liked. He was a member of Kappa Nu, the Everett Athenæum, the Harvard Union, the Hasty Pudding Club, O.K., and Zeta Psi. During his senior year he was president of the Harvard Dining Association and was elected third marshal of his class. Being one of only three southerners in his graduating class of 177 men proved no barrier to popularity.

The proudest and in some ways defining moments of Babcock's life came from pulling the number four oar for the Class of 1882, especially during a race on the Charles River on May 14, 1881. Some background information may help explain why that race held such lifelong significance to him.

Competitive boat racing began in England during the early-nineteenth century, crossed the Atlantic, and became the rage at Harvard, situated on a near-ideal river for the sport. Harvard students organized boat clubs, which the faculty tolerated despite the resulting rowdiness until 1850 when some oarsmen clashed with police. The faculty forbade new clubs and by 1852 only one, the Oneida Club, remained. It was therefore the Oneida Club that responded when Yale students challenged for a race. On August 3, 1852, the first formal intercollegiate competition of any kind in the United States took the form of a race between Harvard students from the Oneida Club and a Yale crew over a two-mile course on New Hampshire's Lake Win-nipesaukee. Harvard prevailed by about two lengths and received the prize of a pair of black walnut oars. In 1857 two crew members, one of whom was future Harvard president Charles W. Eliot, bought crimson Chinese silk bandanas to distinguish theirs from the other 13 crews at a regatta. Thus began the tradition of colors for college teams.

Eliot championed crew during his long presidency even as Harvard added other sports. He considered crew and tennis the only clean sports. He railed against football as "a fight whose strategy and ethics are those of war," against basketball as "too rough ... [with] too many chances for cheating," and against baseball since "a curve ball is thrown with a deliberate attempt to deceive." Rowing and tennis, Eliot averred, "are the only sports in which honorable play altogether is practiced. You can no more cheat in those two sports than in a game of cards; you would be crowded out of society if you tried."[12]

Crew became increasingly sophisticated. Hydraulic rowing machines were introduced for strength training. Major races were preceded by six to eight weeks of rigid dietary and conditioning regimens. Competitions and rigorous training were not limited to the varsity. In 1879 the classes began to compete against each other in two-mile races between eight-oared shells. The class oarsmen took the twice-yearly competitions as seriously as their varsity counterparts, training for five to six months, working on rowing machines during the winter, and getting ready for races by adhering to a strict diet, limiting water intake, and reducing body weight further "by forced sweating under feather beds and by running in heavy flannels as if training for a prize

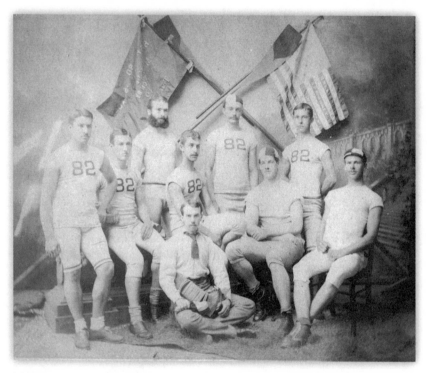

The Harvard Class of 1882 crew. Babcock is second from right, back row. *Courtesy:* Arthur St. J. Simons II.

fight."[13] By the early 1880s the class crew races excited more interest on the Harvard campus than any other event, including the Harvard-Yale race.

James Woods Babcock '82 tried out for the class crew his freshman year, when the first such competition took place, but quit because of the senior captain's tongue lashings. The Class of '82 came in third in a race that included the four classes and also the law school. The '82 crew finished second in the 1880 spring race but last in the same year's fall race. Babcock joined the crew in time for the spring race scheduled for Saturday, May 14, 1881. The *Boston Globe* began its coverage and handicapping of the four classes six days in advance. The seniors were "almost certain of first place," while the juniors were "not expected to come in better than third."[14]

The juniors, however, had a not-so-secret weapon in their coach, the famous oarsman William Amos "Foxy" Bancroft. Then a senior in law school, Bancroft went on to become the unsalaried head of Harvard rowing for five years, a four-term mayor of Cambridge, a brigadier-general during the Spanish-American War (the only person thus commissioned who had not

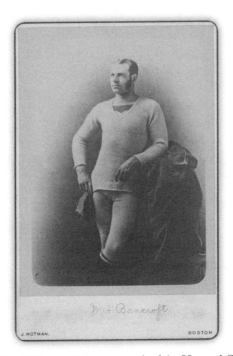

William Amos ("Foxy") Bancroft (1855–1922) of the Harvard Class of 1878, generally considered the greatest collegiate oarsmen of his generation.
Courtesy: Harvard University Archives, HUP Bancroft, W.A. (1b).

been a member of the regular army), and, as president of the Boston Elevated
Railway Company, the highest paid chief executive in New England. According to Babcock he was known as "Foxy" (or "Foxey") because "he made it his
business to know intimately the habits of the men under him."[15] Bancroft
trained the juniors for six months, insisting on wholesome diet, adequate
sleep, regular use of the "rowing weights," and attention to schoolwork. As
the race approached, the *Globe* reported that "betting was fast and furious."
The Class of '82 was "generally regarded in Cambridge as the poorest of the
four." However, insiders reported the '82 oarsmen had covered the course
within the previous week "in somewhat less than the winning time last year,"
and that "they row well together, with a lively catch, though they are inclined
not to pull the oar clear through."[16]

     As spectators flocked to the banks of the Charles River on a fair Saturday
afternoon, the class of '82 oarsmen grew fidgety. Their stroke, Xanthus Henry

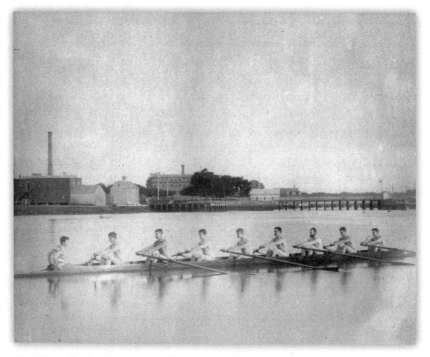

The Class of 1882 crew on the Charles River. Babcock is fourth from right. All
of these men succeeded in later life, perhaps none more than the 108-pound
coxswain, Henry Thomas Oxnard, who pioneered the beet sugar industry in
southern California and for whom a city is named.
Courtesy: Arthur St. J. Simons II.

Goodnough, had sore hands, had not rowed for several days, and his availability was uncertain. "All the college including our own friends & classmates," Babcock reminisced, "considered us out of the race. Our stock was at a discount and we knew it. . . . We were all so nervous we could hardly keep still." The captain appealed to Bancroft for last-minute advice. The famous oarsman "walked up & down the flat with an inscrutable grin for which he was famous." He looked them over and finally spoke: "Well, I suppose you expect that the strongest crew is going to win this race. You have been working on that theory six months. You and all the rest of the world who think like that are wrong. That crew is going to win this race that can bear the most pain. Boat races throw up the ability of crews to bear pain. If you can endure more pain than the 24 other men you will beat them. That's all I've got to say."[17]

With Bancroft's words "ringing in our ears," the juniors took the lead three strokes into the race and held off the other boats. The seniors, the *Globe* reported, made "a splendid struggle for first place, but all in vain, for '82 crossed the line first amid tumultuous bursts of cheers." The winning time was 11 minutes and 18 seconds, 10 seconds better than the second-place seniors, in a race under near-perfect conditions and "decidedly one of the prettiest ever seen on the Charles."[18]

Babcock's lasting impression was of neither the cheering at the finish line nor the "dollar supper" at Revere House two nights later. It was Bancroft's exhortation: *boat races test the capacity to endure pain.* And there was more to the story.

Goodnough, the stroke, had "rowed with one hand in utterly unfit condition, and only sheer pluck sustained him in setting the stroke." We infer that Goodnough persevered despite a hand raw from ruptured blisters. Equally astonishing was the feat of Henry Reese Hoyt, the number-two oar. Hoyt's sliding seat broke as the boat exited the sluiceway. He slid back and forth on the iron runners yet somehow managed to keep pace and rhythm.[19] The Class of '82 in its green and white racing colors successfully defended its title the following year.

Babcock remained close to many classmates and spoke at their twenty-fifth reunion dinner on "The Time I Wasted in College—What it had Done for Me."[20] He never regretted his father's advice to precede medical school with a liberal education, which helped sustained him through many trials. The oars from the two spring races reminded him the rest of his life of Bancroft's truism: *Success depends on the ability to endure pain.* Sixteen years after the race, when a fellow asylum superintendent prevailed against political opponents, Babcock rejoiced with "feelings that had been almost dormant

since I was on the winning crew of a boat race!"[21] Twenty-eight years after
the class race of May 1881 he told a packed audience at the University of
South Carolina, to frequent applause, that competitive sports teach student
athletes "self-reliance, confidence in his associates . . . and that a sacrifice
hit is sometimes greater than a home run with the applause of the grand
stand."[22] After his death press clippings of his class crew's victories were
found "neatly folded in a pocket of an old wallet."[23]

Harvard Medical School

Babcock graduated *cum laude* from Harvard College with an honorable
mention in natural history. He was one of twenty classmates who chose
medicine, writing in an autobiographical sketch (that may have been part
of his medical school application) of his "long cherished ambition of practicing medicine intelligently for the good of my fellow man."[24] Accepted
by Harvard Medical School, he arranged to stay in Hollis on the Harvard
Yard only to be notified by the bursar to vacate his room on two days' notice
because of an alleged infraction.[25] This led to his only documented tête-à-
tête with Charles W. Eliot. The incident demonstrates an ability to manage
stress and seek appropriate help during a crisis.[26]

   The charge was as follows. Some members of his class had planned a
disturbance for Commencement Day. Babcock left Cambridge to avoid
trouble and returned to the campus at midnight, "supposing all would be
quiet." He learned that a bonfire was about to be kindled and agreed to
watch it with some friends. When the blaze began in front of Hollis, the
watchman, a Mr. Gibson, "ran up and attempted to extinguish the fire." A
classmate started throwing back the pieces of wood as quickly as Gibson
could throw them off. The two men came to blows. Babcock, who at 158
pounds was 21 pounds heavier than the average for his graduating class, tried
to separate them. An onlooker, a Mr. Jackson, implicated Babcock as the
primary culprit. Babcock sought the advice of President Eliot, who told him
he stood accused by Jackson, Gibson, and a Mr. Knapp. Knapp and Gibson
later denied giving testimony against Babcock. He petitioned the faculty to
"clear me of this unjust charge by allowing me to enter the Harvard Medical
School without protest, and by declaring my room agreement valid and by
restoring my room to me."[27] He was cleared and the bursar later verified it
was not Babcock who had attacked the watchman.[28]

   Babcock was again a beneficiary of the vision of Charles Eliot, who
made medical education a top priority. "The whole system of medical

education in this country," Eliot wrote in his first annual report, "needs thorough reformation." Harvard, typical of that era's proprietary medical schools, required students to pay their professors for a five-month course of lectures during two successive years before entering the wards. Three-fourths of entering students had only a high school diploma. In November 1869 Eliot shocked the medical school faculty by assuming the chair at a meeting—and then kept the chair for 40 years. He built a case for a progressive four-year curriculum. He overcame opposition from conservatives who favored the time-honored apprenticeship model of undergraduate medical education. In 1871–72 Harvard Medical School had only one endowed professorship. In June 1881 the faculty voted to enlarge the scope of the school, whereupon twenty-five new appointments were made.[29] Thus when Babcock entered in 1882 there were four named professorships, twenty-five full-time faculty, sixteen instructors, and eight clinical instructors. Eliot had successfully moved the medical school into the university. The faculty included such great names as Charles S. Minot in embryology, Henry P. Bowditch

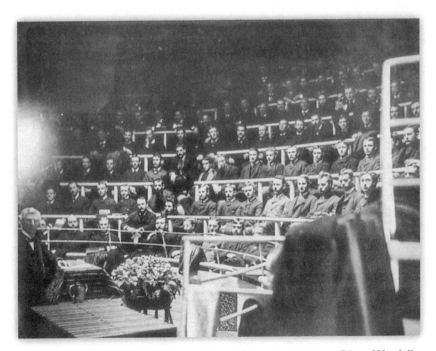

Babcock was almost surely present on November 28, 1882, when Oliver Wendell Holmes Sr (1809–1894) gave his farewell lecture to Harvard medical students.
Courtesy: The Harvard Medical Library in the Francis A. Countway Library of Medicine.

in physiology, Reginald H. Fitz in pathological anatomy, Francis Minot in the theory and practice of medicine, and John Collins Warren in surgery.[30]

The most famous faculty member was Oliver Wendell Holmes Sr., the Parkman Professor of Anatomy. Holmes had pioneered microscopy and histology to North American medical students, had anticipated the germ theory in his 1843 essay on the contagiousness of childbed fever, and was probably the school's most popular teacher. As one student put it, "Every muscle, bone, or organ suggests some witty story." He was also America's best-selling author on both sides of the Atlantic as "the autocrat of the breakfast-table." In Boston he was a celebrity; it was he who coined the term "Boston Brahmin" and nicknamed the city "the Hub." Unfortunately for Babcock, Holmes was resigning from the medical school faculty. The stated reason was his publisher's urging him to devote full time to writing, but Eliot's vision for the medical school may have had something to do with it since Holmes had been one of the old guard who opposed university encroachment on faculty autonomy.[31] Babcock had been a medical student for exactly three months when, on November 28, 1882, Holmes gave his farewell address to Harvard medical students.

Still, Babcock may have benefited, if indirectly, from Holmes's interest in the emerging fields of psychology and psychiatry. Holmes supported what historians call "the first great psychiatric revolution," inspired in France by Phillipe Pinel. More conspicuously, Holmes anticipated by a generation what is now called "depth psychology." In his 1857 Phi Beta Kappa lecture at Harvard, Holmes spoke of the unconscious flow of thought. In his 1867 novel *The Guardian Angel* he wrote: "The best thought, like the most perfect digestion, is done unconsciously." In an 1871 essay on "Mechanisms in Thought and Morals" he wrote that we "know very little of the contents of our minds until some sudden jar brings them to light" and that in our dreams we "do battle with ourselves, unconscious that we are our own antagonists." He used such terms as "latent consciousness," "unconscious celebration," and "the reflex action of the brain." Babcock maintained an interest in Holmes's writing, and it does not seem far-fetched to suggest that Holmes piqued Babcock's interest in psychiatry.[32]

Aside from Holmes, psychiatry had a low profile in the Harvard Medical School curriculum. The early history of neurology and psychiatry at Harvard is primarily the story of two men, James Jackson Putnam and Morton Prince, neither of whom is likely to have had much influence on Babcock. Putnam, an 1870 graduate of Harvard Medical School, was mainly a neurologist. Prince, an 1879 graduate, eventually became the leading experimental psychiatrist in the United States but during Babcock's training was pursuing otolaryngology.[33] Although Charles F. Folsom had become "Lecturer on Mental Disease" in 1876, and although the Danvers Insane Asylum was opened for instruction of medical students in 1879, there is no evidence that Babcock was exposed to either. "Mental Diseases" were not included in the curriculum until the fourth year, which was optional. The faculty recommended a fourth-year curriculum that resembled what later became the rotating internship, but observed that "until further notice the degree of Doctor of Medicine will continue to be given upon the completion of three years of study." The "further notice" did not come until 1888.[34] The learning objectives for the fourth-year elective in mental diseases offered by Folsom were simple, and the recommended textbooks did not include one on mental disorders.

Needing the money—"I did not know very well how I was to pay my next week's board"[35]—Babcock spent the summer after his freshman year at the State Infirmary in Tewksbury, Massachusetts, a small village between the Concord and Merrimack Rivers in the northeastern corner of the state. At the Tewksbury Almshouse, as it was commonly known, he realized a talent for psychiatry that set the course for his life's work.

The Tewksbury Almshouse had opened in 1854 as one of three whereby the state of Massachusetts assumed responsibility for its destitute, notably the Irish immigrants who streamed into Boston but could not find jobs. Built for 500 occupants, it held more than 800 within three weeks. In 1866 it began accepting "pauper insane" and by 1874 approximately 40 percent of its occupants were diagnosed with mental illness of one kind or another. In 1875 a physician, Charles Henry Sanborn, led an investigation that supposedly brought about reforms. Still, residents feared for their lives on an almost daily basis. Among these was Anne Sullivan, who overcame four tortured years there to become famous as Helen Keller's lifelong teacher, friend, and companion. By Babcock's arrival in 1883 it was a large complex with approximately twenty-five buildings and the object of still another investigation. To be sure, the Tewksbury Almshouse had not yet received the international notoriety that ensued a decade later when in 1893 investigators explored rumors of sexual perversions and cannibalism, wholesale selling of corpses to Harvard Medical School, and the tanning of human skin. Babcock's letters make no mention of trouble at Tewksbury. Possibly, his superiors shielded him from the worst of it.

Understaffing enabled him to assume responsibility for "the male department, all white males" even though he had completed only one year of medical school.[36] A letter to his brother Brooks, who had become engaged to a "quiet, sensible lady," affords a rare glimpse into Babcock's life during this period and his relationship with his family back in South Carolina. He regarded his younger brother as a "full-handed man of practice" and himself merely "a supported theorist." He hinted that Brooks should be patient with their father's irritability, since "we have made very cold returns for the sacrifice he has made in our behalf." Tewksbury was "hard work, but I like it," and he had "gained some valuable experience, been deprived of the necessity of spending money, and therefore saved what I have earned." He nevertheless took advantage of cultural opportunities, writing home that he had gone to Boston by train to take in a comic opera with one of the assistant physicians. On the return trip the conductor failed to stop at Tewksbury, landing them in Lowell five miles away. The conductor apologized and "tried to hire a team to bring us over but the stablemen were sleepy and would not come. We were therefore forced to work our passage back on a hand-car."[37] Babcock, a friend recalled after his death, could name nearly every actor, including those who played minor parts, of every play he had seen.[38]

His "no end of work" did not go unnoticed. At the end of the summer the patients lamented his departure with a formal letter:

Mr. J. W. Babcock

We the undersigned patients and Inmates of Ward 19 having learned with profound sorrow and deep regret of your immediate departure from amongst us. We deem it a duty to show our appreciation of the valuable services Rendered by you to us in the double capacity of Doctor and nurse in which you were always untiring and zealous.

Now that you are called upon to resume and prosecute your studies which are essential to the treatment of those that are or in time may become afflicted as we are, we would therefore recommend you to any community where it may please providence to cast your lot.

Would that we were able to offer more tangible evidence of your work, but poor wards of the state as we are, we cannot do more than this attest to the many great qualities you possess as a sober, honest, punctual, orderly, patient, and cheerful man, kind to all, partial to none.

[Signed by seventy-five patients][39]

Babcock had found his calling: to be an asylum doctor.

Two years later, on August 29, 1885, he was notified that he had passed all examinations required for the M.D. degree at Harvard.[40] He elected to forego the optional fourth year and was immediately in demand. In September he was offered the position of second assistant at the Boston Lunatic

Asylum at a salary of $500 per year. In November he was offered the position of Assistant Resident Physician at the State Almshouse of the Commonwealth of Massachusetts, the administrator stating emphatically: "Dr. I <u>want you</u>." Babcock declined; the administrator begged him to reconsider. Babcock applied for the position of second assistant physician at the McLean Asylum, then located in Somerville, Massachusetts. One of his references described him as "a gentleman in all that the word implies." On January 4, 1886, he was notified of acceptance.[41]

McLean Asylum

"The rise of the asylum," writes Edward Shorter in *A History of Psychiatry*, "is the story of good intentions gone bad."[42] Good intentions date at least to the great Islamic societies of the ninth and tenth centuries, where institutions known as *mauristans* cropped up in Baghdad, Cairo, Fez, and Damascus based on the belief that insane persons were divinely inspired and, being holy, deserved comfortable accommodations. Similar asylums appeared in parts of Europe under Islamic rule, notably in fourteenth-century Spain. Sadly, most asylums devolved into horrific chambers of incarceration. St. Mary of Bethlehem Hospital in London, built in 1247, became by the eighteenth century the notorious "Bedlam," its name synonymous with brutal conditions for the mentally afflicted. Two Frenchmen, Philippe Pinel and his pupil, Jean-Etienne-Dominique Esquirol, receive much of the credit for the reappearance of good intentions during the early nineteenth century.

Pinel and Esquirol considered mental illness largely functional (that is, psychological) rather than structural (that is, organic). They proposed a kinder, gentler alternative to the therapeutic aggressiveness of many doctors, of whom the most notable in the United States was the Philadelphian Benjamin Rush (who in 1965 was designated the "father of American psychiatry" by the American Psychiatric Association). Rush based his theory of the "unity of disease" in part on his now-discredited conclusion from his own experience during the 1793 Philadelphia yellow fever epidemic that bloodletting helps treat that disease. He asserted that mental illness begins in the blood vessels of the brain. Bleeding, by reducing tension in the walls of blood vessels, presumably helped. Pinel and Esquirol offered a psychosocial alternative to Rush's biomedical model of mental illness. They and others such as William Tuke in England promoted asylums as therapeutic communities offering hope, reassurance, positive examples, counseling, exercise, useful work, and confidence-building pastimes.

Asylums over the course of the nineteenth century became representative of societal attempts to impose massive architectural solutions on difficult social problems; other examples include almshouses, penitentiaries, reformatories, and orphanages. Asylums came to be convenient places to warehouse inconvenient people. Cure rates plummeted.

To these generalizations McLean Asylum was a notable exception. It opened in 1818 as the Charlestown Asylum, organizationally the psychiatric wing of the Massachusetts General Hospital.[43] Three unforeseen events saved it from the fates of most of that era's asylums. In 1823 a childless Boston merchant named John McLean left $123,000 to the Charlestown Asylum. Then, two public asylums opened in the greater Boston era: the Worcester State Asylum in 1833, sponsored by a progressive young state legislator named Horace Mann, and the Boston Lunatic Asylum in 1839. Those who could pay for institutional care increasingly chose McLean, as the Charlestown Asylum was renamed, and McLean went private.

McLean, unlike its public counterparts, prospered well into the twentieth century and beyond. As told in a recent history entitled *Gracefully Insane*, McLean's eventual 240-acre campus in Waverley (now Belmont), Massachusetts, resembled an elite preparatory school or small private college, complete with Tudor mansions, red brick dormitories, an indoor gymnasium, tennis courts, and a nine-hole golf course, all on grounds designed by America's foremost landscape architect, Frederick Law Olmsted.[44] The move to Waverley did not occur until 1895, four years after Babcock left. Still, he found in Somerville a cottage-style campus more suggestive of a suburban community than a mental facility.

McLean benefitted from a series of progressive superintendents. Rufus Wyman, who ran the institution almost single-handedly for seventeen years beginning in 1818, endorsed Pinel's ideal of a therapeutic environment based on "a judicious moral engagement" that "should engage the mind, and exercise the body" through such activities as "swinging, riding, walking, sewing, embroidery, bowling, gardening, mechanical arts; to which may be added reading, writing, conversation, & c., at stated times, and conforming to stated rules in almost everything." He required "the greatest kindness in the attendants upon a lunatic."[45] Wyman's successor, Luther V. Bell, was even more skeptical than Wyman about the value of medical interventions for mental illnesses. A third reformer was Edward Cowles, who took over in 1879 and became Babcock's mentor.[46]

Cowles had learned hospital administration during a Civil War trial-by-fire, including a stint in Grant's Army of the Potomac. Later, as medical superintendent at Boston City Hospital, he oversaw a building program and founded a training school for nurses with the aid of Linda Richards, the first woman in the United States to hold a diploma as a trained nurse. A short, genial man who was a bit obstinate but with "intellectual vitality of a high order," Cowles led McLean to the forefront of psychiatry. He replaced the bars on some of the windows with unobtrusive screens. He experimented with unlocked doors. In 1882 he opened a laboratory, hired a consulting pathologist, and established the McLean Asylum Training School for Nurses—perhaps the first formally organized such school in a mental hospital in the world. He stressed respect and dignity toward patients: "Once within the hospital, the conduct of physicians and nurses toward the patient should show that he is regarded as simply ill, as having no reason for being ashamed of his illness. . . . he should always be called a 'patient,' not a 'boarder,'" as is the custom in some hospitals." Cowles spent a sabbatical studying psychology at Johns Hopkins and came away sufficiently impressed that he hired a physician experienced in that discipline. McLean's academic flavor was further enhanced by a new library and weekly seminars at which staff members were expected to present cases, review the pertinent literature, and suggest potential avenues for research. Cowles had implemented the now-familiar triad of patient care, teaching, and research.

Babcock could not have timed his coming to McLean more propitiously. He again shined in a new setting. In 1887 a patient expressed his appreciation, adding: "I sincerely regard Dr. Babcock as my Savior (if I may be permitted to use the word)."[47] He also gained experience teaching. He lectured on infectious diseases to the nursing students, one of whom, Kate Guion (the future Mrs. Babcock), kept her notes for posterity.[48] In 1888 he went to Europe and visited various asylums. One of his medical school classmates had written him that patients in Vienna were considered "material" and exhibited "as so many trained animals" and even "without a rag of clothing over them," a practice that "neither the patients nor the public would stand" in the United States.[49] Whether Babcock gained similar impressions of European asylums is unknown—few details of his 1888 trip survive other than that he went to Paris and while in London visited the House of Commons[50]—but surely he considered himself fortunate to train at McLean under Cowles.

Any reservations he may have had about McLean probably revolved around his father, who was not well. In March 1890 Babcock returned to Chester and considered resigning from McLean. Cowles begged him to "let me waive any formal consideration of your resignation" and "to let it have another month, and the conditions will appear clearer to you." He related that the male patients "all miss Dr. Babcock dreadfully." Cowles reassured

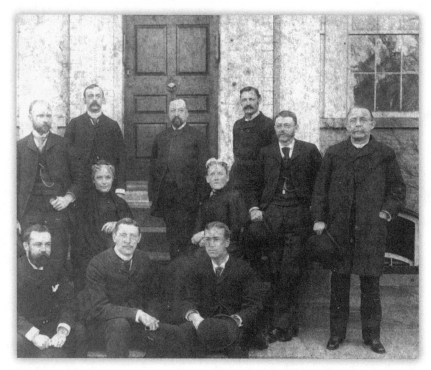

The staff at McLean asylum, circa 1890. Babcock is second from left, back row. At the far right is Edward Cowles (1837-1919), one of the most progressive asylum superintendents of that era.
Courtesy: Arthur St. J. Simons II.

him to "let it be an indefinite leave of absence—for six months if need be," since "we all want you to come back."[51]

For his future peace of mind, Babcock would have done well to stay put. He would almost surely have become a top candidate for the superintendent's job in 1904 when Cowles reached mandatory retirement age. Cowles's successor was one of Babcock's fellow assistant physicians, George T. Tuttle, a short, frail man of modest ambitions who "left few traces of himself behind" and who made "practically no imprint on the character of McLean, let alone on the broader field of American psychiatry."[52] Five years after Babcock left McLean, an administrator told him of the "great regret among the Board of Trustees" at Babcock's departure. The administrator further confided that Babcock "had one characteristic that he had never seen equaled in the McLean Asylum, that of knowing all about the patients you were asked about," and of seeming to be "acquainted with them personally."[53] This would not be possible in his next position: superintendent of the woefully underfunded and overcrowded South Carolina Lunatic Asylum.

Coming Home against Better Judgment

If McLean ranked among the best asylums in the United States, the South Carolina Lunatic Asylum was surely among the worst. It was McLean's polar opposite: public, underfunded, and a political football. In 1891 the state legislature appointed a committee to investigate shortcomings, which led to inquiries concerning Superintendent Peter E. Griffin. Dr. Griffin was promised the chance to cross-examine witnesses and offer rebuttal. However, the committee finished its work, adjourned, and gave Griffin a copy of the testimony. Griffin complained that the committee had not kept its promise and that his case had been prejudiced before the public. He dashed off an epistle to the governor of South Carolina, Benjamin Ryan Tillman, likening himself to the "victim who stood in chains before the Spanish Inquisition" and to the "culprit condemned unheard under the tyrannical procedure of the Star Chamber of England." Tillman was not amused. He told Griffin that he alone would decide Griffin's case. Tillman offered Griffin an opportunity to come before him and defend himself. Griffin balked. Tillman sought and secured Griffin's resignation.[54]

On May 23, 1891, Babcock's younger brother Brooks informed him that he had "been mentioned as a probable successor of Dr. Griffin" who had been "put out in a shabby manner." Brooks offered to lobby for him; this, however, was unnecessary since Babcock was already being promoted by Thomas N. Berry, a Chester life insurance agent with political connections. Brooks told his brother that "Mr. Berry told . . . [the governor and the members of the asylum's Board of Regents] as much as he could, but they said it was largely a question of 'execution ability.'" Their father, Brooks continued, was pleased that "your name should have been mentioned" but "does not seem to think much of your accepting the job even if you have the chance. He thinks you would worry yourself to death over the miserable 'niggers.'" Babcock told his brother that news of his candidacy was "altogether a surprise," and that he understood "the asylum problem in S.C." to be "a grave one" that "should be trusted only to the most experienced humanitarians." Moreover, "I do not think I am capable of assuming such responsibilities. Besides this, I am not an office seeker. Brooks then played his trump card: "Father is not a bit strong. He has had some trying [medical] cases recently, and I wish he would go away [on vacation] again."[55]

Tillman later boasted that it was he who "discovered" Babcock, but correspondence suggests Berry, the life insurance salesman, sold Tillman and then Babcock on the idea. To Tillman he glossed over Babcock's lack of administrative experience. To Babcock he hyped the extent to which administrative responsibilities could be delegated. Berry advised Babcock that Tillman expressed his desire for "a practical business man as well as a good physician. I know your modesty will not allow you to claim this combination but from what I can gather I know you do and simply ask you to give such references as will allow me to get the information in shape for the Governor."[56]

Berry worked to close the deal. He wrote Tillman: "In our hurried conversation the other evening I don't think I gave you what information I had in reference to Dr. Jas W. Babcock." After reciting Babcock's résumé he asserted: "He is a practical and systematic business man. He doubtless has superior executive ability—as he was always a leader among the boys in Chester and also a leader among the students at Exeter & Harvard."[57] This was of course a textbook example of puffery, an exaggeration to make a sale.

Tillman, who considered asylum superintendent "the most important office in the State," sought other opinions. He asked John S. Withers of Chester about Babcock's qualifications, stating bluntly: "Executive ability, firmness, tact, business sense are needed rather than skill as a physician." Withers responded that he had verified Babcock's executive ability with two people who had known him. Dr. S. M. Davega, "the most prominent physician of this place [Chester]," described Babcock as "one of the most complete men to be found anywhere, having combined with finished education fine Executive Ability, tact, firmness, and business sense." A Mr. Paul Hemphill described Babcock as "a born leader of men [,] firm but not obstinate."[58]

Tillman exercised due diligence. He wrote Babcock's supervisor at McLean, Edward Cowles. Cowles confirmed that Babcock "has ability of a high order associated with conscientiousness and modesty that are marked traits of his character" but conveyed Babcock's own reluctance to take a job for which he felt unqualified: "He [Babcock] has decided for himself, without my advice, that he does not possess certain of the qualifications you seek and need in the head of your institution, viz:—business and executive experience." Although Cowles was "greatly interested in promoting his return to his native state to do the work for the insane" he agreed with Babcock's self-assessment that he was "not yet prepared to respond to the requirements you have properly named."[59]

Tillman nonetheless offered the job to Babcock, perhaps because he had no better option and, like everyone else, stood in awe of Babcock's impeccable academic credentials. Besides, Babcock's relatives were Tillman supporters.[60]

Berry still needed to work on Babcock, who told him that "on the business side I know that I should be a disappointment to all concerned." Babcock had by now "looked over a file of the S.C. asylum reports" and saw "many sides of the problem that appeal to me strongly—the building of a new asylum for the Negroes, a better nursing service, etc. But my training here has not yet fully prepared me for the business management of an institution." Berry exhorted Babcock that the job was a once-in-a-lifetime opportunity, an opportunity that might not come again, to make a difference in his native state. Berry suggested that "if it be the wish" of the superintendent, "the Regents will relieve him of the business part of the work subject to such supervision as he may deem proper to give it. This of course will lighten the work."[61] Such hype, along with the declining health of his father, who would die the next year,[62] led Babcock to accept the position. He received a certificate appointing "James W. Babcock Superintendent of the Lunatic Asylum of this State, to take effect on the first day of August, 1891; This appointment to continue in Force during the Pleasure of the Governor."[63]

Babcock thus bade farewell to McLean against his better judgment. A patient expressed a "deep sense" shared by "many others, of your peerless and invaluable ministrations . . . professional skill, and social excellence," adding that the "beneficial results of your medical practice . . . will be a lasting memorial."[64] Babcock shared the patient's wistfulness. When in 1914 he, like Griffin before him, resigned under pressure and started his own private asylum, he named it "Waverley" after Waverley, Massachusetts, McLean's new location.

CHAPTER 2

Superintendent

Hoping, Moping, and Coping

JAMES WOODS BABCOCK RETURNED to South Carolina in 1891 as the state's first fully-trained psychiatrist or, to use the then-current term, "alienist." He had attained at age 35 what was then a psychiatrist's highest ambition: to be an asylum superintendent. However, the South Carolina Lunatic Asylum was an extreme example of the deterioration of public asylums into convenient places for inconvenient people. Meager state appropriations could not keep up with the steady influx of patients, whose diagnoses commonly included such conditions as alcoholism, epilepsy, imbecility (mental retardation), senility, or terminal illness of any kind. Babcock's idealism, energy, and vision could not compensate for his lack of administrative experience and his reluctance to press the legislature for more money. The Bylaws gave him little power over his staff physicians. As conditions slowly but inexorably worsened, he tried on several occasions to leave. In the end he stayed, sublimated through hobbies and community activities, and became a much-admired public figure despite the dismal conditions at his asylum. His twenty-two-year career at the helm illustrates the mot that top administrators often pass through three stages: hoping, moping, and coping. His was hardly the best of times to be a state asylum superintendent or, for that matter, to be a psychiatrist.

Psychiatry in the Late Nineteenth Century

What is now the American Psychiatric Association began in 1844 when thirteen men formed the Association of Medical Superintendents of

25

American Institutions for the Insane, the first organization of medical specialists in the United States. They were called "alienists" on the premise that mentally disturbed patients were alienated from reality.[1] Most superintendents lived on campus. They saw their institutions as therapeutic environments for the newly-minted social and community psychiatry. They acknowledged both psychosocial and biological dimensions of mental illness, recognized the role of heredity, and occasionally suggested that mental illness might someday be reducible to neurology. In their optimism they launched the *American Journal of Insanity*. Their optimism was short-lived. With rare exceptions such as McLean, the position of asylum superintendent was by 1891 hardly an enviable job. In the social hierarchy of American physicians they ranked somewhere near the bottom.

What went wrong? Historians identify several factors, of which the most important was the sheer numbers of patients flooding asylums during the late nineteenth century. Families and communities caught up in the Industrial Revolution welcomed institutional alternatives to home care. Overwhelmed by overcrowding and underfunding, superintendents put Phillipe Pinel's "*le traitement moral*" on the back burner if they found time for it at all. Asylums became little more than jails for the mentally ill and other "undesirable" people. And the superintendents operated in political minefields. They were high-profile public figures in states strapped financially by growing welfare systems.

Finally, nineteenth-century advances in medical science had largely bypassed psychiatry. Bacteriology empowered generalist physicians to diagnose what had formerly been just "fevers." Anesthesia and aseptic techniques empowered surgeons to operate without pain and prohibitive risk of infection. Psychiatrists meanwhile were stuck with such quaint diagnostic terms as melancholia, idiocy, dementia, mania, and monomania—broad categories for which there was neither specific diagnosis nor effective therapy. And psychiatrists were losing turf battles to the more-prestigious neurologists, who had begun to appropriate functional disorders such as "neurasthenia" that lent to lucrative practices.[2] Psychoanalysis had not yet taken off. Psychiatrists had few career options.

Babcock assumed a highly-visible public position at a time when the power and prestige of psychiatrists in the United States was at its all-time nadir. And his impression from afar that "the asylum problem" in South Carolina was "a grave one" that "should be trusted only to the most experienced humanitarians" turned out to be correct.

The South Carolina Lunatic Asylum

An asylum, according to the first definition in the *Oxford English Dictionary*, is "a sanctuary; a place of refuge and safety." Churches and monasteries offered refuge from at least the fourth century onwards, and we still speak of "political asylum" for those whose lives would otherwise be in danger. Large asylums for isolating disadvantaged or persecuted people—including not only the insane but also the incurably ill, the poor, and the criminal—cropped up during the Middle Ages and the trend accelerated. The term "lunatic asylum" increasingly held negative connotations as the nineteenth century wore on, as did its *fin de siècle* substitute, "state hospital."

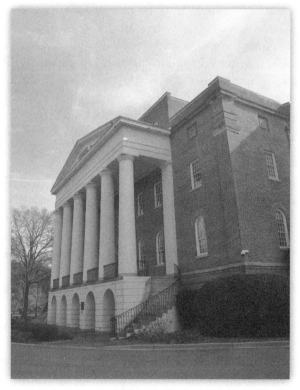

The iconic original building of the South Carolina Lunatic Asylum, known as the Old Building during Babcock's era and now as the Robert Mills Building after its architect.
Author photograph.

The history of the South Carolina Lunatic Asylum (which in 1895 at
Babcock's instigation became the South Carolina State Hospital for the
Insane) has been told several times, most recently by Peter McCandless
in his acclaimed *Moonlight, Magnolias, & Madness*.[3] McCandless calls the
1821 enabling legislation a "propitious moment" during which social activists, economic prosperity, and political willpower combined to make South
Carolina the first state in the Deep South and only the third in the nation
to boast such a public institution. Babcock's notes, articles, and sustained
interest in the asylum's history, regulations, and governance made him a
repository of institutional memory. He was the South Carolina Lunatic
Asylum's first systematic historian.[4]

He recorded, for example, that the original building had been designed
by Robert Mills, the first native-born American to train specifically for
architecture and now known mainly for state and federal government buildings and monuments, including his crowning achievement, the Washington
National Monument. An omnivorous reader, Mills took ideas from other
asylums to which he added some of his own. His ambitious plans caused
cost estimates to soar from $28,932 to $91,000, prompting his dismissal
as supervising architect.[5] Construction ground to a near halt. The asylum
was not completed until 1828—six years after the cornerstone had been
laid. Babcock's notes include a clipping from a November 1829 address by
Governor Stephen D. Miller, who exhorted: "If there be any tax which a
benevolent people ought cheerfully to pay, it is that which provides a safe
retreat for the unfortunate human beings who have lost their reason."[6]

Babcock studied the previous superintendents. The early ones, of whom
there were four during the first eight years, were lay administrators, as was
common practice in American asylums during the eighteenth and early
nineteenth centuries.[7] Their patients were few, making duties light for part-
time physicians James Davis and Daniel Heyward Trezevant. A visitor called
the South Carolina asylum "large enough to contain all of the lunatics in the
United States."[8] When in 1836 John D. Parker became the first physician-
superintendent, he found only forty-six patients. On the positive side, the
institution was self-sustaining and, Babcock noted, "Its conditions then
gave promise of fully realizing the benevolent intentions of its founders."[9]
Occupancy increased under Parker. Conditions deteriorated during the
Civil War. Some 1,200 captured Union officers were temporarily housed at
"Camp Asylum" on the grounds; they were evacuated before Sherman took
Columbia only to be replaced by homeless citizens seeking shelter after the
resulting fire destroyed much of the city.[10] Parker stayed on as superintendent

until "ousted during the administration of the notorious carpet bag governor, Robert T. Scott."[11]

Babcock made lists of all previous regents, assistant physicians, and chaplains. Two regents were of special interest. Thomas Cooper, an early president of South Carolina College, was a regent for only a year but "manifested his interest in behalf of the insane as well as his restless energy" by translating from the French a treatise *On Irritation and Insanity* by the controversial Parisian physician François Broussais.[12] Published in Columbia, this was one of the earliest works on mental diseases printed in the United States. Broussais attributed most diseases to "irritation," which justified bleeding by opening a vein or applying leeches to the skin. Daniel Henry Chamberlain served as regent for two years before becoming in 1874 the last Republican "carpetbagger" governor of South Carolina. Chamberlain opined that while "this institution deserves the generous support of the State," lack of funds continued "to embarrass all our public institutions" and hence "efficiency" became the order of the day. Babcock editorialized that Chamberlain's "view of expense vs. proper care of the insane was advocated

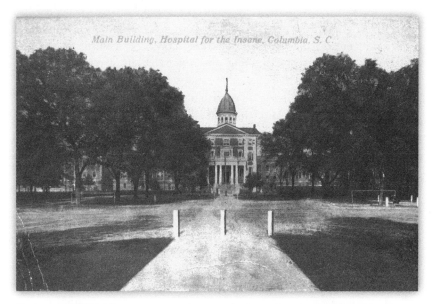

Early twentieth-century postcard showing the Main Building or New Building (now the Babcock Building). Like the Old Building, its design reflected the latest thinking in asylum architecture but ultimately proved disastrous.
Courtesy: South Caroliniana Library, University of South Carolina, Columbia, S.C.

by some regents and legislators well into the 20th Century, as this writer knows from abundant and nauseating experience."[13]

He reviewed the evolution of the physical plant. The influx of patients during Parker's administration prompted a second large brick building, begun during the 1850s but not completed until 1885. It was known as the Main Building, or New Building to distinguish it from the Old Building designed by Robert Mills. Architecturally it followed an invention by Thomas Kirkbride of Pennsylvania. Kirkbride's model featured symmetrical pavilions flanking a central administration building which often served as residence for the superintendent and some of the staff. The New Building, like the Old Building before it, incorporated the latest thinking on mental illness. The separate pavilions allowed segregation of patients by gender and placement of the more disturbed patients at the peripheries. By the 1890s, massive "Kirkbrides" dominated most public asylum complexes in the United States.

The South Carolina Lunatic Asylum by Babcock's arrival was in many ways typical of the vast mental institutions found in nearly every state, their spacious grounds and cupolaed dormitories now suggesting abandoned college campuses.[14] White female and male patients occupied the north and south wings of the New Building, respectively. Black women occupied the Old Building. Black males—who before, during, and after Babcock's administration received the least resources—were housed in a cluster of wooden buildings behind the New Building. The asylum had its own farm, kitchens, bakery, laundry, sewing rooms, machine shops, workshops, and electric plant. It could justifiably be called a self-sufficient community, or, in a darker light, what sociologist Erving Goffman called a "total institution."[15] The near-total control of inmates' lives was, as events played out, made worse by inadvertent flaws in both the Mills design and the Kirkbride model. Babcock and others came to realize that patients would have been better served by smaller buildings—separate pavilions or a "cottage plan."[16]

Flawed though it was, the asylum complex bulked large in the landscape of Columbia, a growing city with, according to the 1890 census, a population of 13,353, of which 57 percent was black and 43 percent white.[17] The asylum commanded the northeast corner of the two-square-mile grid that had made Columbia the first planned capitol in the Americas. Elmwood Avenue, originally known as the Upper Boundary Street, ran east-to-west past the Old Building, ending at Pickens Street, which ran north-to-south past the New Building. The asylum fronted the city to the west, where it faced Bull Street, and to the south, where it faced Lumber Street (now Calhoun Street). To the north and east the property sloped off into farmland. The asylum was one of the city's three major public institutions, the others being the state capitol and South Carolina College (re-chartered as the University of South Carolina in 1906). More important to Babcock, the asylum was a big-ticket item in the state budget, making the superintendent a conspicuous public figure.

In Columbia's medical community, Babcock as asylum superintendent could stand above the fray of competition for patients and petty politics but could expect little intellectual stimulation. The asylum was the only hospital in the state west of Charleston, at a time when most seriously ill people were cared for in their homes.[18] The Columbia Hospital (now Palmetto Health Richland) did not open until 1893 and then as a twenty-five-bed, for-whites-only almshouse.[19] Columbia's small coterie of physicians competed fiercely for the carriage trade—that is, patients who could pay well. The educator John Andrew Rice, in a witty memoir entitled *I Came out of the Eighteenth Century*, gives this description of one of Columbia's leading doctors, Alexander N. Talley: "The most splendid of these ancient dandies was [Dr. Talley], who wore a gold-headed cane in the medical tradition of the eighteenth century. The rest of his get-up was a concession to the nineteenth, but early Victorian. His long black coat was a stopping place for germs from three generations of the best people. . . . To this conventional costume he added an unusual tonsorial touch, which was called, I think, 'military': he parted his silver hair in the middle from forelock back over the crown and all the way down to the nape of his neck. He was Columbia's most admired physician, for what he lacked in medical knowledge he made up in pomposity, the only gift a man needs for success in the world."[20] When in 1899 a Dr. Francis D. Kendall, allegedly quoting the same Dr. Talley, criticized another physician, it caused such turmoil in the Columbia Medical Society that no scientific papers were presented during the next four years. The "Kendall affair" dominated the monthly meetings, sometimes as the only topic.[21] Columbia's medical community was a far cry from Greater Boston's.

Had Babcock summarized the administrative fates of previous superintendents, it would have read: William Hilliard (1832)—*resigned under pressure*; Archibald Beaty (1828–32)—*forced to resign*; E. W. Harrison (1832–36)—*resigned under pressure*; John D. Parker (1836–70)—*dismissed*; Joshua F. Ensor (1870–76)—*resigned under pressure*; Peter E. Griffin (1876–90)—*forced to resign*. Babcock's accepting the job was a triumph of hope over institutional experience. He prepared as best he could, trusting that strategies he'd used at Phillips Exeter and elsewhere—notably, diligence, self-reliance, and amiability—would work in the new environment.

Taking Charge—More or Less

Babcock postponed his arrival date by two weeks to visit asylums in other states.[22] He came to Columbia ready to take charge. He took inventory and set priorities. Yet the record suggests disparity between what the new superintendent *said* and what the members of the governing Board of Regents *heard*.

His agenda for change was limited. Visitors from the State Board of Health described the new superintendent as "active and energetic," "fully alive to all the duties and responsibilities that devolve upon him," but "disposed to make only a few minor changes at present."[23] He had indeed praised the condition of "many departments of the institution." He had singled out the New Building with its facilities for white patients. "The people of South Carolina," he reported, "should take pride in this institution as a retreat for afflicted white men & women." However, he clearly stated his top two priorities, priorities that would dog him the next twenty-two years. First, the asylum should house only persons who could profit from psychiatric care. Idiots (that is, the mentally retarded) and the "harmless insane" should be housed elsewhere. Second, the asylum should provide "better wards for the colored patients especially the men." Other priorities included a workshop, a training school for nurses, the presence of interns from the Medical College of the State of South Carolina in Charleston, and separate pamphlets for the procedures for admission and for the Bylaws.[24]

To what extent, if any, did Babcock's spoken words and body language betray private opinions? One can fault him for not being more insistent or "in your face" to the regents and the state legislature, especially on overcrowding and better facilities for blacks. Alternatively, one can assign his failure to become a more effective agent for change to his nonconfrontational personality, his desire to get along, to embody what Harvard's president Eliot called "the character of a gentleman"—a "disinterested laborer in the service of others" who is "generally quiet, and for the best of reasons—namely, that effectiveness requires steady, close attention, and that attention implies stillness and a mind intent."[25] The minutes of the Board of Regents suggest he never lost focus, but the results tell another story.

To summarize much of what follows, Babcock eventually succeeded at most things within his power but largely failed at things requiring substantial support from the state legislature. He made good on his pledge for better housing for black males, but, as we shall see, largely through his own drive and creativity. He made good on his pledge for a training school for nurses. He made good on publishing and disseminating the procedures for admission and the Bylaws, compiling these documents for the regents' review within two months of arrival.[26] He offered a rotation for students and interns at the Medical College in Charleston but withdrew the offer when it became obvious the students and interns considered it "rather as a joke."[27] He failed miserably at limiting admissions to persons with bona fide psychiatric conditions. And he no doubt concluded from his review of the Bylaws that his authority was limited.

The nine members of the Board of Regents to which Babcock answered were, like the superintendent, appointed by the governor. The board, not the superintendent, held power to hire and fire the assistant physicians. Babcock had little enforceable power over the doctors who were nominally

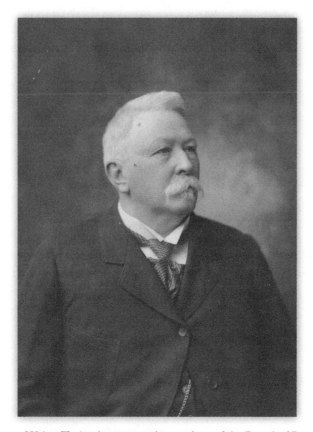

Dr. Benjamin Walter Taylor (1834–1905), president of the Board of Regents when Babcock became superintendent of the South Carolina Lunatic Asylum. *Courtesy:* Waring Historical Library, Medical University of South Carolina, Charleston, S.C.

his subordinates. The agenda for the monthly meetings followed a template: the superintendent's report, the first physician's report, reports by one or more of the regents (usually including an inspection of facilities and operations), and new business, if any. The board could go into executive session without the superintendent, who had to seek the board's permission for just about everything. Babcock never challenged the board's authority, even during his last months as superintendent when its members with one exception had turned against him.

Such deference was understandable during the early going. The board's membership reflected the state's political power structure. Returning from "up north," Babcock certainly did not want to storm in as a know-it-all. He recognized that most if not all of the board members knew more about running an asylum and especially *this* asylum than he did. He recognized that the board's president was one of South Carolina's most admired doctors and beloved citizens, Dr. B. Walter Taylor, who was simultaneously a physician, a surgeon, and a farmer. Taylor's ability to inspire confidence is evinced by his having become at a young age the second highest-ranking physician in the Southern Armies, as Medical Director of the Cavalry Corps of the Army of Northern Virginia. And Taylor was a kindly man, a gentleman of whom it was remembered that "although his life was a strenuous one ... he held out to the end endeavoring to relieve the afflicted who sought his aid."[28] He represented the third generation of his family to serve the asylum. His grandfather, Colonel Thomas Taylor, had owned much of the property on which Columbia was built and reputedly gave land for the original asylum. Babcock's confidence in Taylor's benevolence was well placed. Later, Taylor's son Julius would be Babcock's staunchest supporter.

Babcock soon realized that while his responsibilities were many his powers were few. Crucially, the physicians on the staff owed their allegiance mainly to the board. The first assistant physician, Dr. James L. Thompson, had every reason to resent Babcock. A native of nearby Fairfield County, Thompson had been at the asylum for ten years, had been acting superintendent before Babcock's arrival, and had been the internal candidate for the permanent job. Thompson's education had been entirely in-state: Erskine College, the Medical College of the State of South Carolina, and a one-year internship at the City Hospital in Charleston before joining the staff of the Lunatic Asylum in 1881. He recognized and even overestimated Babcock's superior training, writing in his memoirs that Babcock besides being a Harvard man had "spent several years in Europe studying lunatic asylums, conditions, etc., and was quite well informed."[29] Thompson also derived

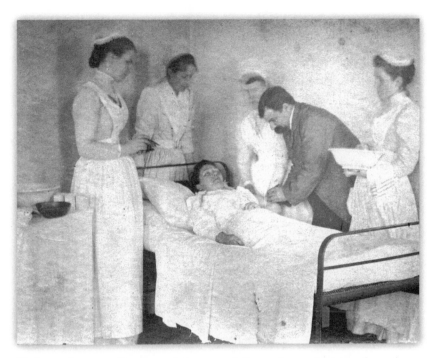

Dr. James Lawrence Thompson (1854–1931), first assistant physician, shown here making rounds.
Courtesy: Arthur St. J. Simons II.

power from his mother-in-law's position as matron or, officially, supervisor of the women's wards. Although there was in the beginning little overt tension between Babcock and Thompson, a courtly man of the old school, some tension surely lurked beneath the surface.

As first assistant physician Thompson gave the medical reports to the Board of Regents. Minutes of the board meetings convey the impression that Thompson, not Babcock, was the asylum's ranking medical officer. This was probably of little concern to Babcock, who had enough to do on the purely administrative side.[30] There were problems with the toilets, the sewage system, and the ventilation. There were problems with employees engaged in petty thieving, transacting business with patients or their families, helping patients escape, or imbibing alcohol on the job. There were problems with the workshops, sewing rooms (separate, for blacks and whites), shoemaker's shop, blacksmith shops, machine shops, electrical plant, and bakery. There were problems on the asylum farm, such as cholera among the hogs, stealing, or hunting on the property by townspeople. There were problems with the manufacture of butter, soap, pillows, mattresses, and coffins. Babcock kept most such problems from escalating into crises, showing firmness when necessary. He clamped down, for example, on the outside private practices of some of the attendants and nurses, who often hired substitutes of variable quality when opportunities arose to make more money elsewhere. He clamped down on the ability of physicians, nurses, and other employees to receive gifts from patients or their friends or families without the regents' approval. He brought in his college classmate and fellow crew member Xanthus Goodnough, who was now Assistant Engineer to the Massachusetts Board of Health, to help with sewage disposal, a health hazard for the city.[31] From today's perspective, Babcock functioned mainly as chief operating officer, not chief medical officer.

Despite his daily hassles Babcock periodically directed the board's attention to long-range planning. Yet he recognized the obstacles to funding any ambitious plans. He concluded within a year of arrival: "Experience seems to show that it is useless to go the General Assembly for a special appropriation."[32]

He reviewed the annual reports of the asylum to the State Board of Health. Of the first report (1880), he observed that "so far as healthy surroundings are concerned, [the asylum was] all that could be desired." Indeed, "Many patients ... live in the open air during the day, engaged in such work as they consent to do in the farm and garden." His predecessors were concerned that patients without mental illness "should not be kept in such institutions in daily contact with the acutely insane."[33] He found no fault with the diet, for the 1888 report claimed: "The diet is ample, varied, and healthy, consisting of fresh beef, ham and bacon, chickens and eggs, and an average supply of 150 quarts of milk daily, cornbread, baker's bread, hominy, rice, and coffee for breakfast and tea for supper, besides vegetables in their season."[34] However, he soon homed in on deficiencies.

At the top of his list was the inadequacy of facilities for African Americans. Closely related to the inadequacy of housing for black patients was the growing menace of tuberculosis, especially in blacks.[35] His thorough study of these issues—tuberculosis and mental illness in African Americans—led to significant publications in the medical literature.

Meanwhile, he forged two lasting relationships. One was with an attractive young nurse, Katherine Guion, who became Mrs. Babcock. The other was with Governor Benjamin Tillman, who would shelter him politically as long as it was in his power to do so.

Kate Guion

There is no documentation of a prior romantic relationship between Babcock and Kate Guion, but the presence of an attractive young southerner among the nurses at McLean could hardly have escaped his notice. He reported at only his second meeting of the Board of Regents that "at Dr. Taylor's suggestion" he had invited Miss Guion to consider heading up a proposed training school for nurses. She was from Lincolnton, North Carolina, which is outside of Charlotte and just sixty-five miles from Babcock's native Chester. She had spent two years at the Government Hospital for the Insane in Washington, D.C., had worked at McLean, and was now taking an additional

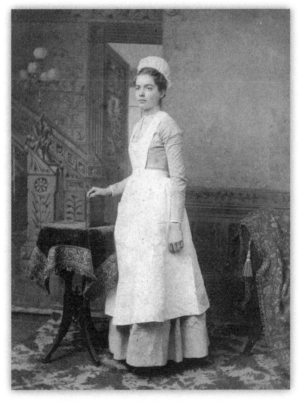

Katherine Guion as a student nurse. Babcock recruited her in 1891 to be the training director for a new nursing school at the asylum; they were married the following year.
Courtesy: Arthur St. J. Simons II.

year of training at the Massachusetts General Hospital, where she had been
a student nurse. With Taylor's backing, Babcock informed Miss Guion that
the position of director of the training school for nurses was hers if she
wanted it. He asked if "on the completion of your training at the M.G.H.,
you would be willing to take the position of Superinten-dent of Nurses in
a training school they wish to inaugurate here." He warned of "very many
obstacles to contend with" but encouraged her that "the enterprise would
prove . . . very interesting, as there is a great opportunity for good work in
this direction here in the South." She thanked him "for the confidence you
have placed in me. . . . I think I realize the importance & the difficulty of the
work but I will try to do the best I can for you although with much misgiv-
ing as to my ability." Babcock confirmed that a nursing school was the "pet
scheme" of the president of the board of regents, Dr. Taylor. She felt that a
salary of $800 per year would be reasonable for a major administrative job
that included starting and running a training school, but accepted the regents'
offer of $500 for the first year, to begin on January 1, 1892.[36]

If Babcock had ulterior motives for offering the job to Kate Guion
without a search process, he nevertheless warned her again about the "many
obstacles," adding: "All innovations are opposed by the so-called conservatives. You will not, I know, be inclined to be too sanguine in your expectations. It is often a satisfaction to make an attempt, even if one does not
accomplish anticipated results. Here, a degree of success very small, as
compared with Dr. Cowles's great achievements, will mean much allevia-
tion of suffering." He warned that she "must not expect too much at first"
and hinted that she could expect opposition from "the matron, Mrs. Carter"
who was "the mother-in-law of the first assistant, Dr. Thompson." Both
were entrenched. As Kate Guion's arrival date drew near, Babcock offered
to advance "two or three hundred dollars or more of your first year's salary"
but reinforced his warnings. "I feel it is my duty to prepare you, so far as
possible, to some very *un*hospital-like customs and surroundings. There will
no doubt be a strong undercurrent of severest criticism of all things connected with the training school." From Mrs. Carter she could expect "not
a little jealous opposition" for "We have to contend not only with ordinary
conservatism, but also with the jealousies and prejudices of people who have
been at the helm for fifteen years." Still, he did not regret leaving Massachusetts and McLean for Columbia and the State Lunatic Asylum," and
expressed a "sincere wish that you may, at the end of four months residence
in Columbia, have no greater reason to regret accepting your charge here,
than I now have, of accepting mine.[37] He signed these letters "Very truly
yours, J. W. Babcock."

They kept the courtship secret. It is unclear whether the regents knew Babcock's intent when they granted him "leave of absence for a few days."[38] The quiet ceremony on August 17, 1892, surprised their friends. She had gone home to Lincolnton, to "River Bend," a plantation on the South Fork River, to visit her parents. He followed. The newspaper reported that "few secrets have been as well kept" but that both "are well known and well liked" and that no couple had "more completely won the friendship and kind wishes of our people than they." The bride was "noted for many lovable traits of character and is a favorite with all who know her."[39]

The bridegroom needed all his interpersonal skills, for Kate was the oldest of twelve children—eight girls and four boys. One of her younger sisters, Connie, wanted to be a doctor. Connie's success in later life—she became a legendary New York City internist and the first female professor of clinical medicine in the United States—prompted a biography of her formative years, with the following account of her first glimpse of the new brother-in-law:

> "What's Dr. Babcock like, Kate?" demanded Connie. "Tell us all about him."
>
> Kate's hazel eyes sparkled and she took a deep breath. "Well—he's wonderful. He's a Southerner, of course. He's handsome and shy and smart. He graduated from Exeter and Harvard Medical School and now he's an alienist."
>
> "My land," said Mrs. Guion, "what's an alienist?"
>
> "It's what you call a doctor who treats mental illness, Mama."
>
> "Alienist," repeated Connie, trying out the word. "Sounds awful. That's one kind of doctor I don't want to be."
>
> When Connie met her brother-in-law-to-be she liked him at once. Dr. James Babcock was a tall, straight man with big brown eyes, dark skin and a heavy moustache. Connie could have done without the moustache, but the rest of him was fine. He was the kind of man who always had a twinkle in his eye and knew just how to talk to children. He was ill at ease with Kate's many relatives gathered for the wedding, but the minute he was alone with the children he told them stories and jokes and had a good time.
>
> "Connie," he said, "Kate tells me you want to be a doctor. Do you know what a doctor is?" Connie shook her head. "A person who has inside information. And do you know what a bridegroom is?"
>
> "No."
>
> "Something they use at weddings."
>
> "Oh, Dr. Babcock, you're a caution."[40]

His wife's connections to the Carolinas became in all likelihood a reason for his staying despite temptations to leave the troubled asylum. Another reason was the arm-twisting of his patient, friend, and political sponsor, Benjamin Ryan Tillman.

Benjamin Ryan Tillman and the Sea Islands Hurricane

Recent historians have seldom been kind to Benjamin Tillman.[41] Some, to be sure, hail him as the populist who founded Clemson College (now University) for men and Winthrop College for women. However, Tillman's populism extended only to whites. Blacks comprised nearly 60 percent of the state's population when Tillman was elected governor in 1890, and he set out to take away their right to vote. He went on to become a national figure through a stock speech on "the race problem" that made him rich and famous. Historians assign him major blame for the exodus of millions of southern blacks to the North and for poisoning whites' attitudes toward blacks throughout the nation during the early twentieth century.

Babcock became Tillman's physician. Tillman became Babcock's friend and political patron. Any assessment of Babcock must therefore include how he came to terms with Tillman's overt racism.

Contrary to the image he liked to project, Tillman did not rise from modest circumstances. He came from a prominent Edgefield County slave-owning family. He became "Pitchfork Ben" not from farming but from a speech in which he pledged to prod President Grover Cleveland "in his old fat ribs" with that implement. Tillman was highly intelligent and a skilled politician. Admirers called him the "Agricultural Moses" who would take them to the Promised Land and make their version of civilization safe for their version of democracy.[42]

Tillman was disabled during the Civil War by an illness that required removal of his left eye. He recovered to the extent that he participated in the 1876 "Hamburg Massacre" during which whites overthrew a militia of African American federal troops and murdered six of them after they surrendered. He attracted political notice in 1885 through a series of speeches to white farmers. In 1890 he was nominated for governor by the Farmer's Association. He appealed to small farmers by sneering at "broken-down aristocrats," but he also appealed to planters, merchants, professional men, and members of a younger generation who cared little or nothing for restoring antebellum values. He prevailed and, as one historian puts it, "for the

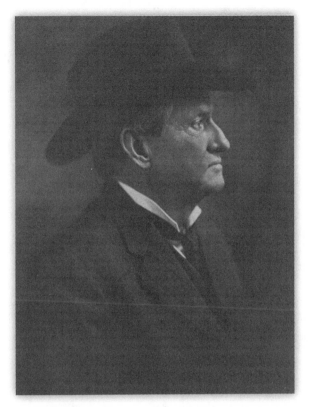

Benjamin Ryan Tillman (1847–1918), who was elected governor of South
Carolina in 1890.
Courtesy: South Caroliniana Library, University of South Carolina, Columbia, S.C.

next decade his word was law in South Carolina."[43] In 1892 he successfully opposed Wade Hampton's re-election to the United States Senate.
Hampton had been one of the South's richest planters before the war, the
state's military hero during the war, and the white's champion after the war
despite losing nearly everything. As a member of the antebellum aristocracy
who knew blacks firsthand, Hampton took more benign positions on racial
issues than some of the politicians who followed him. By prevailing over
the beloved Hampton, Tillman consolidated his triumph over the "Bourbon"
aristocracy.[44] Tillman was himself elected to the United States Senate in
1894 but continued to keep a tight rein on South Carolina politics. He
was the power behind the state's constitutional convention of 1895 that
disenfranchised blacks,[45] later boasting that his "many monuments in South
Carolina" included the convention that relieved "the people of the State of

the menace of negro domination by the organic law under which we live."[46]
In 1900 Tillman proudly maintained: "We have done our level best [to keep
blacks from the polls] . . . We stuffed ballot boxes. We shot them. We are not
ashamed of it."[47] In 1908 he argued for "the fundamental proposition that
the Caucasian race is the superior on the globe; the flower of humanity; the
race responsible for the history of the world; for the achievements of the
human family in a large degree." He proclaimed that "every South Carolinian
worthy to be called a South Carolinian" should endorse white supremacy.[48]
Thus, the task of a Babcock biographer includes giving the reader enough
information to reach his or her own conclusion about the extent to which
Babcock reconciled his humanitarian impulse with Tillman's politically-
charged racism.

Although Tillman had seen in Babcock "an accomplished and thoroughly educated specialist,"[49] a closer relationship between the two men
began after the governor asked Babcock to investigate the aftermath of what
is now known as the Sea Islands Hurricane—the second of three storms
during the most disastrous hurricane season in the state's recorded history.[50]

On August 27, 1893, what began as a tropical storm east of Cape Verde
struck near Savannah, Georgia, with a force at least that of a Category 3

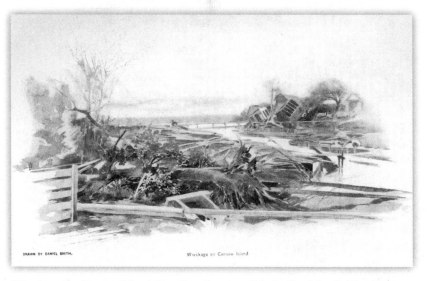

DRAWN BY DANIEL SMITH.   Wreckage on Coosaw Island

Wreckage on Coosaw Island, Beaufort County, after the Sea Islands Hurricane
of 1893 (From Joel Chandler Harris, "The Sea Island Hurricanes: The Relief,"
Scribner's Magazine 15, no. 3 [1894]: 277).
Courtesy: National Oceanic and Atmospheric Administration/Department of Commerce.

hurricane. The barrier islands of Beaufort County, South Carolina, had a population of about 35,000 people, nearly all of whom were black as a legacy of the large labor forces on long-staple cotton plantations. The storm surge killed between 1,000 and 5,000 people, according to various estimates. It damaged beyond repair nearly every building in its path, leaving some 30,000 people homeless. The estimated death toll probably ties it with Hurricane Katrina (2005) as the fourth deadliest in U.S. history. The storm destroyed crops and dealt a near-fatal blow to Beaufort County's phosphate industry, a major employer.[51] Those affected were mainly black and poor. The crisis demanded a response from the governor.

A week after the storm Tillman asked Babcock "to go immediately to the scene of the trouble & report as soon as you can the state of affairs & your opinion as to what is the best thing to do & the probable requirements of the people who are suffering."[52]

Babcock went to Beaufort County, the southeastern tip of South Carolina, along with August Kohn, a 25-year-old Columbia reporter for the Charleston *News and Courier*. Together they toured the county island by island.[53] Initial rumors had not been exaggerated. There had been extensive loss of life and property. "With a few exceptions," Babcock noted, "the dead were buried in hastily prepared coffins, and on account of the water-logged condition of the soil the graves could not be dug deeper than two feet, and the effusive fumes of the decaying bodies is fearful."[54] He looked for infectious diseases such as malaria and diarrheal illness, treated some seventy surgical injuries, and made recommendations for relief committees.

The consensus among historians is that Tillman did not act with sufficient urgency out of concern that crowds of blacks would get out of hand and because Beaufort County held no political value for him. Solidly Republican, Beaufort County in 1893 was hardly Tillman country because of its unique history. Early in the Civil War, in 1861, Union forces liberated the Sea Islands and their main harbor, Port Royal. Slaveholding whites fled, leaving behind thousands of blacks on 195 plantations. Northern whites came down to start the Port Royal Experiment, a model for what Reconstruction might have been had all gone according to plan.[55] Many Northerners stayed on after the war and assumed leadership positions. Beaufort County had a huge black majority backed by white sympathizers.

Tillman had cautioned: "We want to guard against those people who, seeing that aid is coming, might do nothing. . . . I do not want any abuse of charity."[56] Although Babcock recommended that "no supplies should be distributed among those who are not willing to do something to help themselves," he also wrote: "Without doubt the negroes on this place will

need assistance. As yet they have been too much demoralized by their mis-
fortunes to rebuild. I advised them to save timber from the drift for rebuild-
ing."[57] Babcock told Tillman that the central relief committee was sending
a representative to Washington to appeal to Congress for aid, and planned
to ask the Surgeon General of the U.S. Marine Hospital Service to identify
several physicians who could be sent to the Sea Islands at short notice.[58]

There is no record that Babcock either clashed or colluded with Tillman
over relief efforts. Recently, Jennifer Fitzgerald took on Tillman's response to
the hurricane for her master's thesis in history. She concludes that Babcock's
dispatches along with those of a quarantine officer, Allen Stuart, helped
persuade Tillman to seek assistance from the American National Red Cross
through its matron, Clara Barton.[59] But it would not be until October 1 that
the Red Cross arrived in Beaufort and established a warehouse to store and
distribute food and clothing.

This shared experience led Babcock to close friendships with both the
idealistic young reporter August Kohn and the wily politician Ben Tillman.
Fortuitously, Babcock and Tillman shared the same birthday. Tillman needed
a doctor and Babcock fit the bill. (Babcock's being a psychiatrist was no
handicap; he was also a generalist physician, and there was then no stigma
about having an "alienist" for a primary care doctor.) Tillman no doubt
showed Babcock a side of his personality strikingly different from his race-
baiting, fire-eating public persona. Tillman was more cultured than he let on
with his white constituency. His largely self-acquired learning undergirded
his articulateness on the stump. He was a keen autodidact of the humanities,
including the classics. He wrote poetry. He found in Babcock a worthy intellectual companion.[60] An acquaintance of Tillman called him "the smartest
man I ever knew"; an acquaintance of Babcock called him "the brightest man
in this country."[61] Tillman would have the Babcock children sit on his knee
while he recited poetry or long passages from Shakespeare.[62] And Babcock
may have had a positive influence on Tillman for, as one contemporary
reminisced, "Those who knew Senator Tillman could see the effect this
gentle soul [Babcock] had upon his rough . . . character."[63] Babcock would
be secure in his position as asylum superintendent so long as Tillman ruled
South Carolina.

How did Babcock reconcile his desire to help blacks with Tillman's dis-
tinctively racist politics? Where did Babcock really stand on race, the central
issue on which some may judge him today? As background, let us examine
two problems Babcock addressed soon after his arrival in Columbia: tuberculosis, especially in black women, and blacks' access to mental health services.

Tuberculosis in Asylums

Before returning to South Carolina in 1891 Babcock "had seen but one patient die of tuberculosis."[64] He soon grasped that "phthisis pulmonalis," as it was often called, was especially common among black women. He told the regents at his second meeting that an effort was "being made to associate such cases in one ward in the old asylum." He asked and received permission to study the problem and to publish statistics gleaned from other asylums. By 1893 he clearly understood the infectivity of the disease. "The most deadly enemy of our patients," he reported, "lurks not in [the] water supply or drainage but enters the air they breathe through cracks and chinks in the walls and floors where the sputa of former patients have been hidden and dried."[65] He was abreast of the new understanding of tuberculosis.

Discovery of the tubercle bacillus by the German scientist Robert Koch in 1882 enabled rapid strides against "the great white plague." We now know that the causative organism, *Mycobacterium tuberculosis*, flourishes in closed environments such as asylums and prisons because of tiny infectious particles known as droplet nuclei. These form when water evaporates from the larger particles expelled by infected patients when they cough. When inhaled by uninfected patients, the droplet nuclei glide past the hairs (vibrissae) in the nasal passages and the beating cilia in the windpipes (the trachea and bronchi) toward their final destination, the air sacs (alveoli) of the lungs. There they multiply and then spread to other parts of the body. These facts

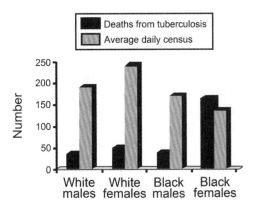

Deaths from tuberculosis at the South Carolina Lunatic Asylum, 1880–1893, by race and gender, compared with the average daily census during this period, based on data tabulated by Babcock.

were not clearly known in 1893. However, Babcock and his contemporaries realized the importance of adequate ventilation and the need to separate infected from uninfected patients. Unfortunately, they could not diagnose tuberculosis in its early stages, since chest x-rays were in the future.

In 1894 Babcock reviewed his asylum's deaths for the fourteen-year period of 1880–1893. Of 298 deaths from tuberculosis, 38 were in white males, 52 in white females, 43 in black males, and 165 in black females. Deaths among black women exceeded by 32 deaths those of all other demographic groups combined, and "this, too, when colored women composed the smallest part of the institution." His analysis of tuberculosis in the South Carolina asylum and others led to a presentation and publication on "The Prevention of Tuberculosis in Hospitals for the Insane."[66]

Worldwide, tuberculosis during the late-nineteenth century caused about one in every seven deaths. In asylums it caused more than one in four. Babcock determined the percentage of deaths attributable to tuberculosis to be 29 percent at the Royal Edinburgh Asylum for the Insane between 1842 and 1863, 35 percent at the Inverness Asylum in Scotland, 25 percent in Palermo, Italy, 33 percent in Vienna, and more than 40 percent in Prague. Surveying 98 asylums in the United States, he found that the mode—that is, the most frequent percentage—ranged between 15 percent and 20 percent, but that the percentage of deaths due to tuberculosis exceeded 20 percent in 39 percent of these asylums. The thirty-eight asylums in which tuberculosis accounted for more than 20 percent of all deaths included South Carolina's. For the ten-year period ending November 1, 1893, this percentage varied between 14 percent and 34 percent, with an average of 22 percent. Black women bore the brunt.

Babcock observed a high prevalence of tuberculosis in some of the wards of the Old Building, occupied "for the most part by colored women." He continued: "The old building ... was the fifth insane asylum built in the United States, and, conforming to then existing ideas, is very like a prison. ... The bedrooms are small, and poorly lighted and ventilated. Judged by modern standards, the whole building is typical, both architecturally and hygienically, of what a hospital should not be." The Old Building, celebrated today as Robert Mills's architectural gem, with its massive Doric columns, rooftop gardens, spiral staircase, resistance to fire, central heating, and timeless visual appeal, had become a death trap.

"In the face of such facts," Babcock elaborated, "are we not forced to raise the question, Whether there does not lurk in some of our institutions a pernicious form of hospitalism which demands rigid investigation into its causation and earnest efforts toward its extermination?" Moreover,

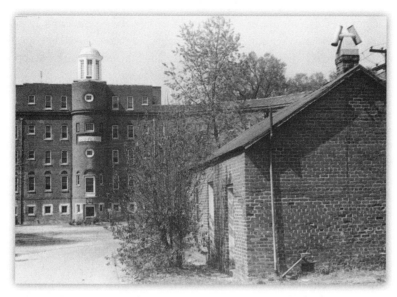

Rear elevation of the Old Building (background), photographed from Lumber Street (later, Calhoun Street) circa 1900.
Courtesy: Records of the State Dept. of Mental Health, Division of Education and Research Services, Historical Research Files (S190093), Box 7. South Carolina Department of Archives and History.

"overcrowding, imperfect ventilation and absence of sunlight, dampness, and defective plumbing and drainage, singly or in combination, have been repeatedly shown to be the predisposing cause or causes of a high death-rate from phthisis in asylums in Great Britain and elsewhere." Babcock like others overestimated the extent to which tuberculosis reflected general sanitation, stating that its prevalence might be regarded as "a test of the sanitary condition of an institution." However, he saw the importance of separating patients with active tuberculosis from uninfected patients. Infected patients should be in single rooms and should receive adequate ventilation, warm clothing, and a nutritious diet.

Tuberculosis then as now was usually a chronic disease, although many patients (somewhat less than a third) died during the first year of symptoms. Babcock found that more than two-thirds of patients with tuberculosis had been in the asylum more than a year. Tuberculosis between 1880 and 1893 had claimed 96 patients with chronic mania compared to 42 with acute mania, and 43 patients with chronic melancholia compared to 22 with acute melancholia. He recognized that heredity was "probably less potent than has been supposed." He urged gymnastics or, for the less robust, "walking parties and tennis, croquet, etc." He urged that "since it appears that cases of chronic insanity and dementia are particularly prone to phthisis they should be forced to exercise out of doors instead of being permitted to mope in corners." He also urged inspection of the dairy herds.

He concluded that tuberculosis was to a large extent a housing issue. He would advocate again and again for better living quarters, with limited success. In 1900 he wrote that "the great white scourge"—tuberculosis— "goes insidiously on decimating the inhabitants of overcrowded insane asylums, because we have not yet learned how to handle it." But he was never able to separate patients with known tuberculosis from those without the disease. In 1907 he reported: "Although the matter has been before you [the regents and the legislators] for thirteen years, very little has been done in the line of adequately handling this problem."[67]

In 1908 Babcock told the regents he considered his paper on tuberculosis his most important contribution to the medicine. He had "disproved the then opinion that the disease was inherited," and his position that it was a communicable disease had been "sustained by the most eminent authorities in the world."[68] Although he claimed no priority in this regard, one of his fellow physicians suggested in 1905 that "Dr. J. W. Babcock of South Carolina was the first to advocate separation . . . for the insane who were suffering from tuberculosis."[69] He had characterized a problem but failed at translating theory into practice at his own institution.

"The Colored Insane"

Simultaneous with his study of tuberculosis, Babcock examined the apparent rise in mental illness among African Americans. This led to an 1895 presentation and subsequent publication on "The Colored Insane."[70] Again, he characterized a problem, compared asylums throughout the United States, and urged better facilities, but made little progress at home.

The observed prevalence of tuberculosis, syphilis, and other diseases including mental illness increased among African Americans after the Civil War. Before the war, southerners and visitors to the South considered mental illness uncommon in blacks, an observation that struck Babcock as "to sociologists . . . scarcely of less interest than it is to physicians." Historians debate the extent to which mental illness in slaves simply went unrecognized.[71] Occasional antebellum physicians described psychiatric conditions they thought unique to slaves. Benjamin Rush of Philadelphia described "negritude" as a rare form of leprosy curable only by becoming white. Samuel

Cartwright of Mississippi and Louisiana described "drapetomania" (a disease that caused slaves to run away) and "dysæsthesia æthiopica" (a disease that impelled them to mischievous behavior), both of which called for the lash, not the lancet. Babcock cited others' data that diseases of the brain in blacks, as compared with whites, had increased "from one-fifth as common in 1850 and 1860 to one-third as common in 1870 to one-half as common in 1880 and 1890." However, he cautioned against placing "too implicit confidence in statistics," especially since "all colored lunatics who had been cared for by their owners became, after emancipation, objects for county and State care."

Babcock harbored no illusions about slavery: "It is doubtful whether in the history of the world any race of men has lived in whom such a degree of inhibitory power has been developed as in the Southern slaves." However, he did not dispute the common and perhaps logical conclusion that enforced labor schedules protected slaves from "much of the mental excitement to which the free population of the union is necessarily exposed in the daily route of life." Slaves did not have to fret over how to pay for the next meal or what to do next.[72] He reported his own observations that blacks, compared to whites, were less prone to melancholia (depression) but more prone to mania. However, the thrust of his paper concerned the flood of patients of both races to asylums, a pressing concern for "the tax-payer, the legislator, and even the asylum officer."

South Carolina before the Civil War had been in the forefront of providing for blacks with mental illness, despite the state's reputation for sponsoring the "positive good" theory of slavery.[73] In 1848, twenty years after the asylum opened, the General Assembly passed legislation "admitting Negro lunatics, idiots, and epileptics upon the conditions previously established for white patients," making South Carolina's one of the few antebellum asylums with facilities for blacks.[74] However, the number of black patients at any one time never exceeded five before the Civil War. After the war South Carolina, like most states where blacks were numerous, instituted segregation. Two wooden pavilions were built for black patients. In 1877 Superintendent Joshua F. Ensor likened them to "miserable cattle stalls."[75] A decade later the regents considered but rejected building a separate campus for blacks, as was done in North Carolina and Virginia. Babcock found a preference for separate facilities in nearly all states with large black populations.[76] He quoted the Jackson, Mississippi asylum superintendent: "The wards are as separate and distinct as the houses on a street ... In the field and in the garden the patients of both races work side by side, harmoniously together under the same supervision," without "wounding of sensibilities" but "with certain well-defined lines of separation which neither class has ever disposed to cross," with the net result being that "we 'dwell together in unity.'" Babcock wrote: "The opinion seems largely to prevail . . . that the separation of white and colored patients in lunatic asylums—in the Southern States, at least— is to the advantage of both races." He saw integration in the workplace as possibly advantageous to blacks but harmful to whites, since white men were reluctant to do the same work they saw black men doing. Opposing racial segregation in the American South was not a viable political option.[77]

Babcock's papers on tuberculosis and mental illness in blacks marked him as a Young Turk among asylum superintendents.[78] Although others addressed these topics,[79] his papers were unusually thorough and devoid of speculation. Unlike some of his colleagues, he resisted the temptation, if he had it at all, which is doubtful, to descend into "scientific racism."[80]

Scientific racism—the use of supposedly objective criteria or "racial anthropology" to assert black inferiority—had a substantial history in the antebellum South. Among its best-known apostles was Dr. Josiah Clark Nott, a native of Columbia, South Carolina, who made his mark in Mobile, Alabama. Nott and a few others used the internal dimensions of skulls to strengthen their argument for black inferiority—a project that today tarnishes somewhat his legacy as surgeon, medical educator, and early advocate for mosquito transmission of yellow fever.[81] Nott and others built an argument that slavery could be defended because blacks represented a separate species; they were supported in this regard by reputable scientists, including Harvard's Louis Agassiz.[82] However, the heyday of scientific racism came after the Civil War, between roughly 1880 and 1930, one of the arguments being that blacks could not compete in a free society.[83] Some even predicted that American blacks would gradually become extinct. In 1904 a Greenville physician asserted at the annual meeting of the South Carolina Medical Association that "from a scientific point of view, the ultimate solution of the race problem" would be "the gradual extinction of the negro . . . through the tireless and resistless forces of natural evolution, and the . . . doctrine of survival of the fittest."[84] Babcock would have none of this.

Babcock's publications, his surviving correspondence, his recorded statements, and his remembrance by others show little if any prejudice toward African Americans. Where did he really stand? The record suggests he was a friend and advocate for blacks or, at worst, an exemplar of a benign, benevolent paternalism. Had he foreseen the extent to which later generations would use the lens of race for their judgments, or if he had cared about the opinions of posterity, he almost certainly would not have returned to South Carolina.

He made sure his paper on "The Colored Insane" was distributed to all state legislators.[85] Nothing came of this effort.

Race and Gender

Babcock's years as asylum superintendent fall within what historians sometimes call "the nadir of American race relations," remembered for highly visible expressions of white supremacy, including violence.[86] Between the fall of the Confederacy and the withdrawal of federal troops South Carolina blacks and their white Republican allies enjoyed political supremacy despite organized resistance by those committed to white supremacy.[87] When the troops left, whites set out to strip blacks of equal protection under the law, equal educational opportunities, and the right to vote. Support for blacks also evaporated at the national level. By the late 1890s even the Republican Party, faced with President William McKinley's conciliatory stance toward white southerners and the Supreme Court's decision in *Plessy v. Ferguson* (1896), which legalized "separate but equal" facilities, had effectively abandoned southern blacks.[88] Loss of the right to vote and equal protection under the law was nowhere more complete than in South Carolina, the first state to secede from the Union and the last to see the federal troops leave. A North Carolina journalist visiting Charleston in 1899 wrote a friend that he would rather be "an imp in Hades" than a black in South Carolina, adding: "One decided advantage that the imp has—is personal safety."[89]

From today's perspective and using the lens of "presentism," racial and gender disparities in allocating his asylum's meager resources constitute the major blights on Babcock's record. Racial and gender disparities continue of course to be serious issues in most aspects of American life and especially in health care; the issue therefore becomes largely one of degree. These disparities aside, Babcock is perhaps best seen as a humanitarian handcuffed by a meager budget and reluctant to push legislators for more money in a financially strapped state.

Perhaps the most direct testimony in this regard comes from Alonzo McClennan, a black Charleston physician who tried to promote interracial cooperation. McClennan published between 1899 and 1900 a monthly periodical entitled *Hospital Herald*. In August 1899 McClennan visited Babcock and concluded that South Carolina was "fortunate in having at the head of this institution a physician who has all the elements that make the good physician and humanitarian." He spoke of "the excellent care and treatment our people receive in this model institution." He said that Babcock "has promised his cooperation in our work and we hope to have one of his nurses take the course at our hospital." Historian Todd Savitt suggests that McClennan did not speak out against the inferior treatment blacks received at Babcock's hospital because he wanted to promote a good relationship between the Charleston and Columbia institutions.[90] Another spin would be that as a realist McClennan knew what Babcock was up against. He felt Babcock was doing his best under difficult circumstances.

Two passages in the previous chapter evince Babcock's humanitarianism toward blacks: his putting the need for "a new asylum for the Negroes" first and foremost in his letter to Thomas Berry, and the letter from his brother, Brooks, expressing their father's concern that if he took the job he would "worry to death" over his black charges.[91] Babcock's daughter Alice wrote years later that "Regardless of color or station in life, all [of the patients] received the same humane attention and kindness from my father."[92] Others made the same observation. Still, the mortality for blacks during Babcock's twenty-two-year tenure as superintendent was nearly twice that of whites, a greater discrepancy than occurred during the years before and after Babcock's years as superintendent (see Appendix 1). Discrepancy was also apparent in the general population; black-sponsored life insurance companies usually failed during this period until they began to base policy contracts on 150 percent of the overall American mortality experience.[93] The lowest mortality occurred among white women, the asylum's largest demographic group.

Babcock neither hid nor apologized for favoritism toward the white women. In 1909 he told a legislative committee: "I honestly admit that I have paid more attention to the white women here than to any other department, but at the same time I do not mean to apologize for it ... I think they were entitled to the best we had."[94] Early during his administration he sought and obtained permission to commandeer one of the black women's wards whenever there was an overflow of white women. He refused to send destitute white women no longer needing psychiatric services back to their counties. "It has never been my opinion," he told the regents, "that the Asylum should send harmless white women back to county poor houses."[95] When a former regent recovered some bonds donated by Dorothea L. Dix, the renowned activist for the indigent insane, these funds were used to renovate a cottage, renamed the Dix Cottage, as "a retreat for our convalescent and quiet white females."[96] Babcock pushed without success for "a separate building for white women of the excited class," since one screaming patient could make the night miserable for the nearly 300 others.[97]

Jane Turner Censer, in *The Reconstruction of White Southern Womanhood, 1865–1895*, points out that by the late 1880s the language of "protection" pervaded southern whites' discussions about their women. White paranoia about black male virility was widespread. "In the late 1890s," Censer writes, "southern women of all classes became more thoroughly enmeshed in the racial tragedy that came to characterize the twentieth-century South."[98] The language of "protection" crops up periodically in the minutes of the Board of Regents. When in 1894 a white girl from Beaufort County, accompanied by her mother, was brought to Columbia by the black sheriff of that county, the regents instructed their president and the superintendent "to call the attention of the Legislature at its next meeting to the danger of thus exposing white female patients to the protection of colored officers."[99] When it became apparent that some of the city's blacks found it a "diversion … to sit and gaze at insane white women," steps were taken to keep the women out of sight.[100] And white women were exempted from the rule whereby all patients were to be sent home with second-class fare.[101] White women could, at the staff's discretion, go first-class on the public conveyances. Women, whether white or black, had their own issues pertaining to equality. Consider, for example, the average salaries in 1909 for attendants: $353 on the wards for white men, $218 for black men, $189 for white women, and $168 for black women.

Babcock showed no personal reluctance to care for blacks. In 1899 he volunteered to take charge of the wards for blacks himself "as a means of making careful study of the question of tuberculosis among the Negroes and also for the sake of economy, as our balance is too low to permit any extra indebtedness."[102] Between 1903 and 1910 he personally took charge of all the black women. The extent to which Babcock may have been ahead of his time on matters pertaining to both gender and race—or, in today's parlance, to exhibit "liberal" leanings—shows at least to some extent in his relationship to, and testimony from, Dr. Sarah Campbell Allan.

Sarah Allan was a native of Charleston and, after being denied admission by the all-male Medical College of the State of South Carolina, a graduate of the Women's Medical College of the New York Infirmary. She achieved the highest score on the first sitting of the newly instituted licensure examination of the South Carolina State Board of Medical Examiners and thereby became South Carolina's first licensed woman physician. On October 1, 1895, she began a twelve-year career as assistant physician on the staff of the South Carolina State Hospital. Thus, it was Babcock, backed by Governor John Gary Evans (and, one suspects, by Tillman) despite strong

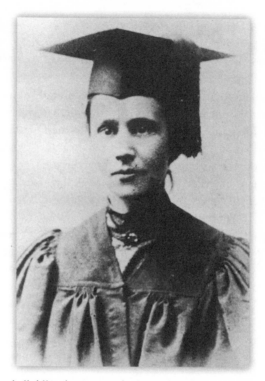

Dr. Sarah Campbell Allan (1861–1954), shown here in cap and gown at
graduation from the Women's Medical College of New York Infirmary.
Courtesy: Waring Historical Library, Medical University of South Carolina, Charleston,
S.C.

political pressure to give the position to a man, who employed the first
woman licensed to practice medicine in South Carolina.[103] A diary kept by
Allan during 1900 attests Babcock's willingness to care for the black women
in the Old Building; for example, "Dr. B. takes the colored women again,"
"I have the darkies again owing to numerous calls on the Superintendent,
"As Dr. B. took darkies back today, I got off to church."[104] Babcock, unlike
Sarah Allan and others, seldom, if ever, used such words as "darkies." In his
paper on "The Colored Insane," for example, he referred to blacks being
"pronounced 'full-blooded' Africans by intelligent men of their own race."

One such intelligent man was Page Ellington. Born a slave, Ellington
became a master brick mason and Babcock's right-hand man for construction. Beginning in 1897 Ellington helped Babcock build, successively, the
Parker Building (for black men), the Taylor Building (for white men of the
"excited or violent class"), the Talley Building (for excited white women),

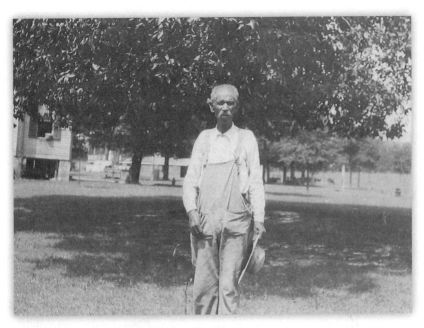

Page Ellington (1835–1912), Babcock's right hand man for new construction.
Courtesy: South Caroliniana Library, University of South Carolina, Columbia, S.C.

and the North Building, as well as a new bakery. According to Babcock's daughter Margaret, Babcock would show pictures of what he wanted to Ellington, who would sketch out plans on butcher's paper.[105] Babcock took keen interest in Ellington and helped him outline a brief autobiography, which reads in part:

> I was born at Wentworth Ct. House, Rockingham Co. [North Carolina], May 30, 1835. My owner was John McCully. Wm. Ellington, he was a Negro trader by business. I was told as late as 1894 that he was my daddy. We left there in Jan '42 in a drove. In Columbia, S.C. we were sold to John McCully—my mother, Henry & Moses twins, Diana and myself—Page. . . . I never had but these 2 owners. . . .
>
> 45-47-48 I was at my master's home. In Sept 49 [I] was messenger in telegraph office . . . While there I was taught from ABC by Mr. Josiah Edwards, they taught me reading, writing & arithmetic. It was necessary for messengers to be able to read as some wealthy white men could not read writing. For these messages I was paid 5-c each—an unwritten law . . .
>
> I stayed at telegraph office till '53.

> I liked my work. My master got the wages—$12 a month—and I got
> the tips—2 or 3 $ a week. The operators treated me well. . . . My old master
> did not want me to learn bricklayer's trade [but] wanted me to be a tailor.[106]

Babcock shared his confidence in Ellington with Tillman, writing: "Page
Ellington asks me to inform you that he has not been able yet to get a competent man to undertake the work you wished to have done. He has two or
three men in view but has not yet got one who is free to make estimates for
you and later to tackle the work, if you should so decide."[107] This correspondence suggests that even Tillman—perhaps like most Southern whites—had
no problems with blacks, indeed got along with them quite well, so long
as they did not cause trouble, show interest in white women, compete with
whites for jobs, or try to vote.

Babcock became a devotee of African American culture. His daughter
Margaret recorded: "A scrap of paper apparently torn out of Page's construction paper and used to jot down some rough words of a song the work-gang
was singing that day, as they mixed cement or toted bricks. Daddy adored
Negro singing and would sit on a keg beaming at the carryings on in laundry,
vegetable house, construction, or in the exercise yards."[108] The song read:

> I was talking to a moaner did not hear
> Moaner I leave you in hand
> Of a kind save ye'
> Farewell I leave in de hand
> Goodbye I leave you in de hand
> Farewell I leave in de hand
> Of a kind save-ye
> John says to leave you in de hand
> Of a kind save ye.

Margaret's son recalled a family story about an elderly African American
vegetable vendor who would arrive at the superintendent's residence in a
mule-drawn wagon. He would announce his presence with a bugle, whereupon Babcock would take his own bugle and join the vendor for a duet on
the back of the wagon. Kate Babcock disapproved of her husband's being
out of step with the social minuet that characterized custom and etiquette
in the South.[109]

Babcock also studied black superstitions and witchcraft. He recorded
the following from his patients:

Just so you live just so you die. The spirit that is in your body will meet the spirit that stays in heaven or hell where you are going. Your sin is higher than you is.

Witches bothers people in the foot. Burns your foot like fire popping on you. The Lord says I will send a sting on you. What does that mean? After you pray the Lord will teach you and send the good spirit to you. After you break up the ground then God will come in.

Old fashioned witches is like people. The witches we got now is made witches. Whenever a cow belches that is a made witch. I've been as big a devil as anybody, but I got religion through prayer.

God sent John & I married him. After John left, the devil come. I didn't know him till I looked at his foot. Then I knowed him . . . John came from heaven. He was a pretty man.[110]

In sum, he took keen interest in blacks and became their advocate, especially for better living conditions, although his efforts always came up short.

Among his major if imperfect achievements was the Parker building for black males. He made this a priority from the beginning. In 1892 in his first annual report he drew attention to "the urgent necessity of . . . permanent and comfortable structures for the colored male patients."[111] In 1892 he added that such necessity "presents strong claims upon our common humanity,"[112] pointing out that the wooden structures behind the New Building were "very unsafe in case of fire."[113] When funds were not forthcoming he experimented with brick making on the asylum grounds. Bricks made by the patients proved unsatisfactory. The eventual success of the brick-making project, accomplished in part through convict labor, shamed the legislature into appropriating $7,500 in 1897. Construction then began in earnest. Babcock served as architect, Page Ellington as engineer and contractor, and black male patients did much of the work. In 1898 the legislature provided another $13,500 and the building was soon completed and occupied.[114] The total cost to the taxpayers for the five-story, 200-bed building, named the Parker Building after the former superintendent, was only $30,000, taking into account the cost of the bricks made by convicts.[115]

Babcock also sought a new building for black women, recognizing that tuberculosis made the Old Building a death trap. He felt such a building could similarly "be erected at little cost." In 1900 the Board of Regents recorded his anger: "We are glad to report that separate wards are being prepared for the isolation of tuberculous Negroes. On this point Dr. Babcock emphatically remarked: 'Such provision is imperative, not only for this, but all public institutions. It is perhaps the burning question today for hospital management in the United States.'"[116] However much he could do for the blacks and for the patients in general, it could never suffice. Patients and problems accumulated faster than his budget allowed, saddled as it was by South Carolina's poor economy.

To what extent, then, were Babcock's attitudes and actions toward blacks progressive or prejudicial? One might ask, "Compared to whom?" As blacks struggled for a semblance of equality during the late nineteenth and early twentieth centuries, even the most progressive or liberal whites modeled what would now be called a benign paternalism. Harvard's President Eliot (Chapter 1) supported better access to education for blacks but sometimes resorted to racial stereotyping.[117] Abbie Holmes Christensen (Chapter 4), probably the most liberal white person to be encountered in the present volume, is considered exemplary of "New South paternalists" who thought blacks still needed guidance from benevolent whites.[118] Joseph Goldberger (Chapter 8) and his associate Edgar Sydenstricker have been criticized for virtually ignoring blacks even though blacks disproportionately got pellagra.[119] Gerald Grob, the authority on asylums in the United States during the nineteenth and early twentieth centuries, writes: "Irrespective of their regional affiliations, psychiatrists tended to share a common belief in the existence of innate racial differences, a view that shaped their attitudes and practices toward black patients."[120] In summary, it seems reasonable to suggest that were Babcock alive today he would, with his humanitarian impulse, agree with charges of racial and gender disparities in his allocation of the meager resources at his disposal. He would also assert that, given the political climate in South Carolina, his only viable solution would have been to leave the state.

As we shall see, he tried more than once to do just that.

Dumping Ground

Although funding for a new building for black women never became available, Babcock and Ellington teamed up on smaller projects. The look of the campus increasingly bore their imprint by the turn of the century. Babcock, whose interests included horticulture,[121] added flowers, shrubbery, and an avenue of magnolias along the Elmwood Avenue entrance. After "some rowdies shot into a room" from Elmwood Avenue, he successfully petitioned the legislature to close the street at its intersection with Bull Street, which was then extended into the country.[122] Electric lights replaced gas lights

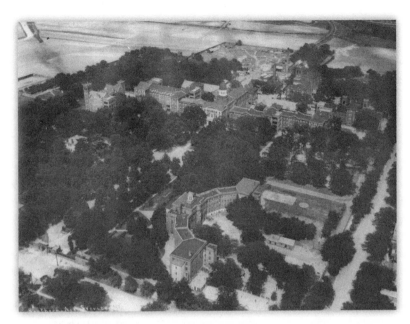

Aerial photograph of the South Carolina State Hospital taken in 1915 (the year after Babcock's resignation as superintendent), looking east. In the foreground is the original asylum (the Old Building), which during Babcock's era housed black women. Behind it is the Main Building (or New Building) with its separate wings for white women (to the left of the cupola) and white men (to the right of the cupola). The cluster of buildings behind the wing for white men includes the Parker Building for black men, built by Babcock and Ellington. In the foreground is Bull Street, running north to south. Lumber Street (later, Calhoun Street), running east to west, is best seen at lower right. A spur of the Southern Railroad brought into the asylum from the east can be seen at upper right.
Courtesy: South Carolina Department of Archives and History. Records of the State Dept. of Mental Health, Photographic File (S190095), folder 2.

throughout the campus. The Southern Railroad extended a spur track to the asylum's east side, where a large storehouse was added. Verandas were added to several wards and infirmaries to several departments. All wards now had running hot water. The regents' minutes reflect much concern over the potential for fire. A new fire house was built, along with fire doors, and although several small fires occurred during Babcock's watch there were no major fires and no loss of human life from fire.[123] A laboratory was organized.[124] Properties adjacent to the asylum were acquired, so that by 1904 the campus consisted of 360 acres, of which 60 were used for the buildings and 300 for farming.[125]

But the main problem was always space and beds. Few sent to the asylum were turned away, and too few recovered or were discharged. Admissions accelerated during the mid-1890s and again after the turn of the century. In 1900 the inspector for the State Board of Health reported that on "the subject of the necessity for relief of the overcrowded Hospital, Dr. Babcock truly and forcibly remarked, 'This Hospital is practically the dumping ground for all the undesirable citizens of the State, who are not criminals, and even criminals who show any mental symptoms are committed to the Hospital.' It is obligatory upon the General Assembly to take steps toward the development of the poor-house system. . . . The State should also make separate provision for inebriates, epileptics, and idiots, who are at present committed to the State Hospital." Relief of crowding was urgent for the "provision of the care for the insane proper, for whom the institution was established and ought to be maintained." Such pleas had little impact. Two years later the health inspector regretted "again to report to report that this *retreat for the insane* is still made the unwilling recipient of idiots and epileptics. . . . care that should be wholly devoted to the insane proper." The inspector, like Babcock, expressed concern especially for black women, whose living conditions constituted "a pitiable spectacle" that was "not only detrimental to their physical well-being" but also "inhuman, unkind, unchristian, and a reproach to us a civilized people." The inspector concluded: "We do not intend any reflection whatever upon the accomplished and faithful superintendent, nor upon the Board of Regents, for these facts clearly prove how their work is embarrassed and frustrated by inadequate accommodations."[126]

Babcock's reports to the regents read like a running jeremiad against overcrowding, especially for African Americans. Thus: "The old cry of overcrowding applies with especial force to the wards for colored patients." And: "The overcrowding is most marked in the colored departments. These figures and conditions are, I know, an old story for you."[127] In 1903 he noted, "Idiots, lunatics, epileptics, inebriates, cases of old age ("dotards") and alleged criminals—[are] all well received. No prospect of other receptacle,"[128] and that the asylum "also plays the part of a large State almshouse, as well as serving as a receptacle for undesirable members of many communities."[129] He found no disagreement from the regents.[130] In the report for 1891–92 Taylor observed that since the asylum was the only hospital in the state outside of Charleston it was "not . . . surprising that patients are often sent here who are not fit subjects for an insane hospital."[131]

Babcock was in a double bind. Recalling his enthusiastic participation in the Golden Branch debating society at Phillips Exeter, he could probably have argued on short notice for either the affirmative or the negative on the proposition "that a public asylum should accommodate all those who are weary and heavy-laden." On the one hand, he took pride that nobody who could establish residence in South Carolina was turned away. On the other hand, he decried the extent to which the asylum had become a convenient place for inconvenient people. All that was needed to send someone to the asylum was two doctors' signatures on a piece of paper. This would generate a court order and off the patient went. Although Babcock could in theory send the patient home after an examination, he knew that political leverage usually trumps professional judgment. Put baldly, if he sent the patient back there would be hell to pay.[132]

James Thompson recalled the case of a patient diagnosed with manic-depressive illness. The patient's father, who lived in North Carolina, removed him from the hospital, promising to take him to that state's asylum if readmission became necessary. When readmission became necessary, Babcock refused the patient on the grounds that he was no longer a South Carolina resident. A committee was formed between the hospitals of the two states, a vote taken, and a resolution passed that the patient should be in South Carolina. The patient was brought back in 1905 where, Thompson wrote years later, "he still remains."[133] The de facto inability to screen patients once they reached the asylum rendered examinations perfunctory. Thompson on one occasion signed commitment papers for a woman from Sumter County without bothering to look at her. The attendant who had brought the patient left hurriedly, leaving Thompson to find a corpse at his door. The woman had died en route.[134]

The asylum's written admission policies, newly approved when Babcock assumed office, reinforced his inability to send patients back home. Probate courses, circuit courts, spouses (or, in their absence, a next of kin), or the combination of a trial justice and two licensed practicing physicians could order admission for anybody found to be a lunatic, an idiot, or an epileptic. Babcock's only option for holding down the census was to press for early discharge. Even then, he had to get the approval of an Examining Committee, the composition of which was nowhere spelled out. In summary, he felt that he had little control over the oppressive patient census. And despite the plethora of patients and his many administrative duties, his nigh-impossible job description required him to be "at all times conversant with the actual condition of each individual case."[135]

He prepared a lecture—probably intended for publication but apparently never published—to educate his fellow physicians. Other states either had qualified "examiners in lunacy" or stipulated that doctors needed to be in practice at least two years before they could sign "a certificate of lunacy."

In South Carolina, any licensed physician would do. "Experience has taught me," Babcock observed, "that this privilege is frequently lightly valued by our profession." Most doctors did not like to deal with mental patients. They were happy to rid their practices of them. Most judges were equally indifferent. Sometimes, Babcock noted, the certificate of insanity was entirely blank except for two physicians' signatures—yet the patient was committed anyway. Even if completed, a certificate of insanity might have little information. Babcock noted that on the certificate "only four classes of facts are called for: (1) what the patient *said*; (2) what the patient *did*; (3) his *appearance*; and (4) *communicated other facts*." He gave twenty examples of poorly completed certificates. One read:

> Patient *said*: "He talked about religion, etc., and about himself."
> *Appearance*: "Not good."
> The rest left blank.

Babcock noted wryly: "If such observation constitutes evidence of insanity, how many of us would be able to keep out of the Asylum?"

In his lecture he urged physicians to present facts clearly and in sufficient detail for "By doing this you will contribute towards the elevation of the standard of psychiatry by the same methods that you are willing to contribute to the elevation of the other medical sciences, that is, by intelligent

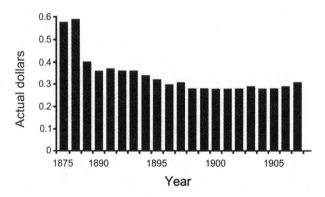

Daily per capita expenditures at the South Carolina Lunatic Asylum (later, the South Carolina State Hospital for the Insane) for 1875, 1880, 1885, 1890, and 1891–1907, in then-current dollars. (One dollar in 1876 was equivalent to about \$21 in 2013 buying power; \$1 in 1900 to about \$27, and \$1 in 1907 to about \$26.)

observation, thought, and effort."[136] The lecture probably fell on deaf ears. Babcock's one suggestion for the "Medical Certificate of Insanity" was to add a provision similar to one used in England: "The said _____ appeared to us to be (or not to be) in a fit condition of bodily health to be removed to the State Hospital." Otherwise, some patients were sent to the hospital in a moribund condition, which contributed to high mortality rates.[137]

Funding only got worse. The patient census rose by 42 percent between 1891 and 1900 and by 127 percent during Babcock's twenty-three-year tenure. The per capita budget steadily decreased. In 1875, under the Republican government, the daily per capita budget had been $9.57 (expressed in 2013 dollars), and when Babcock took office it was $7.95. By 1904, it had declined to $6.10.

Babcock drew praise for making do on a shoestring. The subtitle of an 1897 newspaper article on "Babcock's Report" reads: "The Hospital for the Insane in Excellent Condition. The Cost Per Capita. Big Reduction in Expense of Patients—The Management Shows Strict Economy." The newspaper elaborated on the "excellent and economical management the institution has been [under] for the past year," as the "cost per capita of the inmates seems to have been reduced to the minimum."[138] Babcock was similarly praised in 1900 as "the efficient superintendent" whose report "should be read by every citizen of the State."[139]

Babcock was doing as his superiors bid him to do. In 1898, for example, the Board of Regents demonstrated "how favorably our per capita compares with other similar institutions in this country" with a table showing the monthly per capita cost for South Carolina ($8.54) to be lower than that of any other asylum for which they had data.[140] "It has been the constant purpose of the Regents and resident officers," Walter Taylor wrote in 1900, "to maintain the Hospital with the strictest economy commensurate with the needs of the patients."[141] All marched to the same tune, to the patients' detriment.

South Carolina was a poor state. The reversal of its fortunes during the nineteenth century is perhaps the most extreme case of economic rise and fall in the history of the United States. South Carolina had once been Britain's wealthiest American colony. It ranked near the top of American states in wealth at the start of the nineteenth century. Repetitive cotton planting exhausted much of its soil before the Civil War, at which time nearly two-thirds of its wealth consisted of slaves.[142] According to two economic historians, the annual per capita income for South Carolinians by 1900 ranked second lowest, with only North Carolina lower ($71 per capita for North Carolina; $73 for South Carolina).[143]

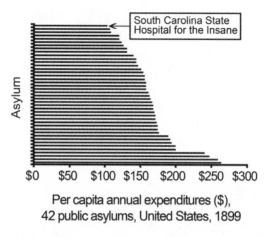

Annual per capita expenditures at 42 U.S. asylums for the year 1899. Each
horizontal bar represents one asylum. The lowest annual per capita cost was at the
South Carolina State Hospital for the Insane ($102.79 in then-current dollars;
the highest was $259.08 at the New Jersey State Hospital).

When per capita expenditures of state asylums are expressed as per-
centages of state per capita personal income, the South Carolina State
Hospital ranks a more respectable eighth of 42 asylums. In this analysis,
South Carolina looks bad mainly in comparison to North Carolina. The
annual per capita expenditures for 1899 were $103 at the South Carolina
State Hospital, $108 at the Eastern North Carolina Hospital for blacks in
Goldsboro, and $124 at the State Hospital at Morganton, North Carolina. In
1900 a psychiatrist wrote the superintendent at Morganton: "Dr. Babcock's
place disappoints me, he has not reached the goal he aimed for when I was
there several years ago, his place has improved very, very much but if Dr. B.
devoted less time to trifles and outside cases his results would be marvelous."[144] The regents were reluctant to press the legislature too hard. Walter
Taylor reported in 1899, "We recognize that many needs are pressing upon
the State, and under present conditions we would not ask that all improvements herein suggested be made in one year."[145]

Babcock was caught in what ethicists call "a conflict of obligations,"
which occurs when two obligations are in tension. He was obliged to get as
much state funding as possible to help the patients. Aren't public servants
obliged to help people? He was obliged to be frugal. Aren't public servants
obliged to help keep taxes low? He resolved the tension in part by deferring
to the regents when it came to lobbying for more funds and by making the
most of the state appropriations that came his way.[146]

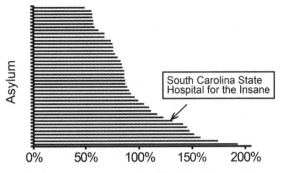

Per capita annual expenditures ($), 42 public asylums, as a
percentage of state per capita income, United States, 1899

Annual per capita expenditures at 42 U.S. asylums (as shown in figure on opposite page) in 1899, expressed as percentages of per-capita personal income for the citizens of the respective states. Each horizontal bar represents one asylum.

He took it upon himself to reduce costs. He became a master bargain hunter. He traveled out of state to government-surplus sales, usually with asylum treasurer John William Bunch. He would stand on his feet all day looking for the best buys. On a 1904 shopping trip to St. Louis, he bought 143 iron bedsteads for $150 (or $27.35 apiece in 2013 dollars), and white duck coats and trousers for five cents per suit (or $1.30 per suit in 2013 dollars).[147] On another trip he and Bunch paid 75 cents each for new khaki suits that the army had rejected for being slightly off color. No one accused Babcock of lack of diligence in this regard. But he found his job increasingly frustrating and began to weigh his options.

Restless Man

In 1897, after just six years at the asylum, Babcock explored two career options. One was at the State Almshouse at Tewksbury, Massachusetts, where he'd been introduced to psychiatry, and the other at the new Lakeside Hospital in Cleveland, Ohio.

It began when the Lakeside Hospital asked Herbert B. Howard, head of the Tewksbury Almshouse, to be its superintendent. Howard declined as he also had an offer from the Massachusetts General Hospital. Howard recommended Babcock to the Lakeside trustees and confirmed to Babcock the attractiveness of the Lakeside opportunity and of Cleveland, where Euclid Avenue was "the most beautiful residential avenue I have ever seen."

The hospital was financially sound and the trustees were "willing to give a man free rein in organizing" the hospital as the superintendent saw fit. The only drawback was that living quarters for the superintendent's family were in a second-floor suite in the hospital rather than a separate building. C. Irving Fisher, superintendent of the Presbyterian Hospital in Manhattan, wrote Babcock that he had written in his behalf for the position in Cleveland. He also related that Howard, who had just visited him, "believes that you [Babcock] can have Tewksbury if you want it." Fisher continued: "You are familiar with the Institution, its people and methods. . . . You would be . . . among friends . . . Here are two good positions [Cleveland and Tewksbury]. A man's chances of success are sometimes better among friends and familiar conditions, than they are to go among strangers . . . Tewksbury is organized and moving. Cleveland means building up from the foundation.[148] Babcock agonized.

He turned to Tillman, perhaps because he wanted to be transparent. Tillman responded: "It makes me very proud to see how other states are trying to get you away from South Carolina but I will never consent for you to accept any of these offers unless things get in much worse shape in the state than they are. You can not have many enemies there—certainly none who can bother you very much—and it would be an irreparable loss to have you go away." Tillman claimed a "right to be consulted in this matter because I 'discovered' you." He cautioned that "you must not forget that you might be subjected to the same animosities and jealousies in another state, in a less limited degree, that you have to combat in ours, and there you would be at the disadvantage of having nothing but your medical knowledge and skill to back you up. Then you are getting along in years enough to feel the need of holding on to the friends you have made. I know you would make friends wherever you go, but new friends are not like old ones."[149]

Within days of receiving Tillman's letter, Babcock received an invitation to visit Cleveland, followed a month later by an offer of the position, the salary to be negotiable. Babcock replied that should he accept, his then-current salary of $3,000 would suffice.[150]

Babcock's agony became public knowledge at least among fellow superintendents. His close friends Theophilus O. Powell of Milledgeville, Georgia, and Patrick L. Murphy of Morganton, North Carolina, expressed their sadness. Powell told Babcock that he "had accomplished so much at the Columbia Hospital," adding: "We cannot give you up without deep sorrow and regret and I still hope you may find it to your interest to remain." Murphy agreed that "I simply don't see how we can give you up for you are doing more for our cause & the cause of our helpless charges than any of us. . . .

I say that deliberately & with full knowledge of the subject. I do trust that you can see your way clear to remain at your present post. . . . I don't feel competent to say anything about the Hospital or the work at Cleveland for I know nothing but you cannot do better work than you are doing, though it may be more pleasant & profitable."[151] Babcock answered that he had all but consummated his agreement with the Lakeside trustees, that he deeply regretted the "breaking up of the pleasant associations" especially with Murphy and Powell, but that the "ignoble intra-mural antagonism arising from Mrs. Carter's influence is the 'last straw' that makes me incline to Cleveland." Babcock asked Murphy, who had just survived an attempt to remove him by the governor of North Carolina, whether he would consider the job in Columbia were it offered.[152]

He stayed. The deciding factors were almost surely his sense of duty to his native state and his family. Kate Babcock was near her relatives and felt responsibility toward younger siblings. The Tewksbury offer brought back memories of cold Massachusetts winters. The Lakeside offer would deprive her of the free-standing cottage the family enjoyed in Columbia. By May 1897 the Babcocks had two daughters, two-year-old Margaret and three-month-old Ferebe. A third daughter, Alice, would follow in 1900.[153] Alice later recalled a near-idyllic family life on the asylum campus: "Margaret, Ferebe and I, Alice, lived normal happy lives at the State Hospital. . . . We lived on the grounds in a lovely old slave-built house, [with] wide floorboards, large and well proportioned rooms with beautiful ceilings and ornate plaster work." Their father often took them "and our dog Fuzzy Wuzzy on his 'rounds' of the hospital grounds. Sometimes we would go to hear the colored women sing spirituals as they peeled vegetables. . . . How they loved his praise." Alice reminisced that "no children had a happier childhood than we three," for which she gave her parents full credit since their "fine intelligent judgments, natural attitude towards our environment, [and] invisible protection" kept them "ignorant that our surroundings were not as normal as any children living outside our beloved red brick walls."[154] The children were happy if their father was not.

Babcock's temptations in 1897 to leave Columbia were not his last. In 1903 he actually tendered resignation. He received a personal letter from governor Duncan Clinch Heyward urging him not to, indeed declining to accept his resignation, begging him "in behalf of the institution and of our State, both of which you have served so well."[155] In 1906 the Board of Regents held an impromptu meeting at the Hotel Jerome in Columbia, urging him not to resign on account of an incident that had occurred earlier that day.[156]

Alienist

He became well known as an alienist. He was often called for consultations by physicians from other parts of the state, and, being the only trained psychiatrist in South Carolina, found it hard to say no. Recognizing that such consultations detracted from his primary responsibility—running a large asylum—he asked the regents' help and obtained in 1899 their approval of a policy requiring him "to decline by authority of this Board any and all calls for his professional services to private citizens."[157] He kept up with the literature in psychiatry but made few attempts to contribute his own clinical observations.

His only published case report was entitled "Communicated Insanity and Negro Witchcraft."[158] The case intrigued him because of an African American root doctor. The patient, "B. S.," was an illiterate but successful white farmer and merchant whose store doubled as the local post office. He was married, quiet but industrious, and temperate. "B. S." began to suspect his brother was trying to kill him and that the "White Caps" were after him. He developed rheumatism. Then: "A negro styling himself 'Doctor' George Darby appeared in the neighborhood, claiming to 'cure disease and to do many wonderful things through the medium power of God.'" Darby used a "Jack" or "Little Solomon" consisting of "a bundle of roots about three inches long, wrapped in a piece of cloth and tied with a string ten inches long and having three knots tied in it." He would suspend the bundle or roots by the string "held between the thumb and forefinger," ask a question, and claim that the answer was affirmative if "the weight of roots inclined to the right" but "sinister results were to be expected" if the roots tilted to the left. Darby told "B. S." that the "Jack" would answer such questions as whether his store was being robbed. Darby then sold a bundle of roots to "B. S." for five dollars, taught him how to use it, and left the neighborhood. "B. S." explored the powers of his new bundle of roots. It warned of plots to murder him. He persuaded his wife, his two young children, and five black men to accept the powers of "Solomon." They kept guard at his house and store. They kept fires burning at each corner of the house to keep away witches who sometimes appeared in the shapes of animals. When the witches wouldn't leave he closed the store. The government informed him that he would be punished for refusing to deliver the mail. The situation deteriorated. "B. S." was perceived as a threat by his neighbors. He sent for his root doctor, who was jailed for practicing medicine without a license. The neighbors, having been unable to take away the weapons from the patient, his family, and his assistants, "finally succeeded in obtaining all the weapons upon the promise of a visit from 'Doctor' Darby." The root doctor "privately expressed the opinion that ["B.S."]'s mind was deranged, because he had studied too hard."

The root doctor was fined for practicing medicine without a license. He moved to another part of the state. The patient was hospitalized and released after improvement, but with his neighbors "prepared at any time to return him to the asylum."

One suspects "B. S." had paranoid schizophrenia, which was not then a diagnostic term. Although we recognize most of the diagnostic labels of the late nineteenth century (Table 2.1),[159] the terms differ substantially from those used today and even those of the early twentieth century. Note from Table 2.1 that "acute mania" was the most common admitting diagnosis, followed by "acute melancholia." "General paralysis" usually referred to "general paresis of the insane," an old term for syphilis involving the brain. The major innovations in psychiatric diagnosis and nomenclature

TABLE 2.1   Psychiatric Diagnoses ("Form of Insanity") for 309 Patients Admitted to the South Carolina Lunatic Asylum during the Fiscal Year 1893–1894*

Diagnosis	Number	Diagnosis	Number
Circular insanity	1	Puerperal melancholia	1
Senile insanity	15	Hypochondriacal melancholia	4
Acute mania	74	Hebephrenia	1
Epileptic insanity	28	Terminal dementia	28
Toxic insanity	8	Primary dementia	9
Post-febrile insanity	1	Senile dementia	2
Chronic mania	9	Hysteria	4
Dipsomania	2	General paresis	13
Puerperal mania	6	Cerebral syphilis	3
Paralytic insanity	2	Imbecility	13
Paranoia	11	Idiocy	9
Acute melancholia	43	(Not insane)	(9)
Chronic melancholia	4		

*Dipsomania = compulsive water-drinking; melancholia = depression; hebephrenia = schizophrenia; general paresis = tertiary syphilis involving the central nervous system

were taking place in Europe. In 1899 the German psychiatrist Emil Kraeplin defined the two major psychoses as manic depression and dementia praecox. He divided dementia praecox (soon to be renamed "schizophrenia" by the Swiss psychiatrist Paul Eugen Bleuler) into three types: hebephrenia, catatonia, and paranoia. Babcock kept up with the psychiatric literature and the diagnostic terminology at the asylum stayed reasonably current.

Babcock tabulated the alleged causes of insanity over fourteen years.[160] Causes were listed for 65 percent of patients. The most common was heredity (19 percent of patients), followed by epilepsy (14 percent), "ill health" (11 percent), domestic affliction (8 percent), intemperance (7 percent), and religious excitement (6 percent). Whites, compared to blacks, were more likely to develop mental illness because of heredity, ill health, or intemperance (for whom 92 percent of the patients were men and 71 percent where white men). Blacks were more likely to develop mental illness because of epilepsy or religious excitement. These data clearly represent a hodgepodge. "Speaking broadly," Babcock elaborated in 1900, "insanity seems to be one of the penalties of civilized life, and the changed conditions brought about in all lives during the last half of the nineteenth century have developed an unheard of proportion of insane."[161]

Although admission to the asylum required a psychiatric or neurological diagnosis, patients typically died from something else. Between 1894 and 1907 (the year pellagra was first recognized at the asylum), tuberculosis

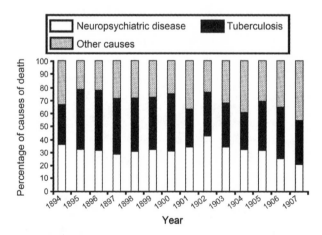

Causes of death at the South Carolina State Hospital, 1894–1907, based on the author's tabulations of data from the original sources. (Data are shown as percentages of all causes of death, since more than one cause was listed in 9.1 percent of the 2,524 deaths.)

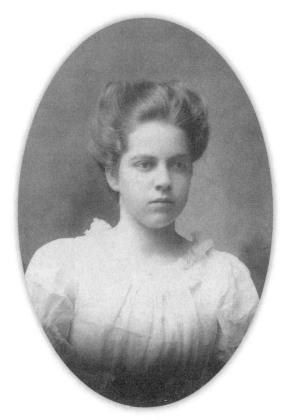

Connie Myers Guion (1882–1971), Babcock's sister-in-law, as an adolescent. She made rounds with him beginning at age 12 and went on to become "the dean of women doctors" in the United States.
Courtesy: Medical Center Archives, New York-Presbyterian Hospital/Weill Cornell.

explained 38 percent of the deaths, neuropsychiatric conditions caused 37 percent, and the remaining deaths were due to a wide variety of medical or other conditions. Of deaths attributable to neuropsychiatric conditions, only 27 percent reflected psychiatric diagnoses as opposed to neurologic conditions. "General paresis of the insane" accounted for 44 percent of the neurologic causes of death (328 of 750 deaths). Mood disorders—acute or chronic mania or melancholia (depression)—accounted for 89 percent of the deaths attributable to psychiatric diseases. Perhaps remarkably, only four deaths during this period were attributed to suicide.

What was Babcock like as a psychiatrist? His sister-in-law Connie Guion beginning at age 12 sometimes made rounds with him during her visits to Columbia, providing the basis for this remembrance:

James Babcock was, by any standards, an unusual man. When he wasn't caring for patients, he sat in his wingback chair and read, wearing eye glasses which he bought by the dozen at the five-and-ten-cent store. He read everything, and—thanks to a photographic memory—forgot nothing. Sometimes he would jump up from studying the writings of a young doctor named Sigmund Freud and go out to talk with a patient. He never stopped trying to unlock the mysteries of a personality, and he was far ahead of his time in understanding Freud's ideas.

Connie often went with Dr. Babcock on hospital rounds and although she was only twelve, she could tell he was a good alienist. He was interested in every detail of his patients' lives. He treated them as normal people and listened carefully to their stories, no matter how fantastic, always trying to give them some feeling of reality. Dr. Babcock told Connie, "Look your patient straight in the eye and listen to every word he says. If you *really* listen, you'll find he's telling you more than he realizes."[162]

Listening then as now was an essential skill for physicians not only for diagnosis but also for enhancing the patient's sense of well-being. In the back of a notebook, Babcock wrote: "If you cannot cure an insane patient, the next best thing is to make him as happy as possible."[163]

James Thompson described in his memoirs some of their patient cases, which usually reflected a mix of psychiatry and general medicine. An elderly woman who had seemed contented stabbed herself in the throat with a table knife. Babcock and Thompson rushed to her aid and dressed the wound. The patient quieted down, remarking "If my 'guzzle' had not been so tough I would not be here now." A severely depressed woman who was dying from anorexia was fed for three months through an orogastric tube. She was able to return home and appeared well at one-year follow-up. A man who had attempted suicide by swallowing an entire bottle of tincture of iodine had his stomach washed out by Babcock and Dr. Eleanora Saunders. He recovered but killed himself seventeen years later with a morphine overdose.[164]

Thompson also described Babcock's diligence and ingenuity. "Dr. Babcock," he reminisced, "never hesitated to take charge of any department where there was a vacancy for a time." Babcock would respond at all hours of the morning for emergencies. On one occasion, a "jar" occurred in the Center Building, the lights went out, and the radiators began to leak. Babcock and Thompson investigated, found a leak in a gas pipe connected to the radiator, and opened the window to the basement. A general explosion would have occurred had they lit a match. The authorities investigated the electric plant and eliminated the gas. On another occasion, the State Board of Health

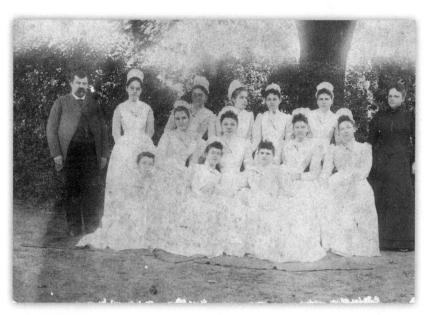

Damaged photograph of the first graduates (1893–1894) of the Training School for Nurses at the South Carolina State Hospital for the Insane. Dr. James L. Thompson is at the left; Mrs. Amanda Carter (Thompson's mother-in-law) is at the right. Although Katherine Guion Babcock (center, back row) was the school's founding director, her position in the grouping and her body language (as the only person not looking at the photographer) suggest her subordinate role to Carter and Thompson. Babcock is conspicuous by his absence.
Courtesy: South Carolina Department of Archives and History.

could not find the source of an epidemic of typhoid fever. Babcock insisted on flushing the water mains and the epidemic subsided.[165]

Of the positive changes that occurred during Babcock's tenure as superintendent, none was more visible than the nursing school. Thompson reminisced that the school brought about "a revolution" in patient care. Previously, the nurses were preoccupied almost entirely with "looking after the insane" and did not understand medical conditions. They could not use thermometers, could not take pulse and respiratory rates, and could not give hypodermic solutions. They were clueless about "what to do with patients suffering from heart conditions."[166] All this changed, according to Thompson. Others were less complimentary. Dr. Sarah Allan questioned the caliber of the nursing students.[167] The school failed to grow. On average, about six students graduated each year between 1893 and 1900, but only about four per year graduated during the next decade. Males stopped enrolling because their opportunities were better elsewhere.[168] In 1897 it became necessary to "borrow" nurses from the North Carolina asylum at Morganton.[169] In 1911 the South Carolina Graduate Nurses Association ruled that graduates of the asylum's school were insufficiently qualified for membership in their organization. They insisted that graduates receive additional training. Babcock's prompt intervention prevented resignation of the entire student body.[170]

The record indicates that Babcock was popular with the physicians and the staff.[171] He and Thompson got along well, at least during the first decade of Babcock's tenure. There is no record of staff opposition to changes he wanted to institute.

He could not change the problem of overcrowding, which grew worse after the turn of the century. In 1902 the chairman of the State Board of Health wrote: "Emphasis is made upon the conditions from overcrowding. ... The competent and self-sacrificing superintendent has no way to meet the difficulty, as patients are still sent to him, and the crowded condition is most inhumane and dangerous to the lives and interest of those unfortunate wards of the state."[172] In 1904 Babcock reiterated: "The lesson to us today is that build as fast as we may we cannot with present appropriations meet present demands upon us without overcrowding."[173] In 1907 a committee found 1,700 patients occupying space adequate for just 1,100 patients, requiring as many as seven to eight patients to share a room, keeping patients in dark, poorly ventilated basement rooms "which were never intended for living apartments," and making it impossible to separate TB patients from others.[174] The Board of Health noted repeatedly Babcock's diligence despite the deplorable conditions.

Babcock's defense for his own mental health was to sublimate—to find other outlets for useful activity when his job caused so much frustration and stress.[175]

Citizen

He sublimated in part through civic activities.[176] Columbia was growing rapidly. Between 1890 and 1900 the population rose by 37 percent and whites became the majority (53 percent). By 1910 the population had risen another 25 percent since the 1900 census, to 26,319, and the white majority had increased to 56 percent. New textile mills opened, so that by 1907 there were six mills employing about 3,400 workers. Paving of the major streets began in 1908. The city needed to improve its infrastructure, and fellow citizens turned to Babcock as a capable man who might help.

His public service began, logically enough, with an 1898 appointment to the City Board of Health. In 1901 he became a member of the Columbia Sewerage Commission, and in 1903 a member of the Columbia Commission on Water and Waterworks, which redid the city's water supply.[177] The newspaper called the latter appointment "a compliment merited by the past services of one of our most public-spirited and best-beloved citizens."[178] It could later boast that "no city in the South has a better system and the gentlemen who so successfully saw that the plans were carried out deserve the highest appreciation of the people of the city."[179] In 1903 Babcock was chosen for the Board of Directors of the newly created National Loan and Exchange Bank.[180] He belonged to a legislative committee created to erect a monument to General Thomas Sumter ("The Gamecock") of the American Revolution, which evolved into a monument to three wartime heroes: Sumter, Francis Marion ("the Swamp Fox"), and Andrew Pickens.

Although hardly a social climber, he was one of fifteen charter members of the Kosmos Club, which included President Benjamin Sloan of South Carolina College and seven faculty members along with seven "town members."[181] His ties with the South Carolina College became closer. In 1904 Sloan informed Babcock of his intent to confer "a proper and significant degree" in recognition of "your attainments in learning and your distinguished services to your State and country."[182] Sloan's successor wrote Babcock: "After coming here it did not take me long to learn something of the high esteem in which you are held by all the people of this community, and the fine example of public spirit which you have set."[183] In 1905 Babcock received an honorary L.L.D. from the college, the citation reading that "South Carolina has produced no more useful citizen before the war or since."[184]

He also sublimated through hobbies. He gardened, collected stamps and Native-American artifacts, and became a connoisseur of antique furniture. *The State* reported that his home was "the fullest and most remarkable" in the city, indeed "a veritable treasure house." "The most casual observer," asserted the journalist, "could not fail to be interested in his [Babcock's] charming colonial furniture, portraits, silver and copper, but to one with the antiquarian instinct, it is like the opening up of Aladdin's cave."[185]

He accumulated this fine collection by attending auctions and by visiting cabins formerly associated with antebellum homes, usually in the company of two close friends, August Kohn and Dr. J. J. Watson.[186] His Indian artifacts were ultimately donated to the University of South Carolina and his collection of Confederate currency to the Smithsonian Museum in Washington, D.C., but he sold some of his rare stamps to pay for his daughters' educations. He enjoyed theater and "had seen the complete repertoire of all the famous old players."[187]

He got the most pleasure from his books. His library with built-in bookcases and niches for statuettes and antique candelabra was among the city's finest and most complete, although ultimately surpassed by that of August Kohn, whom Babcock had encouraged to take up book collecting.[188] Kate Babcock complained that her husband spent entirely too much money on books. But he did not hoard them. One contemporary observed that "a friend could never leave his home without one or more books that had been graciously forced upon him"; another mused that "the size of Dr. Babcock's library varies from day to day, as he has an incurable habit of giving his friends almost every book for which they show a fancy."[189] He bought a complete set of Dickens's works and took them home one at a time in his overcoat to hide the extravagance from his wife. One of his daughters accidentally discovered the ploy.[190]

Was he paying *too* much time and attention to outside activities? Over time, he probably withdrew to some extent from the concerns at the asylum. He spent more time downtown with his friends. These included a regular group that met at Gittman's Book Shop on Main Street. On January 15, 1903, he was downtown when Lieutenant Governor James Tillman (Ben Tillman's nephew) gunned down N. G. Gonzales, editor of the *State* newspaper, in broad daylight. Babcock reached and remained at the side of the unarmed and mortally-wounded editor. At the ensuing trial Babcock recorded some of Gonzales's dying words, such as "I sent no messages." Babcock testified that Gonzales told him he tried to avoid the conflict.[191] Although James Tillman was acquitted by a Lexington County jury, the up-and-coming politician Coleman Livingston Blease (a political ally of James Tillman) developed a grudge against Babcock.

In May 1907 Sarah Allan returned to Charleston to care for her seriously ill father. Her replacement was another woman, Dr. Eleanora Bennette Saunders, valedictorian of her class of twenty-one students at the Medical College of South Carolina in Charleston.[192] She took responsibility for the white female wards on the North Wing of the New Building. Her destiny at the asylum would be tightly bound to the superintendent's.

CHAPTER 3

Founder of the Movement

Zeists and Anti-Zeists

IN DECEMBER 1907 BABCOCK RECOGNIZED a symptom complex consistent with pellagra, widely thought not to exist in the United States. He was unaware that George H. Searcy of Alabama had made the same observation earlier that year. Over the next two years, Babcock with his Columbia colleagues verified that the disease was pellagra, convened two conferences, organized what became the National Association for the Study of Pellagra, and helped mobilize the U.S. Public Health and Marine Hospital Service to investigate. He accepted the prevailing view that pellagra was somehow related to a diet based mainly on corn—a position known as the zeist theory (after the Latin word for corn, *Zea mays*).[1] He did not think the disease was infectious or communicable. He prescribed a generous diet but did not posit a specific dietary deficiency, as vitamins were then unknown. In 1909 a colleague wrote that "to Babcock . . . belongs the credit for the most complete study of cases yet presented in this country, and for stimulating the observations of others in various sections."[2]

What We Know Now

Although our knowledge of pellagra and of niacin, the deficient vitamin, remains imperfect, we can summarize part of what we know as follows: *Pellagra is to a large extent an electron transport disorder that strikes at the heart of human metabolism.*[3] Let us review briefly (1) the principal forms of niacin, (2) two molecules known as NAD+ and NADH, and (3) ATP, the "molecular currency of life."

Browse through any textbook of biochemistry, or, for that matter, of high school biology, and one finds repeatedly the abbreviations NAD+ and

NADH. "N" is for *nicotinamide*, one of the two principal forms of niacin; the other is *nicotinic acid*.[4] In 1937 researchers at the University of Wisconsin used these molecules to cure a disease in dogs known as "black tongue," a model for human pellagra.[5] Others then cured human pellagra,[6] ending the hunt for Joseph Goldberger's elusive "pellagra-preventing vitamin" or "vitamin P-P," presumed and now confirmed to be present in brewer's yeast. Food additives containing either nicotinic acid or nicotinamide, conjoined under the new name "niacin,"[7] stopped the red plague of pellagra.

The near-universal importance of NAD+ and NADH to metabolism helps explain why generations of doctors struggled with the diagnosis of pellagra, especially in its early stages.

NAD+ and NADH are coenzymes—molecules that activate enzymes—abundant in all living cells. They participate in chemical reactions involving exchange of electrons between one molecule and another—that is, oxidation reactions and reduction reactions.[8] The coenzyme pair NAD+/NADH drives at least 200 enzyme-dependent reactions. These include key enzymes in the Krebs cycle and the electron transport chain, both of which operate within mitochondria, the tiny organelles within cells. Mitochondria are called "cellular power plants" because they produce ATP, short for adenosine-5'-triphosphate. The main purpose of cellular respiration—the process by which cells use oxygen and nutrients to provide energy—is to make ATP, the "molecular currency of life."

ATP powers just about everything our bodies do—for example, transmitting nerve impulses and contracting muscles.[9] It is a highly unstable molecule and cannot be stored. We possess only about 50 grams of ATP at a given time. To assure a constant supply we recycle each ATP molecule 1000 to 1500 times a day, producing (or turning over) approximately our own weight in ATP every day. Cellular respiration can churn a single glucose molecule into up to 38 molecules of ATP. This process depends critically on an adequate supply of nicotinamide to make NAD+ and NADH.[10] In summary, we need niacin to make ATP, the body's chief energy source. And niacin participates in other key processes such as protein synthesis, adrenal hormone synthesis, repair of DNA, and neutralization of toxins.

Foods contain both principal forms of niacin. Certain vegetables are rich in nicotinic acid; certain meats and dairy products are rich in nicotinamide. Nicotinic acid cannot be changed into nicotinamide in humans, but both can be used to make NAD+. Niacin is not a vitamin in the strictest sense—something the body cannot make at all—because the liver can make nicotinamide from *tryptophan*, one of the essential amino acids. However, it takes on average about 60 milligrams of tryptophan to make one milligram

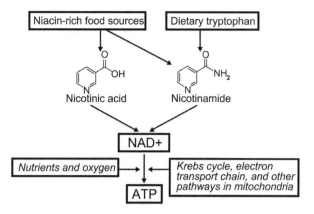

The principal forms of niacin are nicotinic acid and nicotinamide. Both are usually derived mainly from food, but the body can synthesize nicotinamide from tryptophan, one of the essential amino acids. Niacin is a component of the coenzymes NAD+ and NADH, the numerous functions of which—including the synthesis of ATP, the "molecular currency of life"—explain the protean manifestations of pellagra (niacin deficiency).

of niacin. Still, dietary tryptophan, sources of which include meat, milk, and eggs, can contribute as much as two-thirds of our daily niacin requirements.[11]

Armed with this information we can explain why the manifestations of pellagra are so diverse and, in early cases, so perplexing. Babcock and his contemporaries recognized far-advanced pellagra as the "disease of 3 D's" (dermatitis, diarrhea, and dementia or severe depression) but were baffled by the bewildering range of symptoms and signs.[12] The impact of niacin deprivation on all human cells explains the protean manifestations of pellagra, including such early, nonspecific symptoms as low energy and loss of interest in everyday affairs.[13]

We can also explain at least in part an observation that puzzled Babcock and his contemporaries: Europeans and North Americans who relied mainly on corn often got pellagra, but Latin Americans, who had relied on corn for millennia, did not. Corn contains niacin and tryptophan in bound form— that is, the molecules are bound tightly to other cellular components and cannot be absorbed by the gastrointestinal tract. Pre-Columbian Indians learned to preserve corn and separate the hulls from the grain by mixing the grain with slaked lime and water in earthenware pots, which were then heated for about eighteen hours. This process, used to make tortilla flour, frees up niacin and tryptophan, allowing these nutrients to be absorbed.[14]

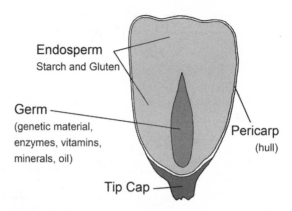

Anatomy of a corn kernel. The germ comprises only about 12 percent of the kernel's weight but contains most of the vitamins. The germ's high oil content causes corn to spoil during storage and shipment. Wide use of degerminating machines during the first decade of the twentieth century converted this dietary mainstay from a whole grain to a highly refined carbohydrate for millions of Americans.

Finally, we can explain at least in part why epidemic pellagra appeared in the United States during the first decade of the twentieth century.[15] The vitamin content of corn is found mainly in the germ. The high oil content of the germ causes corn to spoil and turn rancid during storage and shipment. Before 1900 most corn consumed in rural parts of the United States was ground locally in grist mills. Then John Beall, an employee of the Union Iron Works Company in Decatur, Illinois, invented a machine to separate the germ from the rest of the grain, patented in 1901 and widely marketed by 1906 as the Beall degerminator. Cornmeal could now be safely stored and shipped long distances. But what had been essentially a whole grain became a highly-refined carbohydrate. Millions of Americans now relied on cornmeal bought and distributed in bulk, unaware that the product had been stripped of key nutrients, including molecules that would later be known as vitamins.[16]

Babcock suggested on several occasions that understanding pellagra might unlock many secrets of mental illness. He was correct to the extent that pellagra was a molecular disease awaiting a molecular solution. Sadly, the relevant molecules were discovered long before the solution became apparent. In 1873 the Austrian chemist Hugo Weidel discovered nicotinic acid. In 1901 the British physician and biochemist Frederick Gowland Hopkins, working at Cambridge with a student, S.W. Cole, isolated tryptophan. Hopkins went on to show that tryptophan and certain other "accessory food factors" were essential to life. In 1906 British biochemists Arthur Harden and William Youndin discovered NAD. However, the terms "vitamin" and "vitamin deficiency" were not in the medical literature in 1907 when Babcock and other Americans encountered pellagra.[17]

What They Knew Then

Historians debate whether pellagra occurred before the eighteenth century and, if so, when and where, including the inevitable speculation that Job of the Old Testament might have had it.[18] However, it is generally agreed that highly endemic pellagra began in Europe when the rural poor of certain areas began living mainly on Indian corn (or maize), newly arrived from Latin America. Corn was easier to grow and yielded more calories per acre than just about everything else they'd known. Among the scores of European physicians who wrote about pellagra during the eighteenth and nineteenth centuries, at least six deserve mention: a Spaniard, a Frenchman, and four Italians.

The Spaniard was Gaspar Casál, town physician of Oviedo in the Asturias region of northwestern Spain. The Asturias with its rugged coastal cliffs and mountainous interior had been occupied successively by *Homo erectus*, *Homo neanderthalensis*, and, since the Lower Paleolithic era, *Homo sapiens*, but population growth took off only after corn arrived in the sixteenth century. Between 1720 and 1735 Casál studied a disease the peasants called *mal de la rosa*, "disease of the red rash." The rash occurred mainly on sun-exposed areas, especially the backs of the hands and feet and around the neck, extending onto the breastbone (the sternum) where it became known as "Casál's necklace." It started out like sunburn, evolved into ash-gray or blackish crusts, and culminated in glistening red, depressed areas of thinned (atrophic) skin. Affected patients were weak, listless, and depressed or at times delirious. Diarrhea and dementia portended death. Casál found it useful to provide milk, cheese, eggs, and meat, but stopped short of attributing *mal de la rosa* to deficiency of these foodstuffs. One of his friends was a vegetarian who lived to a ripe age without *mal de la rosa*. Still, he correlated pellagra with poverty—as Joseph Goldberger, who duly acknowledged Casál, would do 158 years later.

Casál's observations drew little notice.[19] The rural poor in parts of Spain and later in France and Italy continued to know a disease they variably called *mal del monte* (disease of the mountains), *leper endèmique* (endemic leprosy),

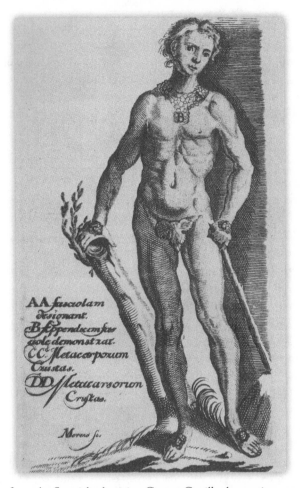

Illustration from the Spanish physician Gaspar Casál's observations on pellagra (1762), showing the symmetrical rash on the back (dorsal) surfaces of the hands and feet and also on the neck, extending down onto the breastbone ("Casál's necklace"). Casál correlated pellagra with poverty and prescribed a generous diet—just as Joseph Goldberger did 158 years later.

or *scorbuto alpino* (alpine scurvy), to name but three of more than eighty known colloquialisms. In 1771 the Italian physician Francisco Frapolli, studying the poor around Milan, used the name that stuck: *pelagra*, later spelled "pellagra," from the Italian *pelle* (skin) and *agra* (rough). Frapolli usually gets credit for calling international attention to the disease, but it would not be until the twentieth century that his monograph was translated into English—by James Woods Babcock.

Frapolli concluded that pellagra was not contagious and could be cured by a robust diet. He observed that it got worse during the summer months and better during the winter, and therefore blamed excessive sun exposure. In 1776 another Italian, Jacopo Odoardi, blamed excessive use of corn. In 1789 a third Italian, Francesco Fanzago, confirmed that victims subsisted mainly on polenta (made of ground cornmeal). Fanzago campaigned for a varied diet. Authorities ordered him to cease and desist, since alternatives to corn, notably wheat, were more expensive. In 1810 a fourth Italian, Giovanni Battista Marzari, proposed that corn lacked something necessary for good health—that pellagra might be a *deficiency* disease. Marzari's idea was revolutionary, anticipating Joseph Goldberger's demonstration by more than a century. He got nowhere with it. The same obstacle that later faced Goldberger stymied these Italians: reluctance by the rich and powerful to buy more expensive food for workers and their families on the basis of a hunch.

A Frenchman succeeded politically where the Italians failed. French doctors recognized pellagra not just among field workers and their families but also among alcoholics, inmates of mental asylums, and people who never ate corn. In 1866 Jean-Baptiste Victor Théophile Roussel published on pellagra and began a campaign to persuade the French government to place limits on corn acreage. He won, forcing people to rely on other grains and vegetables, especially potatoes.[20] Although pellagra remained a problem in parts of Italy and Eastern Europe, it virtually disappeared from France by the turn of the twentieth century.

In retrospect, each of these Europeans held one or more pieces to the puzzle. Casál observed the benefits of a balanced diet. Frapolli realized the disease was not contagious and that sun exposure played a role.[21] Odoardi, Fanzago, Marzari, Roussel, and others surmised that near-exclusive reliance on corn was the main problem. Marzari inferred the cause to be *deficiency* of something rather than the *presence* of something. A key but often overlooked observation—an exception that proved the rule—was that some people who never ate corn got pellagra.[22]

Two unfortunate additions to the small pile of puzzle pieces seriously distracted early twentieth-century researchers. These were (1) the idea that pellagra was caused by corn that had been spoiled by one or another germ or fungus; and (2) the idea that pellagra was a specific infectious disease, perhaps transmitted by an insect. The leading proponents for these ideas were, respectively, Italy's Cesare Lombroso and Britain's Louis Sambon, both of whom had large reputations and expansive personalities. Their ideas were variations of the germ theory, generally credited to Louis Pasteur in France and Robert Koch in Germany. The germ theory had sparked a frenzied

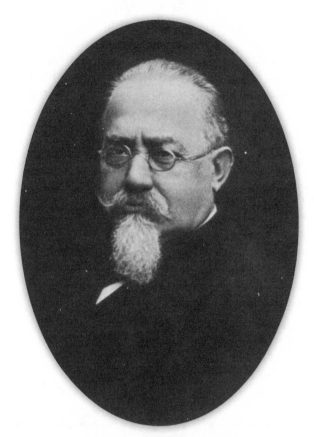

Dr. Cesare Lombroso (1835–1909) of Italy, remembered as "the father of modern criminology" because of his work in forensic psychiatry, championed the idea that pellagra was caused by a toxin in spoiled corn. This was a variant of the zeist hypothesis (that is, pellagra was somehow related to corn).
Courtesy: Photo Researchers/ScienceSource.

pursuit for infectious causes of diseases of then-unknown etiology, with fame awaiting the winners.

Cesare Lombroso, born in Verona, was famous in his day for describing "the born criminal" recognizable by such features as a sloping forehead, large ears, facial asymmetry, and protruding jaw. Lombroso's efforts to correlate criminality with anatomy have been long discredited, but he is still revered as the "founder of modern criminology" because he shifted the focus from the crime to the criminal. He wrote extensively on such then-novel subjects as political and financial crime, juvenile delinquency, and the relationship of

crime to socioeconomic status.[23] Lombroso in his later years became obsessed
with pellagra and the spoiled-corn hypothesis, which had been around since
the 1850s. He claimed a specific fungus, *Sporisorium maidis*, caused corn
to make a pellagra-causing toxin which he named *pellagrozeïn* (from the
Latin, *zea*). When injected into animals the toxin caused abnormalities he
claimed were analogous to those of patients with pellagra. Lombroso thus
embellished the idea that the problem was "bad" corn—not "too much" corn
or "little else besides corn." Lombroso's massive 1892 treatise became the
standard text on pellagra. His reputation and winsome personality—he was

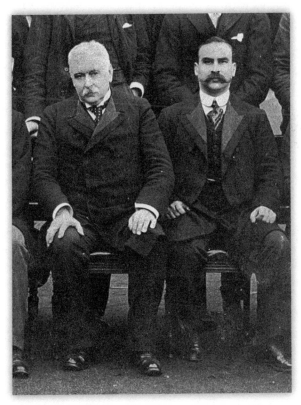

Sir Patrick Manson (1844–1922) and Dr. Louis Sambon (1865–1931) at the
London School of Tropical Medicine in 1902. Sambon proposed that pellagra
was caused by an infectious agent (possibly a protozoan) transmitted by an
insect (possibly a *Simulium* species). Note Sambon's upright posture, direct gaze,
and clenched fists—features that are also present in other group photographs
containing Sambon.
Courtesy: London School of Hygiene and Tropical Medicine.

idealistic, generous, compassionate, energetic, intellectually omnivorous, and persuasive—drew many Zeists into the "zeitoxic" camp.

Louis Sambon, born Luigi Westerna Sambon in Milan, suggested in 1905 that pellagra had nothing to do with corn. Pellagra was caused by a specific infectious agent (probably a protozoan parasite) transmitted by a specific insect (probably a fly of the genus *Simulium*, which includes buffalo gnats, sand flies, and black flies). He based his argument on the seasonal occurrence and geographic distribution of pellagra in northern Italy. Pellagra seemed to occur mainly among people living close to fast-flowing streams teeming with *Simulium* flies and their larvae.[24] Sambon like Lombroso became infatuated with his own idea. It will be argued here that Sambon's intricate speculation more than anything else slowed Americans' scientific assault on pellagra, leading to thousands of deaths that might have been prevented.

When Babcock and other Americans became involved in pellagra, Louis Sambon enjoyed a wide scientific reputation buttressed by flamboyant charm and backed by the great Sir Patrick Manson, "father of tropical medicine." A cosmopolitan almost from birth—his mother was of English and Danish ancestry, his father of French and Italian—Sambon received his MD degree from the University of Naples and started out as a gynecologist in Rome. He became interested in infectious diseases and made contributions to the study of malaria and other parasitic diseases. He moved to England and courted controversy at the Royal Geographical Society by proposing that parts of Africa were "the white man's grave" not because of the climate but because of parasites, notably the trypanosomes that cause sleeping sickness.[25] This idea resonated with Manson, who had become almost obsessed with finding parasitic causes of diseases of then-unknown origin. Manson welcomed into the London School of Tropical Medicine the colorful and supremely self-confident Sambon, who further ingratiated Manson by proposing the name *Schistosoma mansoni* for one of the parasites that cause schistosomiasis.[26] Many admired Sambon's powers of inductive reasoning. An editorialist wrote: "Apart from Manson perhaps no one working at tropical medicine has given us so many new ideas as Dr. Louis Sambon."[27] Unfortunately for the American pellagra effort, insect transmission of pellagra became one such idea.

Babcock and his American colleagues would have done well to concentrate exclusively on the early Europeans such as Casál, Frapolli, Roussel, and Marzari. Many Americans including Babcock grasped the essential points: (1) pellagra was not contagious; and (2) it could be cured, if caught early, with a varied diet. The newer hypotheses championed by Lombroso and Sambon ultimately required massive expenditures of time, talent, and money to disprove. Meanwhile, searching for a causative toxin or germ enjoyed more public and political support than providing better food for the disadvantaged. Babcock would spend countless hours perusing and when necessary translating the early European literature on pellagra. It is unclear whether these efforts made a difference in the long run. Students of pellagra were seriously divided between the Zeists, including those who favored Lombroso's spoiled-corn hypothesis, and the anti-Zeists, who increasingly followed Louis Sambon (Table 3.1).

TABLE 3.1   Zeist and Anti-Zeist Hypotheses of Pellagra during the Pre-Goldberger Era (Before February 1914)

	Zeists	Anti-Zeists
Premise	Indian corn (*Zea mays*) has a definite causal relationship to pellagra.	Indian corn has nothing to do with the cause of pellagra.
Adherents	Most students of pellagra before 1900	An increasing number of students of pellagra after 1900
Major variations	Corn contains one or more harmful substances or, more broadly, corn taken in excess is somehow harmful. Corn sometimes harbors a specific infectious agent (germ), such as a mold or bacterium. Corn causes the body to produce a harmful substance ("autointoxication"). Damaged or moldy corn produces a toxic substance (the "zeitoxic" hypothesis, championed by Cesare Lombroso). Corn is an insufficient nutrient because it lacks one or more substances necessary for health (Giovanni Batista Marzari, 1810).	Pellagra is not a specific disease but rather a symptom complex (syndrome) occurring in persons suffering from alcoholism, insanity, or other depressed states (this idea was held especially by French researchers prior to 1900). There is possibly a hereditary component. Pellagra is a specific infectious disease transmitted by something other than corn. Pellagra is caused by a specific infectious agent (possibly a parasite) transmitted by a specific insect (possibly a fly of the genus *Simulium*) (Louis Sambon, 1905).

First Cases

The historian Charles E. Rosenberg suggests that epidemics can be considered as four-act plays, as follows: progressive revelation (Act One), managing randomness (Act Two), negotiating a public response (Act Three), and subsidence and retrospection (Act Four).[28] Babcock's role in the pellagra drama was major in Act One ("What's happening?") and important in Act Two ("Who's getting it, and why?").[29] Joseph Goldberger assumed center stage in Act Three ("How do we solve it?"), although Babcock and his American colleagues—to continue the metaphor—had installed the props and painted the backdrop. Act Four continues to this day, as social historians and others find in the pellagra story broader issues that still concern us.

When Act One opened in 1907 pellagra was generally thought not to exist in North America. William Osler, the most famous physician in the English-speaking world, said as much in the sixth edition of his *Principles and Practice of Medicine*. He described pellagra as a "disease due to the use of altered maize, which occurs extensively in parts of Italy, in the south of France, and in Spain," adding: "It has not been observed in the United States." Osler was apparently unaware of occasional American case reports. Treatment consisted of a "change in diet, removal from the infected district, and, as a prophylaxis, proper preservation of maize."[30]

The American pellagra epidemic was first recognized at the State Hospital for the Colored Insane at Mount Vernon, Alabama, a small town in northeast Mobile County where much of the population is still below the poverty line. In 1901 Alabama's African American psychiatric inpatients were transferred from Tuscaloosa to Mount Vernon. Physicians at the Mount Vernon asylum began to see each summer a few cases of a mysterious and usually fatal illness. Numerous cases during the summer of 1906 prompted the superintendent to invite Dr. George H. Searcy of Tuscaloosa to investigate. In April 1907 Searcy reported that during the late summer and early fall of 1906, from a population of about 600 patients, there had been eighty-eight cases of a disease he identified as pellagra, with fifty-seven deaths. Eighty of the eighty-eight patients were women. The average age of affected patients was 34. Two-thirds of them had been in the hospital longer than a year, and 80 percent had been in good or at least fair physical health before the illness.

Searcy, like other Americans who followed, came close to getting it right. He wrote: "The disease occurs among the poorer classes and in institutions where the diet is at times limited." "No nurses had the disease. They handled the patients, slept in the halls near them, and the chief difference in their way of living was in the diet.... [which had] "a little more variety." "I believe that when it becomes generally known that pellagra may occur in this country we will have more cases reported, especially in the South, where corn bread and grits are so largely used." Following Lombroso's lead, now enshrined in Osler's textbook and elsewhere, Searcy hewed to the line of "bad" corn as opposed to "too much" corn or "little else besides" corn. He sent a sample of corn billed as "the best western meal" to a plant pathologist in Washington, D.C., who declared it "moldy" and "wholly unfit for human use." Searcy bought the viewpoint "generally accepted now ... that pellagra is caused by eating a substance formed by the growth of certain organisms in corn."[31]

Babcock and his colleagues at the South Carolina asylum were unaware of Searcy's report when, while discussing various types of insanity during a staff meeting in the late fall of 1907, someone mentioned "pellagrous insanity." Babcock suggested they immediately look up the subject in a reference handbook. "With three recently admitted cases before him," he later wrote, "all of which represented the triad [of] skin, intestinal, and nervous symptoms ... the writer [that is, Babcock] at once recognized the description applying to the disease which for a year had been to him a mysterious complex of symptoms."[32] On December 30, 1907, he submitted to the South Carolina State Board of Health a report entitled "What Are Pellagra and Pellagrous Insanity? Does Such a Disease Exist in South Carolina, and What are its Causes?" He told the regents that pellagra "although not commonly recognized in America, is apparently affecting certain classes of the citizens of the State and patients are frequently sent to this hospital on account of its effects upon the mind."[33] The report was published in the February 1908 issue of the *Journal of the South Carolina Medical Association*.[34] Characteristically deferring to the Board of Regents, Babcock put the names of the board's two physician members, W. W. Ray and Julius H. Taylor, ahead of his own on the list of authors. He also included as coauthors his three staff physicians, James L. Thompson, H. H. Griffin, and Eleanora B. Saunders. An editorialist prefaced the article as "worthy of more than passing interest" and praised Babcock as "a man whose zeal, ability, and conscientious attention to details of his duties make him pre-eminently a man to occupy his position as superintendent of the State Hospital. By pain staking and able investigation he, with the assistance of his associates in that institution has succeeded in identifying, conclusively it would seem as pellagra, a condition heretofore unrecognized and undiagnosed in this part of the country." The editorialist added that Babcock had been denied due credit for being the first to urge "the isolation and modern care of tuberculosis patients in institutions," and expressed hope that in the case of pellagra "the record will be kept in straighter shape" so that "credit shall go to whom it properly belongs."[35]

Babcock reported that colleagues and acquaintances had seen from time to time perplexing cases of depression or delirium with rash on sun-exposed parts of the body and severe diarrhea. Affected patients came from various sections of South Carolina, but especially from the upstate or Piedmont section. He was satisfied that his patients presented "conditions very similar to those presented by true pellagra" as described by the Europeans, but added that as to the "the real nature of the disease, especially as to its etiology, we are in doubt." He strongly suspected that he was dealing not with a new disease but rather with a newly recognized old disease, for "the older members of the staff" could recall similar cases. He urged the need to direct "the attention of general practitioners to its symptoms and thereby gain a fuller knowledge of its distribution, causation and prevalence."

He then gave a textbook account of pellagra: its definition, its history, its symptoms, the principal ideas on causation, and grounds on which to make the diagnosis. His first case report of what soon became the leading cause of death at his asylum reads as follows:

CASE I. M. C., admitted to the State Hospital for the Insane, December 9, 1907; white, female, American, housekeeper, age 30 years, married 11 years, three children no miscarriages. In this State one year. Previously, for three years, in Cleveland County, N.C.

Previous history: Family very poor, but patient was healthy up to five years ago when menses ceased. In spring three years ago rash appeared on back of hands like sunburn, which spread in spite of treatment. Got better in cold weather but never entirely healed. Family produced all the corn they used. None of family or neighbors have had "eczema," but family physician said he had had a similar case. Patient developed symptoms of mental depression two or three years ago. Bowels have been constipated with occasional diarrhea, which has been constant and severe for three months before admission.

On admission: Extreme adynamia, stupid appearance; reluctance to exertion. Sat with bowed head and spoke in monosyllables, and only when spoken to; muscular system fairly preserved; axillary and suprapubic hair present; poor appetite, but intense thirst; temperature 97 degrees; pulse 30, regular and full; respiration 20; urine normal, as shown by repeated examinations; blood examination showed a relative increase of lymphocytes and a moderate degree of anemia. Gastro-intestinal symptoms: Abdomen flat; exhausting diarrhea, sometimes as many as twenty stools a day, light yellow to copper color; hookworms and eggs found by several observers. Skin: Slightly jaundiced; eczematous condition covered forehead, also alae nasi, malar bones, and chin, as well as dorsal surfaces of hands and feet; very scaly and rough on exterior surfaces of elbows and knees; no sores or scars over shirts; (most of these regions were chapped and fissured); anaemic and puffy about eyes. Mouth: Foul breath; tongue deep red, and clean, straight and not tremulous. Lungs: Normal. Heart: Accentuated aortic second sound.

Nervous and Mental Symptoms: Tendon reflexes exaggerated; tabetic gait; stiffness of muscles; dull and melancholy; suspicious about food; occasionally mildly excited; pupils react to accommodation and slightly to light. Has slightly lost ground physically and mentally since admission. Has become more and more paretic, so that she had to be put to bed. Temperature varies between 96 and 99 degrees. January 1, 1908, she was given thymol, grains 15. Repeated January 12. Has made an assault on an old woman sleeping in room with her.[36]

The second case was that of a 30-year-old African American man with progressive mental decline, seizures, incoherent or profane speech, a mind that "ran much on religion," diarrhea, and a rash on the hands, and who "died from exhaustion" on the twenty-first hospital day. Also rapidly fatal was the third case, that of a 34-year-old African American woman whose family produced "the corn they used, except a little grits" and who "died of exhaustion" caused mainly by intractable diarrhea. He briefly told of six other cases from Columbia, pointing out that pellagra was not confined to asylums.[37]

Babcock like Searcy had described a more aggressive disease than was usually seen in Europe. American victims were more likely to die quickly and less likely to enter remission during the winter months. The diagnostic problem was lack of a confirmatory test. Pellagra is a *syndrome*—a diagnosis based on a stereotypical combination of symptoms and signs. What should be the "diagnostic threshold" for deciding whether a patient did or did not have the disease?[38] As the pellagra epidemic in the United States evolved, physicians would gradually relax their insistence on the classic triad of dermatitis, diarrhea, and dementia (or severe depression), typical of the late but not the early stages.

This landmark paper contains three noteworthy observations. First, Babcock made it clear that Searcy, not himself, had been the first to recognize epidemic pellagra in American asylums. Second, he emphasized: "Whatever its nature the disease is not infectious or communicable." Finally, the usual treatment was "to prohibit corn in any shape and form as food" if at all possible and to encourage the use of other cereals. Like Searcy and others, influenced as they were by Lombroso, he bought into the idea that the problem was likely to be "bad" corn, not "too much" corn or "little besides" corn.

The editorialist in the *Journal of the South Carolina Medical Association* commented that Babcock's report combined with the efforts of his colleagues constituted "a long step forward in the progress of scientific medicine in the United States," and predicted that the disease would be found in other parts of North America.[39] The local newspaper's announcement of pellagra in South Carolina followed by only a few days a report that hookworm caused much of the anemia among textile workers.[40] Pellagra and hookworm soon became regional embarrassments.

Travels with Tillman

On March 19, 1908, Senator Tillman suffered a stroke with left hemiparesis—loss of much of the use of his left arm and leg. Three years earlier, he had sustained what we would now call a "transient ischemic attack" or "reversible ischemic neurologic deficit," with full recovery.[41] The 1908 attack was more severe. It was not until the fifth day that he sat up in bed, at which time he could not walk unassisted.[42] He gradually improved and was advised to take an extended trip to Europe.

Tillman, fearful of another stroke in a country where he did not speak the language, invited Babcock to go and to pay Babcock's expenses.[43] When Babcock accepted, Tillman cautioned: "You may think you are going to study Pellagra but I shall depend on you to act as guide & antiquarian [,] historian & interpreter."[44] Babcock also took Tillman's dictations of a travelogue, which were forwarded to August Kohn for release to the newspapers. For Babcock it was a working vacation but a vacation nonetheless—his first since becoming superintendent.

Senator and Mrs. Tillman, accompanied by Dr. and Mrs. Babcock, sailed from Boston on May 16 on the SS *Canopic*. They landed at Gibraltar and went briefly to Morocco where, Tillman dictated, a "saunter of an hour and a half through the narrow, filthy streets . . . gave us all the idea of Moham-medan and Moorish life and civilization that we wanted." They enjoyed Spain, especially the sights of Granada, Seville, and Cordova. Letters from home about "hot parched conditions in South Carolina," helped them appreciate all the more "the marvelous Spanish climate . . . in June, where oranges flourish and hot house plants grow in the yards." They took a steamship from

Spain to Italy. By June 25 Babcock could report that Tillman had become a "gay bird" with no signs of his stroke. They spent twelve days in Rome and then took in Naples, Florence, and Venice, at which point Babcock began to observe pellagra as seen by the Italians.[45]

Beginning in 1784 the Italians had established special hospitals for patients with pellagra, or *pellagrosari*. On July 10 Babcock visited the Rio Instituto Pellagrosi in Mogliano, near Venice, where he was "received with much consideration by Doctor Caldano and Sister Speranza." Most of their patients were children. From Venice the party went to the industrial city of Milan, from which Babcock and Tillman visited the large asylum in Mombello. The members of the medical staff "did everything in their power to show us their pellagrous patients and demonstrate the disease in all its forms." Babcock learned that they had treated 2,858 patients with pellagra between 1879 and 1906 in their asylum, which usually had about 2,200 patients. He made detailed notes on nine patients, eight of whom had the typical rash. The other patient had no rash, introducing Babcock to a variation known as pellagra *sine* pellagra ("pellagra without the rash"). His observations in Mogliano and Mombello were "sufficient to confirm my opinion that the disease I have observed in South Carolina is identical with the disease described as pellagra by the physicians and writers in Italy." As to treatment, "None of the products of Indian corn should be given pellagrous patients. The basis of treatment is good food, especially meat, cheese and wine."[46]

On July 25, Babcock sent from Milan an Associated Press dispatch at the insistence of acting consul William Bayard Cutting, Jr., who had become interested in the disease. Babcock verified (1) that pellagra as he recognized it in the United States was basically the same disease that occurred in Italy; and (2) the Italians treated the disease with a wholesome and varied diet. They also used various drugs including arsenic preparations.

The Tillman-Babcock party proceeded to Austria, Switzerland, Holland, and France. In Paris the two men lingered in "those queer little book stores one sees on wheels lined up along the banks of the Seine."[47] They crossed the channel to London, where they exchanged silver-headed canes engraved with each other's initials. The Babcocks returned to the United States while the Tillmans continued on to Scotland. Before leaving London, Babcock had an audience with the foremost authority on pellagra in the English-speaking world, Dr. Fleming Mant Sandwith.[48]

Although Babcock and Sandwith apparently never met again in person, their collaboration became important to the American pellagra effort. Fleming Sandwith was a "very quiet" man who could be a bit cynical,[49] but

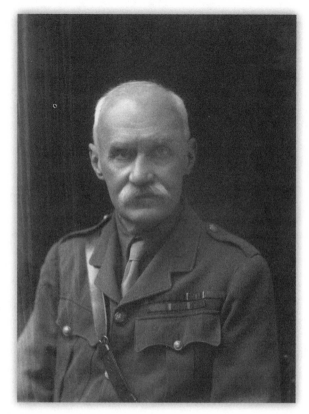

Dr. Fleming Mant Sandwith (1853–1918), the only authority on pellagra in the English-speaking world in 1907 when American physicians began to recognize the disease.
Courtesy: National Portrait Gallery, London.

his career exemplifies the adventuresome spirit of many Britons during the Victorian and Edwardian eras. He served as an ambulance surgeon during the Turco-Serbian war of 1876 and again in the Russo-Turkish campaign of 1877–78, in which he saw some of the heavy fighting in the Battle of Shipka Pass in the Balkan Mountains. In 1883 he went to Egypt to help out during a cholera epidemic. He spent most of the next twenty-two years in that country, interrupted by a stint in South Africa to serve in the Boer War. Egypt had only recently opened up to tourists who wanted to see the pyramids and other sites. In 1889 Sandwith published a travel guide for his fellow countrymen.[50] He became vice director of the Egyptian Public Health Department, physician to the Kasr El Aini Hospital in Cairo (then as now one of the major teaching hospitals in the Arab world), and chair of

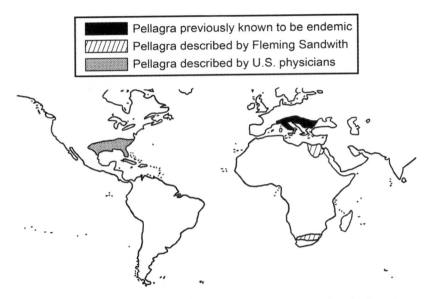

Areas of the world where pellagra was epidemic or highly prevalent (endemic) by the end of the first decade of the twentieth century included parts of central and eastern Europe (where it appeared after corn became a dietary staple), Egypt and South Africa (where it was recognized by Fleming Sandwith), and the southeastern United States (where it was recognized by George Searcy, Babcock, and others).

medicine at the Cairo Hospital. In the course of these experiences, Sandwith described endemic pellagra in parts of Egypt and South Africa.

When Sandwith began his studies, the English literature on pellagra consisted mainly of occasional accounts by travelers. Notable among these was an account by the physician Henry Holland, who in 1817 described pellagra in Lombardy, its noninfectious nature, and its relationship to "a deficiency of good nourishment."[51] In 1893 Sandwith began seeing patients in Lower Egypt with a symptom complex that included dermatitis, diarrhea, and melancholy, which he could not attribute to the highly prevalent hookworm on which he was an authority. He went to Italy to verify the diagnosis, as Babcock would do.[52] His description of a red, smooth tongue in the later stages of pellagra is still known as "Sandwith's bald tongue."[53] He later described pellagra in South Africa. In 1904 he left Egypt to become lecturer at the London School of Tropical Medicine. Sandwith had long suspected that conditions in parts of the United States were ripe for pellagra. He was pleased that Babcock, Searcy, and others had now confirmed it.

Babcock became Sandwith's main source for keeping up with the American literature on pellagra. Sandwith kept Babcock abreast of his thinking on pellagra and wrote papers at Babcock's request for the subsequent national pellagra conferences.

Babcock was not the only North American, nor indeed the only Columbia, South Carolina, physician to visit Italy in the summer of 1908 for the purpose of confirming the diagnosis of pellagra. The other was his close friend Joseph Jenkins Watson, one of Columbia's best doctors.[54] Watson met Lombroso and received from the great man himself instruction in how best to examine corn for soundness.[55]

While Babcock was away an election took place for the presidency of the University of South Carolina. Babcock, promoted by his friend August Kohn, was one of nine undeclared candidates who received votes at a meeting on May 27, 1908. According to an official history of the university, Babcock was "the man most favored," even though "he had not sought the position," but that "when it was learned that he was unwilling to leave his profession, the board turned to other possibilities," including the eventual nomination of Henry Nelson Snyder, president of Wofford College.[56] After the election Kohn confided: "Every member of the Board expressed the very highest feelings as to you and the highest regard for your ability, and the only objection I heard was that it would appear ridiculous for the Superintendent of an Asylum to be called to the Presidency of the State College."[57] Undergraduates joked that were the asylum superintendent elected it might be necessary to change their mascot from "the Gamecocks" to "the Lunatics" or "the Loonies."[58]

The First Pellagra Conference— Columbia, South Carolina, 1908

The first conference on pellagra held in an English-speaking country took place on the afternoon of October 29, 1908, in the assembly hall (also known as the amusement hall) of the South Carolina State Hospital for the Insane.[59] Highlights included reviews of the prevailing theories, reports suggesting a wide distribution, and the presence of Claude Hervey Lavinder of the U.S. Public Health and Marine Hospital Service, the first step in the federal government's involvement.[60] The proceedings were published as a booklet and also as a symposium issue of the state medical journal, making this the first monograph on pellagra in English.

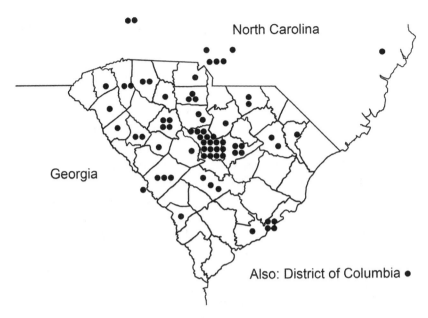

Physician attendees at the pellagra conference in Columbia, South Carolina, on 29 October 1908—the first conference on pellagra to be held in an English-speaking country—came mainly from South Carolina. (Each dot represents the hometown of one of the 72 physician attendees; about 200 laypersons also attended.)

Babcock had planted the idea for the conference just two weeks earlier by suggesting to the executive committee of the State Board of Health that there were "a sufficient number of cases ... in the State Hospital to furnish material for an interesting clinic on pellagra."[61] The board's secretary, Dr. C. Frederick Williams, moved with haste because of the upcoming South Carolina State Fair, during which two medical meetings in Columbia had already been scheduled.[62] He invited physicians in South Carolina and neighboring states and placed an advertisement in the state medical journal.[63] The meeting exceeded expectations.[64] Seventy-two physicians, most of them from South Carolina, and some 200 laypersons attended. Dr. Robert Wilson Jr. of Charleston, chairman of the State Board of Health, called the meeting to order. Governor Martin F. Ansel and Tillman gave introductory remarks, Tillman telling about the trip to Italy. The overarching significance of the meeting was that Americans *met* to discuss pellagra. Nothing presented would have struck an Italian doctor as novel, but for the first time an assembled group of Americans discussed and resolved to study the disease.

The first group of speakers staked out the various positions of Zeists and anti-Zeists. According to *The State* newspaper, many of the papers "were devoted to the causation of pellagra, the maize theory and the germ theory each being warmly defended."[65] Dr. Noel Moore of the Medical College of Georgia summarized the divide in a single sentence: "As Dr. Babcock has suggested, the association with Indian corn is too constant to be ignored; and yet, certain resemblances between pellagra and some of the protozoal diseases suggest, according to Sambon, the possibility of damaged maize bearing a somewhat similar relation to pellagra that stagnant water does to malaria."[66] Dr. Edward Jenner Wood of Wilmington, North Carolina, tried to reconcile the hypotheses by suggesting that corn whether sound or spoiled might form a culture medium for the "organism which is the specific cause of the disease."[67] The next three speakers had probably been asked to summarize on one or another hypothesis. J. J. Watson spoke on Lombroso's version of "the Italian maize theory," praising Lombroso for methods of "prevention and treatment of pellagra [used] in every country today."[68] James Thompson reviewed a variant known as "Roumanian theory," intended to explain pellagra in people who ate only apparently-sound corn.[69] Julius H. Taylor summarized Sambon's "protozoan theory" without committing to it.[70] Nobody brought up Marzari's "deficiency" hypothesis, now nearly a century old and all but forgotten.

Other speakers illustrated the value of clinical observations. Isaac M. Taylor of the Broadoaks Sanatorium in Morganton, North Carolina, reported on eight patients, only one of whom survived. Four suffered from alcoholism, including a 20-year-old farmer who "had been drinking steadily for a year of the poorest quality of corn whiskey." Five ate little or "almost nothing" after admission to the asylum. One of these was a 26-year-old "lady of highest culture" whose illness might now be diagnosed as the anorexia-bulemia syndrome. Although Taylor was unaware of damaged corn at his asylum, he assumed "the liability of all our people from the universal use of corn products as food." Still, he like others considered the best preventive measure to be "rigid inspection of corn offered for sale for men and beast."[71] In retrospect, these speakers had shown that alcoholism, anorexia, and reliance mainly on corn all promote *deficiency* of essential nutrients.

Harvey E. McConnell, a general practitioner from Chester, South Carolina, presented the first case series (and probably the first report) of pellagra as an emerging disease among Southern textile workers. He also staked a claim for being the first to diagnose pellagra in South Carolina.

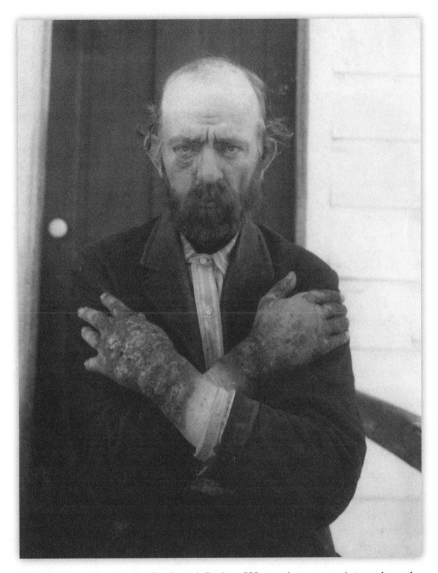

This photograph, taken by Dr. Joseph Jenkins Watson (1872–1924), is perhaps the most frequently reproduced illustration of pellagra, at least in English-language accounts. Pellagrins, wrote Dr. Harvey E. McConnell of Chester, South Carolina, "almost always have a frown of their foreheads" and the "erythematous eruption on the hands . . . the most constant and diagnostic sign. . . . needs to be seen only once to be recognized, and if you ever shake hands with one of these patients, you never forget the sensation."
Courtesy: Waring Historical Library, Medical University of South Carolina, Charleston, S.C.

For at least four years he had seen sporadic cases of "a peculiar condition or disease among some of my patients in a mill village near town" with rash, sore mouth, and diarrhea that usually appeared in the early spring. He consulted his textbooks to no avail. He then chanced upon a brief account of pellagra translated from a French medical journal and "realized at once" the diagnosis. McConnell wrote: "If the claim to priority in recognition of the disease in this State is of any significance, I am certain I diagnosed it as early as 1904, but, unfortunately, did not report my cases, though I called the attention of my doctor friends to the disease." All seven of his female patients were dead; all three of his male patients were living. Thus, "men withstand the disease better than women; and . . . women are more prone to the disease than men." One man allegedly "cured himself by drinking corn whiskey, and plenty of it." Another man went into remission after a regimen consisting of various drugs and a diet with "plenty of milk, eggs, and vegetable broth." McConnell's pithy descriptions bear the mark of a careful clinician. McConnell related that Babcock had spent a day with him and confirmed the diagnosis in several cases.[72]

Other reports included a suggestion by a Clemson veterinarian that pellagra might be causally related to "blind staggers" in horses.[73] Babcock went last. He reviewed cases he had seen in Italy, how he and Watson had independently confirmed that pellagra in South Carolina was the same disease "described as pellagra by the physicians and medical writers of Italy," how the staff of the State Hospital for the Insane had diagnosed pellagra unaware of Searcy's report, and how the disease was now being recognized in the asylums of other states (North Carolina, Georgia, Florida, and Mississippi) and in an orphanage in Tennessee. He did not address causation. He was mainly concerned with diagnosis and treatment.

"After familiarizing oneself with a number of cases," Babcock said, "the diagnosis is not difficult, since no other disease presents the syndrome of dermatitis, diarrhœa, and depression." Babcock concluded that the "pellagroid" (that is, "pellagra-like") disease in the Southeastern United States resembled the Italian and Egyptian forms of the disease, but with important differences: the overwhelming preponderance of females, the high death rate early in the disease, and the presence of rash in areas normally covered by clothing, such as the inner thighs and the skin around the genitalia and anus (which like "Sandwith's bald tongue" may have been due to coexistent riboflavin deficiency). With regard to treatment, he echoed others' conclusions: "Diet: As a rule, the patient should not be allowed any food derived from Indian corn. It is best to deny the products of maize known to be sound, in view of the possibility of introducing a new supply of the unknown poison.

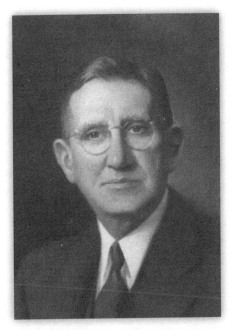

Dr. Charles Frederick Williams (1875–1948), head of the South Carolina State Board of Health, worked with Babcock to organize conferences and collect statistics on pellagra. He later became superintendent of the South Carolina State Hospital for the Insane.
Courtesy: Waring Historical Library, Medical University of South Carolina, Charleston, S.C.

A generous dietary should be given, including fresh meats and vegetables." He was in the main a Zeist, endorsing Lombroso's "spoiled corn" hypothesis without vigorously defending it.[74]

Claude Lavinder of the U.S. Public Health and Marine Hospital Service wrote the Surgeon General that "the energetic and progressive manner in which the medical profession of the State [of South Carolina]" pursued pellagra was to be commended. He reported that the regents of the Columbia asylum had passed a resolution asking for help "from the Public Health and Marine Hospital Service, or some similar scientific body" and that Babcock had confided to him that "if one of the Service officers would be detailed at the Hospital for the study of the disease, the Hospital would place at his disposal the cases and all reasonable means for a scientific study of them, equipping laboratory, etc."[75] Thus began the journey of the U.S. Public Health Service (as it was renamed in 1912) toward the eventual conquest of pellagra.

The First Statistics and the First Laboratory, 1909

The October 1908 conference sounded the alarm. Dr. Robert Wilson Jr. later wrote that "as a result of this conference and its published proceedings, general interest [in pellagra] was awakened in many states, and gradually the inference of a widespread malady was confirmed by its recognition in Northern and Western as well as Southern states." Wilson attributed the conference "almost wholly" to Babcock, who was supported by the state health officer, Frederick Williams.[76] Two days after the conference Williams mailed a questionnaire to all South Carolina physicians asking if they had seen pellagra or something like it. The 29 percent response rate was disappointing, but one-third (89 of 269) of those who responded answered yes. The 187 cases came from thirty-two of South Carolina's forty-two counties. Williams extrapolated from the response rate that there were at least 500 cases of pellagra in South Carolina exclusive of patients in asylums. He wrote that these data, the first to hint of a wide distribution, should "stimulate every physician in the State to take renewed interest in the subject of pellagra, so that in the future we may lay before the world data of sufficient accuracy to form a foundation for investigations that will lead to solving the problems of the origin, prevention, and cure of the disease."[77]

The year 1909 would be Babcock's *annus mirabilis* in that it solidified his place in the history of pellagra. In January Governor Ansel commended him to the South Carolina Senate for "a very important contribution to medical science in the study he has made and the paper he has contributed on the disease known as pellagra."[78] Events that year included the federal government's sending Lavinder to Columbia to study pellagra; a publication by Lavinder, Williams, and Babcock showing that pellagra was widespread in the United States; and a fall conference in Columbia that prompted formation of a National Association for the Study of Pellagra. The year 1909 would also be Babcock's *annus horribilis* because of a legislative investigation of conditions at his asylum, the subject of the next chapter.

Claude Lavinder arrived in Columbia in May 1909, thus beginning his underappreciated role in pellagra research.[79] Lavinder was a University of Virginia medical graduate and had chosen public health on the suggestion of his mentor Dr. Henry Rose Carter.[80] In 1897 Lavinder entered the U.S. Marine Hospital Service.[81] He spent the next decade working mainly as a quarantine officer in various seaports. While serving in Wilmington, North Carolina, he helped several local physicians diagnose pellagra. Unlike his successor, Joseph Goldberger, he had no real track record in research. Lavinder was given two small rooms in the Old Building to set up a laboratory.

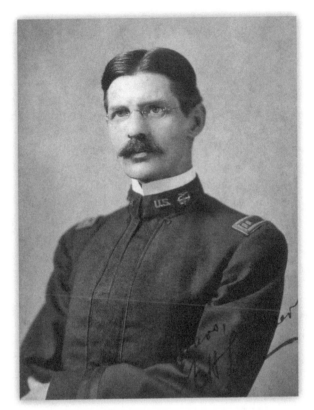

Dr. Claude Hervey Lavinder (1872–1950) was the first physician assigned to pellagra by the U.S. Public Health and Marine Hospital Service (renamed the Public Health Service in 1912).
Courtesy: National Library of Medicine.

Neither room had running water or gas. The regents asked Babcock "to aid Dr. Lavinder in every possible way ... to find something of the causes and if possible a remedy by scientific investigation of the new disease pellagra." Although Lavinder stayed in Columbia less than five months, he and Babcock became close and continued to collaborate.[82]

Lavinder accomplished much in Columbia despite meager facilities and lack of support staff. He wrote the surgeon general that "the opportunities to work here, while leaving many things to be desired, are nevertheless large." He inoculated chickens, rats, rabbits, and guinea pigs with blood, spinal fluid, and spleen pulp from patients with pellagra. The results were negative. He studied twenty-five patients in detail. He made numerous cultures, with negative results. He examined blood smears and autopsy specimens. For therapy he tried giving salts of mercury and arsenic, or serum from recovered patients, without success.[83] Lavinder's main contribution during this period came from two brief assignments to go elsewhere—to Nashville, Tennessee, Chicago, and Peoria, Illinois. In Chicago he confirmed pellagra in three women at the Cook County Hospital for the Insane (the Dunning Asylum), and the physicians there told him at least six patients had died of the then-mysterious disease the previous year.[84] At the Peoria State Hospital he found forty cases of pellagra, and the physicians told him that in retrospect they had seen the disease for at least five years. A nurse had been dismissed in 1904 on accusations she had "boiled" a patient to death. The nurse was reinstated when the patient received a retrospective diagnosis of pellagra.[85]

Lavinder, Williams, and Babcock teamed up to write on "The Prevalence of Pellagra in the United States—A Statistical and Geographical Note, with Bibliography" for the June 18, 1909, issue of *Public Health Reports*.[86] This, the first publication on a vital topic, announced that pellagra was a national problem—not just a southern problem. The article included results of a survey Williams had sent to asylum superintendents and others. To 164 inquiries he received 120 replies, "about 20 being in the affirmative." The reports suggested at least 1,000 cases of pellagra in thirteen states. More than half of the patients were in mental institutions. The Georgia State Sanitarium in Milledgeville reported the largest number of cases (225), followed by the Mount Vernon Hospital in Alabama (156 cases) and the South Carolina State Hospital (125 cases). Lavinder reported conservatively that 1,500 cases of pellagra had occurred in the southern states since 1906.

Doctors took note of what was happening in South Carolina. In May 1909 Dr. William Sydney Thayer of Johns Hopkins visited Babcock for two days to study pellagra.[87] Fleming Sandwith of London asked Babcock for the print version of the 1908 Columbia conference, as did a Cairo physician.[88] Local medical societies began to hold their own conferences, as doctors wanted to learn more about the new disease. They often invited Babcock to speak.

On August 7, for example, the medical society in Abbeville, a small community in upper South Carolina, held a meeting that attracted 125 people, including 79 physicians and medical students. Babcock spoke last. He credited Harvey McConnell for being the first South Carolinian to recognize the epidemic. The newspaper reported that Babcock was "decidedly pessimistic" about prognosis. Some speakers made stray observations that added to the confusion about causation. Dr. Isaac Taylor of the Morgantown, North Carolina, asylum reported that all of his cases of pellagra had occurred in the "well-to-do class" and were clearly not "victims of malnutrition." Did this not point away from dietary deficiency? Dr. John Lyon of Ninety-Six, South Carolina, told of patients who had largely recovered only to relapse immediately after eating a small quantity of corn bread. Did this not point toward a pellagra-causing toxin or microorganism?[89] All the while American physicians labored under the penumbras of Lombroso and Sambon with their respective spoiled-corn and insect-transmission hypotheses.

Lavinder meanwhile worked on a comprehensive article on "The Prophylaxis of Pellagra," published later that year.[90] How could pellagra be prevented when the cause was unknown? Like Searcy, and indeed like some of the early Europeans, he came tantalizingly close to getting it right. Pellagra was caused by faulty diet. It was not communicable. The best way to prevent it was "the education of the people to the dangers of spoiled corn and the healthfulness of a varied diet and better living conditions." Pellagra was declining in some areas of Italy for precisely these reasons: "The laborers and peasants now can eat better food than ever before; numbers of the rural population are employed in industrial institutions, where they receive a varied diet ... [and] demand and get better food and living conditions; the consumption of meat is increasing, and wages are higher." His conclusions were forceful: (1) "There is no evidence that pellagra is a communicable disease"; (2) "Quarantine measures ... would appear unnecessary"; (3) "Unless we can disprove it, we must for the time being at least accept the existence of some connection between corn and pellagra"; and (4) "In our efforts at prophylaxis we must take cognizance of the alleged effect of this grain as a human food." Lavinder was open minded but, like most of his contemporaries, framed the causation of pellagra as a disagreement between Zeists and anti-Zeists.

The First National Conference on Pellagra, 1909

The first National Conference on Pellagra took place in the assembly hall at the State Hospital for the Insane on November 3–4, 1909, and was attended by 394 physicians and an untold number of laypersons. Columbia did not have enough hotel rooms for such a large meeting. Some of the delegates were therefore housed at the asylum in the New Building's wing for white women.[91] The *State* took pride in its coverage.[92] The meeting shared headlines with the first of fifty-one consecutive "Big Thursday" football games between the University of South Carolina and Clemson.[93] Perhaps nothing of comparable national significance had taken place in Columbia since Sherman came through forty-four years earlier.

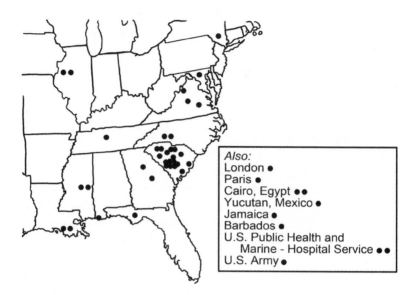

Residences of the speakers at the National Conference on Pellagra held
November 3–4, 1909 in Columbia, S.C. Each dot represents the hometown of
one speaker.

Elizabeth Etheridge in *The Butterfly Caste* calls the 1909 Columbia
conference "the most dramatic event in the early years of the antipellagra
campaign."[94] Sixteen of the forty-one speakers were from South Carolina,
but eleven other states, two branches of the federal government, and six other
nations were represented. Opinion on causation and treatment centered
on Lombroso's version of the zeist hypothesis, but most positions found a
hearing. The Committee on Resolutions hailed Babcock "whom we justly
recognize as the father of the movement for the study and control of pellagra
in America, for his valuable labors and his many courtesies to this body
during our session." The proceedings were published as a 297-page book.[95]
When Goldberger first wrote on "The Etiology of Pellagra" in 1914, he drew
his first three observations directly from these proceedings.[96]

The conference began with Governor Ansel welcoming the delegates
and praising Babcock as the first to recognize pellagra in the United States.
Babcock immediately corrected the governor. He pointed out that American
doctors had through the years published case reports on pellagra, that Dr.
Searcy of Alabama had described epidemic pellagra in an asylum, and that

he did not "wish to be placed in the false position of making any claims as to having discovered or made any early observations upon pellagra, because such is not the case, and credit is due to all of the gentlemen whose names I have mentioned, and perhaps there are others." Babcock underscored his certainty that "every one of us is interested in bringing out the whole truth with regard to the pellagra problem." The minutes of this meeting are entirely devoid of the acrimony that would characterize pellagra meetings beginning in 1914, when Joseph Goldberger became involved.

Babcock read introductory remarks submitted by his new London colleague Fleming Sandwith, who congratulated and encouraged "the many physicians in the Southern States who are now working at the various problems connected with pellagra." These Americans had "provided us with a literature on the subject in the English language," of great interest to Sandwith because "until I began to write on pellagra, there were apparently no literary contributions in our tongue, if we except two or three accounts by travelers to describe cases they had seen in Italy. The English textbooks were either silent on the subject or frankly ignorant." Still a Zeist, Sandwith like Babcock and most others embraced diet as a cornerstone of therapy: "The treatment of early cases, without mental symptoms, can be successfully accomplished by putting the patient on a liberal diet, excluding maize and by ridding him of the hookworms which are so often co-existent, but the pellagrous symptoms return if he is allowed to resume a diet of musty maize. ... Pellagra is essentially a disease which cries for preventive measures." Sandwith closed with a prophecy: "We are now waiting, in the confident hope that some of the pellagra problems, so long unsolved, may be successfully mastered in the United States."[97]

The large number of papers prompted a resolution to restrict presentations to fifteen minutes with an additional five minutes for discussion, a format for scientific meetings that became common by the second half of the twentieth century. Most of the speakers were Zeists but a vocal minority represented the emerging anti-Zeists. Babcock did not give a paper. Several South Carolina doctors expressed embarrassment about having nothing new to say, stating they were on the program at Babcock's insistence.

Summarizing the zeist position was Assistant Surgeon General J. W. Kerr of the U.S. Public Health and Marine Hospital Service. According to Kerr, the "belief that there is some relation between pellagra and the use of corn as food would seem too universal and too profound to permit of rejection except in the case of demonstrative proof to the contrary," although the "nature of this relation awaits final solution."[98] Kerr preached the doctrine of "bad corn" for which he found a choir of supporters among the practicing doctors in the audience. Dr. J. J. Watson of Columbia asserted: "Ordinary corn does not produce pellagra. It is when corn is damaged that we get pellagra."[99] Dr. W. H. Dial of Laurens, South Carolina, likewise asserted that "sound, properly cured corn is one of the greatest and best of our food products." Dr. J. D. Jones of Sweet Water, Alabama, allowed that "pure, fully developed, hardened corn—hardened by the rays of the noonday sun—will never produce pellagra."[100] Others speakers reminded the audience of the economic implications of blaming corn, especially "good" corn.

The U.S. corn crop was of global importance. Sandwith suggested that the United States produced "at least three quarters" of the world's corn and therefore "the cultivation and curing of this cereal are of supreme importance to every American citizen."[101] Ebbie J. Watson, commissioner of South Carolina's Department of Agriculture, Commerce, and Industries, pointed out that corn was grown on 80 percent of the farms in the United States, and that if the ears of the U.S. corn crop were placed end to end they would encircle the earth at the equator over 1,100 times.[102] He lamented that South Carolina had no inspection law and was getting much of its corn from markets in Nashville, St. Louis, Cincinnati, and Richmond. Other states were dumping damaged corn on the Palmetto State. South Carolinians need to grow more of their own.[103] Kerr pointed out that the manner in which corn was prepared or processed had "excited investigators like Dr. Carl L. Alsberg" of the U.S. Department of Agriculture. Toward the end of the conference, at a time when many participants were no doubt heading home, Dr. J. S. De Jarnet, superintendent of the Western State Hospital in Staunton, Virginia, gave a summary paper entitled "The Corn Curse."[104] He claimed the "disease is never found except among a corn-eating population," and that treatment was to discontinue all corn products and substitute a mixed animal and vegetable diet. Thus, the Zeists were of two general camps: those who would eliminate corn altogether and those who would eliminate only "bad" corn.

Anti-Zeists were also of two camps. Some were anti-Zeists because of their natural inclination toward skepticism. Others favored a specific infectious agent. A Maryland physician asserted: "Pellagra is a specific infectious disease, due to a parasitic fungus, namely, the *aspergillus fumigatus*."[105] J. J. Watson of Columbia asserted: "Pellagra is an endemic disease attributed to eating Indian corn infected with certain hyphomycetes."[106] Various bacteria, fungi, and parasites were suggested as potential causes, but Louis Sambon's version of the infection hypothesis was beginning to work its way to the fore. Julius Taylor of Columbia, echoing his previous paper on Sambon's hypothesis, disputed the spoiled-corn hypothesis and pointed out that it had not been "yet shown that a protozoan element does not play a part."[107]

Lavinder reported on the other hand that his examination of numerous blood smears and tissues at autopsy had shown "nothing resembling a protozoal parasite."[108]

Dr. Hiram Byrd of Jacksonville, Florida, understood the meeting's broader implications. He pointed out that the conference "has taken upon itself the character of an international body. Every part of the world, where pellagra is an important problem, is represented here either in person or in sentiment." Since the "proceedings of this conference will be read by the entire world" he felt it best not to go "on record that corn is the cause of pellagra." Byrd built a powerful case for skepticism: "We better say, we do not know. This is a scientific body. It ought not to accept anything short of absolute proof which the most exact science can furnish. So far as corn is concerned, the least we can say is, it is unproven that it is the cause of this disease, and let us not put ourselves in the humiliating position at some future time of having to take back what we say in this conference." Byrd's comments drew applause but did not dim the enthusiasm of those anti-Zeists who favored an infectious etiology.

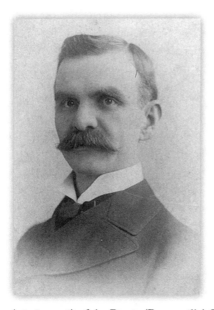

Dr. George A. Zeller (1858–1938) of the Peoria (Bartonville) State Hospital in Illinois reported epidemic pellagra in the American heartland. Zeller endeared himself to Babcock as a fellow "asylum doctor."
Courtesy: Mental Health Historic Preservation Society of Central Illinois.

The anti-Zeists received a boost when the United States Army assigned Drs. Joseph F. Siler and Henry J. Nichols to study pellagra. They evaluated 70 patients with typical pellagra and 150 with possible pellagra at the Peoria State Hospital in Illinois. A "surprisingly small" percentage of patients had relied mainly on corn before entering the institution. None had used corn continually "as an article of diet." However, the food given the inmates was "necessarily limited as to variety and component constituents." They determined that amebic parasites were more likely to be found in the stools of pellagrins than in patients without pellagra. In retrospect, this finding almost surely reflected an epiphenomenon—that is, a secondary manifestation of the disease having nothing to do with its cause.[109] Thus began Joseph Siler's pursuit of an infectious cause of pellagra, which ultimately became a disappointing detour in Siler's highly productive career.

Also presenting data from the Peoria State Hospital was George Zeller, one of that era's most progressive asylum superintendents.[110] Zeller described the emergence of pellagra in the American heartland: "Seeing it develop in every ward of my institution and to the larger extent in the tent colonies for consumptives where the most nutritious diet of milk and eggs is given, seeing it develop in men and women of splendid physique as well as among those showing more marked mental and physical decline, I can only await its dread appearance in the citizenship outside the institutions."[111] Babcock and his fellow southerners welcomed Zeller's confirmation that pellagra was not just a southern problem. Babcock hailed Zeller as a fellow "asylum doctor." When Zeller came under attack during a discussion period, Babcock rose to defend him: "I think Dr. Zeller, like all asylum doctors, including myself, is here absolutely in the interest of truth. I do not think Dr. Zeller or myself represents any particular school, as to the theory of the development of pellagra. We are all here to learn the truth, and to confer together in the interest of truth."

Babcock went on to praise Zeller as a sterling example of "the often maligned asylum and the asylum doctor." He reminded the audience that "as far back as twenty-five years ago we were asked by so great a light as Weir Mitchell what contribution had the asylum doctors made towards the progress of medical science?" Now, asylum doctors, and notably Zeller, had rebutted in spades the denigrations of Mitchell and other neurologists. Encouraged by another round of applause, Babcock added that as "it has been my pleasure to serve as a private in the ranks with men for twenty-five years, whose position is like nothing else on earth, I will say that there are some men whose prime characteristic is moral courage. In all my experience with asylum doctors, I have known of no one of them who has shown the high degree of moral courage that Dr. Zeller has in reading his paper from this platform this afternoon, and if I may presume on this occasion to thank Dr. Zeller personally, and in behalf of asylum doctors throughout the length and breadth of the United States, then I want to return our humble thanks to him for standing here in South Carolina and reading us that magnificent paper."[112]

With hindsight it seems reasonable to suggest that the cause, treatment, and prevention of pellagra might have been solved sooner had people paid more attention to the data coming "out of the asylums." The three physicians sharing data from the Peoria State Hospital—Siler, Nichols, and Zeller—observed that no nurse, physician, or employee had contracted pellagra, just as Searcy had reported from Alabama.[113] And the observation that pellagra was occurring among asylum inmates, condemned to dwell far from fast-flowing streams, constitutes in retrospect a strong argument against Sambon's insect-borne parasite hypothesis.[114]

Among the sidebars to the debate between Zeists and anti-Zeists was a report by Drs. Herbert P. Cole and Gilman J. Winthrop of Mobile, Alabama, on "Transfusion in Pellagra." Having experimented with blood transfusions in dogs, they postulated that blood from patients cured of pellagra might benefit active cases because of the "possibility of the existence of a specific curative agent, of the nature of an antitoxin." They gave blood to nine patients. Six of the nine patients recovered. Three died, one shortly after the procedure and the other two several weeks later. In retrospect, they had given small amounts of niacin to their patients but had exposed them to the risks of transfusion reaction.[115]

As the meeting drew to an end it was resolved to found a National Association for the Study of Pellagra. Babcock was elected president.[116] Dr. Robert Wilson Jr. of Charleston, on behalf of the State Board of Health, acknowledged "the work which Dr. Babcock has done and is doing in furthering this cause," adding to applause that "Dr. Babcock's enthusiasm has been an inspiration and the conference was largely due to his activity."

The applause did not stop there. From Chicago an editor of the *Journal of the American Medical Association* observed that a "striking feature was the purely scientific, humanitarian spirit which pervaded the meetings and which influenced those who took an active part in the proceedings. There was no disposition displayed to seek personal gain or aggrandizement. It seemed that every delegate had come with a desire to learn more about this disease which has been attracting not only the medical professional of the world, but the laity." The conference had indeed "assumed both a national and an international character," and the editor credited Babcock, Williams, and the State

Board of Health "for calling this national conference to discuss this very vital topic."[117] Sandwith congratulated Babcock on the "splendid success" of the conference and "on becoming the first President of the National Association of the Study of Pellagra. This is obviously your proper place." Many delegates and their wives privately thanked Kate Babcock for her hospitality.[118]

In pellagra Babcock had found a welcome diversion from the cares of an asylum superintendent in a less-than-prosperous state. He had acknowledged to the Board of Regents just before the conference: "I recognize that upon pellagra I am often a bore."[119] While he busied himself with the new disease, his many problems at the South Carolina State Hospital for the Insane now included a highly public investigation.

CHAPTER 4

How Bad It Was

"All Who Enter Here Leave Hope Behind"

Tнᴇ 1909 NATIONAL PELLAGRA CONFERENCE in Columbia was in many ways the high-water mark of collaboration, good will, and civic pride in the public response to the epidemic. As it became increasingly apparent that the disease struck mainly in pockets of poverty and deprivation, pellagra like hookworm became for many southerners an embarrassment they preferred to ignore. As historian Edward Beardsley puts it, "The South preferred to embrace paternalistic fantasies rather than uncomfortable realities."[1] While Babcock busied himself with the first national pellagra conference he could not ignore the uncomfortable realities in his backyard. The sorry conditions at the State Hospital for the Insane triggered an investigation by the state's progressives, led by State Senator Niels Christensen Jr. of Beaufort County. Babcock's lack of executive ability ultimately became the focus, leading to a recommendation that he and also the regents be dismissed. Babcock survived the investigation but not without further erosion of what little power he had over his subordinates.

The Allegations

While Babcock toured Europe with Tillman in 1908, a Columbia attorney named A. Hunter Gibbes had as a client a young man who had been jailed for fraud and then committed to the asylum on certificates from two physicians. The client wanted out but could not get a release. Gibbes talked with other inmates with similar complaints. He offered to get them out for $35 each.[2] He snooped around the asylum and wrote a long letter to the legislature. As "one interested in the welfare of suffering humanity," he felt

113

it his duty "to call your attention to some instances of mismanagement in the affairs of the State Hospital for the Insane."[3] Gibbes spared no detail.

Negligence and brutality were the rule, not the exception. Gibbes charged "that many of the keepers or so-called nurses employed in the Hospital for the Insane are cruel to patients, grossly ignorant as to their duties and unworthy of their trusts." A 65-year-old Confederate veteran "was cruelly and severely beaten and kicked by a keeper," prompting relatives to take him home where he died within two hours. Another man "was assaulted by a so-called nurse, severely beaten on the head and face and kicked in the groins . . . [and] so completely disabled he was placed in the hospital ward." Two nurses had been indicted on a charge of using counterfeit money made by a patient in the asylum. The nurses would "not infrequently require, under force of very effective persuasion, the patients committed to their charge to do their work," whereupon the nurses would "idle away their time in bed or in other ways more congenial than the performance of the duties assigned to them."

Filth was everywhere. Some of the nurses would "bathe as many as twenty or twenty-five patients one after another in the <u>same water</u>, because forsooth the nurses are too lazy and indolent to take the trouble to change the water." Gibbes added: "When it is borne in mind that some of these patients have loathsome diseases it is impossible to imagine conditions more filthy and horrible." Because "most of the cooking . . . is performed by filthy Negro patients . . . the food is frequently unclean, improperly prepared and a positive source of danger to life and health." The asylum dairy was "for the most part under the control of patients positively dirty, and who are totally ignorant as to the hygienic care in handling the milk used by patients."

Patients became de facto prisoners. A patient admitted in a drunken state might be "retained in custody for months at the expense of the State and people" after he sobered up. It was "common practice . . . not to release a patient, after he regains his sanity, unless some friend or relative voluntarily sees fit to interest himself in his behalf and agrees to be responsible for the patient's future good conduct. In consequence of this practice 'all who enter here leave hope behind.'" The patient without friends or relatives might be doomed to "pass the remainder of his life within [the asylum's] walls, no matter how complete, no matter how sure, his mental soundness may be." And because many "of these so-called lunatics are required to work in the dairy, on the farm, in the laundry, and in other departments," for which they sometimes but not always received nominal payments, "practically a system of peonage exists." Gibbes argued that if patients were "sufficiently sane to work for the State as menial servants, as hewers of wood and drawers of water, as a matter of common sense it necessarily follows that they are sufficiently sane to be released and allowed to work for themselves and their families."

The main problem as Gibbes saw it was poor administration. The asylum had not been investigated for nearly twenty years, and, Gibbes suggested, "lack of general efficiency" inevitably crept into an institution "under one management for a long term of years." But the problems of "this particular institution" included "a lack of business methods, a lack of system and proper organization, and a failure in the proper conception of the duties imposed upon the management by the laws of South Carolina." Much of the "flatteringly good showing" of the administration's financial performance had been "at the expense of human flesh and blood," since the patients were required to work, especially on the asylum farm, like criminals or bondsmen. The administration also tolerated widespread petty thieving among certain employees and allowed perquisites from the asylum farm for those not entitled to them.

It was not the first time Babcock had come under fire before the legislature. Twelve years earlier, in 1897, a dismissed employee ranted about conditions, including Babcock's lax administrative style. "The Superintendent spends much of his time upstairs investing in old postage stamps," she claimed, "and can scarcely be found in his office . . . . He visits the wards so seldom that there are many patients whom he does not know." A legislative committee completely exonerated Babcock, confident that his administration was "far superior to that of many of the other public institutions" of which they had knowledge, and the regents expressed "entire and complete confidence" in Babcock's management.[4] Hunter Gibbes, "actuated only by motives of humanity" and using lawyerly language, was not so easily dismissed. His letter spurred the legislature to convene a Committee to Investigate the State Hospital for the Insane, triggering a highly public showdown between the old guard conservatives and the new progressives led by State Senator Niels Christensen Jr. of Beaufort County.

Niels Christensen Jr.

The Progressive Movement—a broad program of political and social reforms in the United States between the 1890s and 1920—is usually traced in South Carolina to the 1903 introduction of the state's first child labor law.[5] The state's conservative traditions and the era's lawlessness[6] put reformers at a huge disadvantage. Also, the reformers focused mainly on the interests of white South Carolinians, as the disenfranchised blacks had little political influence. Despite these obstacles a handful of politicians identifiable as progressives achieved limited success. Prominent among these was Niels Christensen Jr.

It would have been hard to find a native-born white southerner with a stronger pedigree for progressivism than Niels Christensen Jr.; a geneticist might quip that he was homozygous. The senior Niels Christensen, son of Danish innkeepers, came to the United States in 1862 at age 22, enlisted as a private in the 145th New York Volunteer Infantry, fought at Chancellorsville and Gettysburg, was wounded twice, participated in Sherman's march, and, of great importance to his social conscience, became captain of the 44th U.S. Colored Infantry in Alabama and Tennessee.[7] His black

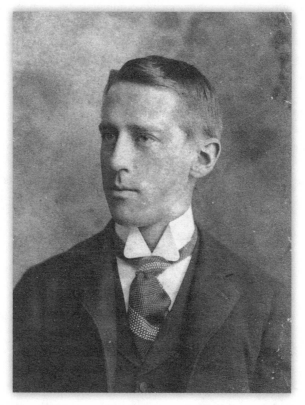

State Senator Niels Christensen Jr. (1876–1939) of Beaufort County, a leader among the progressives in the legislature, chaired the Committee to Investigate the State Hospital for the Insane.
Courtesy: Anne Christensen Pollitzer.

charges, contemporaries agreed, rivaled their white counterparts in drill and discipline. After the war Christensen and another officer tried farming with "shared wage" contracts with freedmen. Unlike the majority of white officers who had commanded black troops, Christensen supported black suffrage. In 1870 he moved to Beaufort to become keeper of the National Cemetery there, part of an effort to honor wartime dead on a scale the nation had never before seen.[8] He endeared himself to southern whites by improving the gravesite of a Confederate general who had fought against him at Gettysburg. In 1878 Wade Hampton, a Democrat, made Christensen, a Republican, a commissioner of elections. Christensen retired from his cemetery position that year to devote his energies to business ventures, in which he succeeded while staying true to his principles. He defended blacks against racist charges in an article entitled "The Sea Islands and Negro Supremacy."[9]

Abbie Holmes Christensen more than matched her husband's advocacy for African Americans. She was the daughter of Massachusetts abolitionists who moved to Beaufort to join the Port Royal Experiment when Abbie was twelve. As a teenager she became steeped in black culture, including folklore. At age 22 she published her first story, "De Wolf, de Rabbit an' de Tar Baby" (1874), which was followed by "Negro Folklore: The Elephant and the Rabbit" and "A Story Teller" (both in 1875) and a compilation entitled *Afro-American Folk Lore as Told 'Round Cabin Fires on the Sea Islands of South Carolina* (1893). Many called her "the Original Uncle Remus." She is still studied as a folklorist who preceded the better-known Joel Chandler Harris. Like Harris she effectively combined trickster stories, dialect, and a fictional narrator—in her case an Uncle Scipio who told stories from slavery and even from Africa to a Miss Alice as she swung "in her favorite hammock on the broad, shaded veranda." However, she thought of herself first as an activist, not a folklorist. Her major accomplishment was the Port Royal Agricultural School (later known as the Beaufort County Training School and to locals as "The Shanklin School"), which she financed in part with royalties from *Afro-American Folk Lore.* Although her activism on behalf of blacks now falls under the category of "New South paternalism"—even in her stories she conveyed that blacks needed assistance and guidance from whites—she is considered one of her era's great liberals. In 1932, at the age of eighty, she was an elector for the socialist candidate for President.

Niels and Abbie Christensen pinned much of their hope for a better future on Niels Jr. He did not disappoint them, although as a Progressive Democrat he found it politically necessary to distance himself to some extent from his mother's liberalism on the issue of black suffrage. Described as

fair-minded, studious, and straightforward, with no liking for small talk—
"earnest" was a frequent adjective—he added to his father's enterprises the
Beaufort Gazette, which he served as publisher and editor from 1903 to 1921.
Elected to the State Senate in 1905, he led a campaign against the state-
run liquor dispensary and succeeded in having it suspended. The dispensary
had been Ben Tillman's brainchild. Christensen railed against Tillman for
having created the dispensary in 1893 "at the cost of riot and bloodshed"
and for having "covered with his cloak" the dispensary's murky affairs. He
doubted whether a new county-administered system would be much better,
for "whatever that trade [the liquor industry] touches it tends to pollute."[10]
In 1908, backed by many newspapers who decried the efforts of Tillman's
supporters to ridicule him, he successfully campaigned for reelection. Now
he took on the woefully underfunded asylum and its popular superintendent.

Christensen held no grudge against Babcock. It seems likely that his
father, as one of seven Beaufort citizens who formed a local relief committee
after the Sea Islands Hurricane of 1893, had interacted with Babcock in a
favorable way. The young state senator approached the superintendent with
tact and respect. In mid-January 1909 he invited Babcock to discuss with
him privately what was about to happen. The superintendent, Christensen
wrote his father, "approved my course, thanked me for seeing him, and
said that if he had been in my place he would have done the same thing."
Christensen next invited Babcock to meet with both him and the governor.
Babcock volunteered to present his own petition asking the legislature to
investigate the asylum. Christensen liked the idea. Babcock with input from
the regents drew up his own petition. Christensen persuaded Hunter Gibbes
to withdraw his petition in favor of Babcock's.[11] It was a good start.

Christensen did his homework. He and other members of the Committee to Investigate the State Hospital for the Insane probed around to the
extent that the regents complained that "the methods of the legislative committee investigation are seriously disrupting the institution."[12] With Wade
C. Harrison, a committee member from the state's House of Representatives,
Christensen toured asylums in North Carolina, Virginia, and the District
of Columbia, gleaning "a lot of data with reference to the management of
institutions of this kind in other parts of the country." The *State* quoted
his "abhorrence for any allegations which might be unfounded," but also
his surmise "from the casual observations made that tremendous reforms
are needed." He realized what he was up against for, as the newspaper put
it, "How best to arrive at results ... without inciting sensationalism now
presents itself as the great question of this investigation."[13] He promised
to be fair.

Eight Days of Testimony

The Committee to Investigate the State Hospital for the Insane began hearings on the asylum campus on April 27, 1909, with Christensen as chairman.[14] The focus was twofold: the allegations by Hunter Gibbes (as emended by Babcock and the regents) and the adequacy of Babcock's administration. First assistant physician James Thompson gave the most damning testimony against Babcock. Drs. Julius Taylor and Eleanora Saunders vigorously defended Babcock. August Kohn, reporting for the Charleston *News and Courier*, wrote the press coverage most favorable to his friend, the superintendent.

Babcock was allowed an opening statement. He pointed out that he and the regents had themselves called for "a special committee . . . to investigate and report upon the condition and affairs of the hospital and its management."[15] He listed twenty-three reasons for an investigation "regardless of any charges." He reviewed how the asylum had been "started in a small way, in a feeble way" by early nineteenth-century legislators William Crafts and Samuel Farrow, had continued as an experiment in the treatment of mental illness, but had devolved into "a dumping ground of every form of humanity that is undesirable in any community." He continued: "We receive feeble, broken-down old men and women, who have worn out their welcome in their homes for no other reason under the sun than they are untidy, and in South Carolina that has been a good and sufficient reason why they should be sent to the Asylum. Our patients are not picked. We take them all." A committee member asked whether such an open-door policy was at the superintendent's discretion. Babcock answered yes, "but I have not turned away three patients since I have been here. We take them and do the best we can, if we have to crowd them until they cut one another's throats." The mortality rates would be much lower if "you let the doctors go to the front gate and pick out such patients as are going to live three or four years . . . . The statutes will have to take care of this." August Kohn reported in the *News and Courier* that "Dr. J. W. Babcock, full of human kindness, has said 'Come along and bring your unfortunates, and we will do the best we can for them.'" Kohn marveled that Babcock made do on a state appropriation of less than thirty cents per patient per day, less than most South Carolina counties paid to keep prisoners.[16] Christensen became frustrated with Kohn's reporting. He wrote his mother that "Kohn has astonished me in the lengths he has been willing to go in suppression and misrepresentation." Witnesses would have to face "Babcock, his Board of Regents, and unfriendly reporters, and unfriendly members of the committee," he told Abbie Holmes Christensen, when "the people need to see the truth—which is that there has been no supervision, but laxity and shiftlessness, and that the plant is deplorably run down."[17]

The first witness was a former inmate from Charleston who had been a patient on two occasions separated by five years. His symptoms suggest paranoid schizophrenia; he had hallucinations in which a divine power ordered him to do such things as spit at people or choke them. He claimed to have seen Babcock only three times during his first hospitalization, which lasted slightly more than a year, and twice during his second hospitalization, which lasted two years. Still, his criticisms were aimed more at the asylum than at Babcock. He had enjoyed the twice-weekly baseball games. He had not seen restraint used except for violence, and had himself been restrained only once, for spitting on an employee. He complained about the diet, about being kept too long, and about the asylum's being behind the times in providing "proper diversion, exercise and fresh air," his point of reference being other asylums where he had been committed. The second patient, a 43-year-old man from Abbeville, had likewise been hospitalized twice, the first time for nine months and the second for about two years. On the second occasion he hired a lawyer to win release. He had seen Babcock only once. It was his impression that Thompson wanted to discharge him but couldn't get Babcock's approval. Like the first patient he complained of poor food, bed bugs, and boredom. These two patients' testimonies accounted for 115 of the 440 pages of printed transcripts.[18]

Both patients as white males had been on Thompson's service, explaining in part why they had seldom seen Babcock. James Thompson was the next to testify, and he would be recalled twice.[19] The worst thing Thompson said was that Babcock was "out of touch" because he seldom visited Thompson's wards. This prompts the question whether Thompson's testimony reflected a grudge against Babcock.

In the present author's opinion, the short answer is no, at least not then. Babcock respected Thompson's desire for autonomy, to manage his wards as he saw fit. Physicians of that era, even more so than physicians today, were highly territorial and did not welcome criticism from peers.[20] Nurses at the new Columbia Hospital later wrote that the doctors "demonstrated an ability to get along with their patients better than with each other."[21] Thompson had every reason to resent Babcock's becoming superintendent (see Chapter 2). A state senator asked rhetorically: "Was not Dr. Thompson disappointed when this brilliant young South Carolinian [Babcock] was brought from Massachusetts and placed in charge of the asylum? If he was not, he was

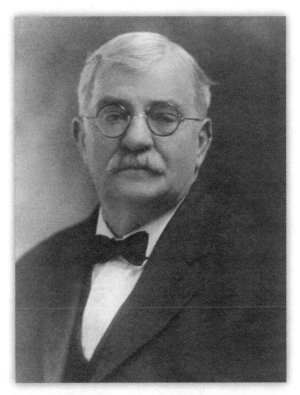

Dr. James L. Thompson, the first assistant physician, reluctantly gave testimony
unfavorable to Babcock during the 1909 legislative hearings.
Courtesy: South Carolina Department of Archives and History. Records of the State Dept.
of Mental Health, Photographic File (S190095), folder 1.

more God than man."[22] The more likely explanation for Babcock's failure to
be conspicuous on Thompson's wards was Babcock's inclination to respect
Thompson's autonomy, to avoid confrontation, and to direct his energies
to areas where he might make a substantial difference. Babcock's price for
staying on amiable terms with Thompson was an unspoken agreement not
to trespass on Thompson's turf.

Thompson in his memoirs wrote that he had criticized Babcock reluctantly: "I was nearly crazed, could not sleep nor eat through the entire
investigation. I would have protected Dr. Babcock but knew the [members of
the] committee were familiar with the conditions, as they had gone through
the Institution and had seen for themselves."[23] August Kohn did not see in
Thompson any maliciousness, writing: "All speak kindly of him. He has a
big heart and is a hard worker." In Kohn's opinion, Thompson told all simply

because "good Presbyterian that he is" he "kept nothing back."[24] Thompson's testimony was straightforward and matter of fact. Still, he gave abundant evidence of the bad conditions and testified that Babcock was by and large out of touch with the wards, at least Thompson's wards, which he had not inspected "for some time to my knowledge."

Thompson was cross-examined by Julius Taylor, who had succeeded his father, Walter Taylor, upon the latter's death four years earlier.[25] Then 32 years old, Julius Taylor was the fourth member of his family to serve the asylum and the third to serve on the Board of Regents. Like Babcock he was a native South Carolinian, had been out of state for much of his education, and was a

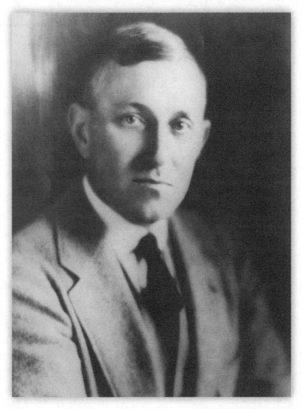

Dr. Julius Heyward Taylor (1877–1938), representing the fourth generation of his family to support the asylum, cross-examined witnesses in Babcock's behalf. He ultimately became the only member of the Board of Regents supportive of Babcock.
Courtesy: Waring Historical Library, Medical University of South Carolina, Charleston, S.C.

scholarly man with a strong humanitarian impulse.[26] Taylor took his duties as a regent seriously and became Babcock's close friend and ardent supporter. Taylor elicited from Thompson that Babcock unlike the staff physicians had seldom taken a vacation, had saved the taxpayers considerable money, and was nearly always available if needed. He got Thompson to agree that "if you want him [the superintendent] you can get him at once." Thompson also agreed that it was unreasonable to expect Babcock to supervise all aspects of the asylum while simultaneously giving "medical attention that is necessary to the colored women." The third time he was called to testify, Thompson admitted that he had never asked or invited Babcock to visit the white men's wards.[27]

Thompson was in many ways complimentary of Babcock, as he would be in his memoirs. August Kohn reported that Thompson "felt the loyalty of the regents and of Dr. Babcock. He [Thompson] has always been treated as having the utmost confidence of Dr. Babcock. He never knew of Dr. Babcock getting any personal or professional aggrandizement. He never knew of Dr. Babcock getting even a bunch of lettuce or radishes."[28] Thompson confirmed Babcock's general rule to dismiss any nurse who had abused a patient. Another cross-examiner tried unsuccessfully to get Thompson to say that Babcock had made an exception to this rule for one employee out of favoritism. Thompson answered: "I don't think so. I don't think it was any favoritism. He never shows any favoritism."

Thompson acknowledged that Babcock worked hard, perhaps unreasonably hard, so hard as to jeopardize his health. However, Babcock mismatched his priorities against the asylum's needs. He did not confer sufficiently with key staff including department heads. He did not delegate sufficiently. Thompson's testimony fed into the idea that as an administrator Babcock was well meaning but ineffective.

Next to testify was J. M. Mitchell, a pharmacist for the male wards hired by Babcock's predecessor, Peter Griffin. Although listed as a supervisor, Mitchell was a poorly educated man. He had taken a course in pharmacy by mail but did not complete it. He testified about the disarray of the pharmacy, the lack of a regular system of record keeping, the lack of cleanliness including an abundance of lice, the absence of a fire alarm, and the nursing shortage. The male wards had in his opinion deteriorated under Babcock. In the beginning Babcock had gone through the male wards twice each week, but "that was before he [Babcock] took charge of the colored women and the Dix cottage [for white women]." Mitchell acknowledged that Babcock was a very busy man, but felt conditions had deteriorated: "Dr. Babcock's management was all right for several years after he came here" [but] "in recent years he has appeared indifferent, and from some cause, I don't know."[29] Mitchell's main complaint was that he was underpaid.

Babcock's most favorable witness by far was Dr. Eleanora Saunders, the 25-year-old assistant physician who had come to the asylum two years earlier after graduating first in her class at the Medical College of the State of South Carolina. Questioning revealed that she had no office of her own, no filing system, and only twelve or thirteen nurses for about 500 women under her care. She did her own bacteriology work. She did a thorough physical examination on each patient, even though it was not required. She defended Babcock against Thompson's charge that some of the patients resented Babcock: "My patients always speak of him in the highest terms. They're constantly telling me how much better he is to them than I am. Dr. Babcock is unusually kind to them, and if I have any complaint to make against him it is his excessive kindness." The transcript of Saunders's testimony runs just 28 pages, less than half the length of the poorly educated Mitchell's testimony, prompting the question of whether the committee preferred to hear unfavorable information. Saunders told, for example, how she and some of the nurses helped make baseball uniforms for the patients.

The next three witnesses confirmed that blacks did most of the work. When asked whether the asylum farm would function better if the races were kept separate, the treasurer, John William Bunch, responded: "My opinion is that if you want to run an economical asylum you had better leave the races together. It is impossible to get any work of any consequence out of the white people, and the Negroes do quite a lot of the drudgery."[30] The dairy manager testified that blacks did most of the milking. The kitchen foreman testified that blacks did all of the cooking. These observations confirm the impressions of other asylum superintendents of that era that white patients, especially white men, were hesitant to do work they saw blacks doing.[31]

Babcock, when finally called to testify, was defensive toward some of the charges but refused to finger point. Responding to questions about the skimpiness of referring physicians' notes, he hedged that "sometimes a doctor does not write out those things." Responding to charges that the asylum accepted too many mentally retarded children (then known as "idiots") and children with epilepsy, he aimed "to administer the institution with the broadest charity, and that it is better to receive those children than to keep them at their homes." Responding to charges of abuse, he told how he had once caught an employee named Kinard abusing a patient, and although "I am a man of peace ... when I caught him I caned him." Kinard was dismissed. Babcock denied knowledge of patients being bathed in the same water. He felt the milk was wholesome. A few cases of typhoid fever occurred each year but there had never been a major outbreak. He acknowledged that he had used female nurses in the male wards, but mainly because of the "difficulty of getting proper nurses for men in all institutions." Asked about the jail-like gratings on many rooms, he answered that it was "better to have the feelings wounded" by gratings than to have to "tramp out in the sandhills chasing a patient who has made his escape because the gratings are defective," as Babcock had done on occasion.[32]

Committee members wanted to know why patients who had substantially improved were not released—the issue that prompted the investigation in the first place. Babcock resorted to anecdote: "I know a case of a colored man and his wife. They got under a religious spell, underwent a period of fasting, and in the meantime felt that they were in close communion with the Almighty, and thought they received orders from him to sacrifice their child. So, they cut the child's throat with the understanding that the child was to be restored to life at the end of three days. They were arrested and [sentenced to be] put to death, and I think properly committed to the asylum" where they remained.[33] The committee pressed on. Babcock deflected the charge that the asylum physicians were "neglectful in regard to the examination of patients in here to ascertain if they are able to get out," but admitted that "with more physicians we could do better clinical work than at least I have been able to do." He felt it best to err toward longer lengths of stay, since "the brain is the most delicate organism of the body" and required ample time to heal. Were one of his own daughters to suffer an attack of acute insanity, he would "want her to remain in [the] asylum for a year to eighteen months after she seemed to be well." It was better to err on the side of overtreatment even if this added to expenses and crowding.[34] In his opinion, "all asylums make the mistake of sending the patients out too early."[35]

He pointed out that the annual per capita funding for his asylum in 1908 was $109.30, compared to $155 and $165 at two North Carolina asylums. Yet he offered little or no defense to charges that he was insufficiently aggressive about pressing the legislature for more money. He had gone before the legislature's Ways and Means Committee "whenever they have asked me." Otherwise, he left the lawmakers alone. He pointed out that his predecessor, Dr. Griffin, "had been assailed on the ground of extravagance." Therefore, "My administration started with the idea that the money that was supplied for this institution must be made to go as far as possible . . . . The money that is sent to the asylum comes from the people, from so many taxpayers, and it is by the special providence of God that you get a penny, and when you get it, get down on your knees and thank God, and make it go as far as possible; but, above all things, don't go to the Legislature and say you haven't

got a plenty of it." When asked what the state appropriation for the asylum
ought to be, he replied that $150 to $160 per capita was "just as low as an
honorable State ought to try to administer to the wants of the insane." But
he was reluctant to ask for more.[36]

Nobody questioned Babcock's dedication. He was asked: "Haven't you
got about three times as much work as you ought to have?" He replied that
"the burden I have taken upon me I have carried as uncomplainingly as a man
can. I have no complaint." At one time, he had personally cared for about
900 patients.[37] Julius Taylor reminded Babcock that he had asked "several
times . . . if it would meet with your approval if the Board of Regents would
ask the Legislature to raise your salary of three thousand dollars to what it
should be, four to five thousand dollars . . . and you have constantly refused
to allow it to be done." Babcock verified Taylor's statement but added: "I
think I am paid all I am worth." He also confirmed his policy that neither
he nor his staff should accept as perquisites food, supplies, fruit, or vegetables
from the asylum farm.

The gist of testimony by both hostile and friendly witnesses was that the
asylum was in bad shape, and that while Babcock worked hard he perhaps
focused too much on keeping expenses down to the detriment of patient
welfare. He denied knowledge of any personal friction with Thompson: "I
had thought that the doctor and I had gotten along here very harmoniously;
possibly a little friction the first year or two, but I certainly felt he was one of
mine. When the troubles came upon me he stood by me and helped me to
bear them. At any time when he has had trouble I did the best I could. The
fact that we were not in touch is a revelation to me."[38] And nobody, including Thompson, denied that Babcock responded promptly when called upon.

Last to testify was assistant physician H. H. Griffin, the 33-year-old
son of the previous superintendent. Griffin, who was in charge of 330 black
male patients, held that there was "absolutely" no friction between Babcock
and the staff, and that Babcock was not guilty of any inefficiency. The basic
problem was clear and simple: lack of funding. "The ideas of economy that
have been forced upon us," he insisted, explained why the asylum had so
many shortcomings.[39]

The Majority Report

Christensen got little public support for blaming Babcock, the regents, or
both for the asylum's shortcomings. One editorialist suggested the South
Carolina Medical Association be placed in charge because "when Dr.

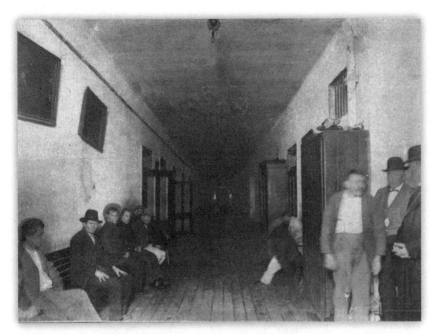

New Building, fourth ward for white men. The caption in the investigative committee's report reads: "Poorly ventilated, heated, and lighted. These patients spend most of their days as well as nights in idleness in this corridor and adjoining porch. Floor in bad condition."
Courtesy: South Caroliniana Library, University of South Carolina, Columbia, S.C.

Babcock has gone before the Legislature to ask for increased appropriations he has practically gone alone." If doctors were in charge, "Dr. Babcock would experience no difficulty in obtaining the needful support for the institution from the state."[40]

Christensen pressed ahead with a full-scale investigation that included outside consultants and in-depth comparisons with other asylums. In the end his committee was sharply divided on where to assign blame. That the decision would not be unanimous was almost preordained; one member of the special committee came from Babcock's native Chester County and another was a physician. The result was in effect a hung jury on whether Babcock and the regents should be held accountable for the appalling conditions. The final product was a 121-page volume containing an 83-page Majority Report signed by four members and a 15-page Minority Report signed by three.[41]

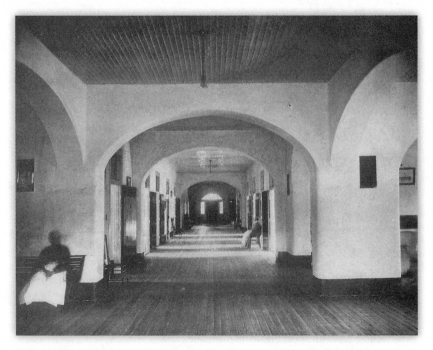

New Building, ward for white women, described as the "best ward," "clean and
well kept, but poorly furnished." Babcock felt obliged to give white women
patients "the best we had."
Courtesy: South Caroliniana Library, University of South Carolina, Columbia, S.C.

Frederick Howard Wines, a Presbyterian minister from Chicago
brought in as an outside consultant, set the tone for the Majority Report.
Wines, an authority on charitable institutions including mental asylums,
began: "Nothing that I may say is intended as a personal reflection upon
any one, least of all on Dr. Babcock, who treated me with great courtesy, and
who is, no doubt, a gentleman, a scholar, and a skilful physician." Yet surely
someone "is to blame for conditions which existed at the date of my visit to
the institution." Even if blame should be assigned mainly to the legislature,
"the Superintendent and trustees may be censurable for accepting the sums
without vigorous protest. If such protest was made and passed unheeded,
they would, in my judgment, have been justified in severing their connection
with the hospital." Wines compared diets at the Columbia asylum and the
asylum at Kankakee, Illinois, near Chicago: "You will see how much more
liberal our allowance is than yours." At Kankakee meat was served with
every meal and fresh beef rather than scraps was used in the beef stew. Two

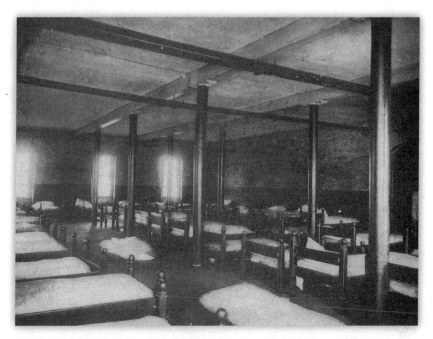

Parker Building, sleeping room for black men. "Overcrowded, mattresses on the floor, poorly heated and ventilated; fifty-two men sleep in this room. The death rate in this building last year [1908] was 28% of the number of occupants."
Courtesy: South Caroliniana Library, University of South Carolina, Columbia, S.C.

vegetables were always served at dinner and fruit at supper. Without realizing he had done so, Wines had identified why pellagra was more common in Columbia than Kankakee.[42]

The Majority Report included rare concessions such as an opinion that "requirements for white patients should be greater than for the colored by reason of their higher standard of living."[43] The report was damning mainly in its comparisons of the Columbia asylum with seven others, of which two were in the South, four in the North, and one in the District of Columbia. However, the forty-six full-page photographs and their captions rendered the text almost superfluous. Consider, for example, the caption to a photograph taken in the Parker Building: "The odor in these wards is almost unbearable." We can only imagine the sights, sounds, and smells that awaited visitors.

The committee laid much blame on the regents, who supposedly had "general control of the administration." The regents were appointed by the governor for six-year terms and were paid $250 per year. In 1910 there were five regents, two of whom were physicians. The law required the regents "to

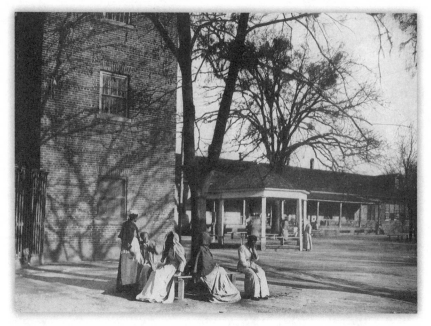

Exercise yard for black women, showing the lack thereof.
Courtesy: South Caroliniana Library, University of South Carolina, Columbia, S.C.

report annually to the Legislature the state and condition of the institution, fully and particularly," but in fact the regents had "not reported to the Legislature the deplorable sanitary condition, the lack of treatment for patients and the economic waste of appropriations, all of which we have found and which are admitted by some of the officials to exist."[44]

The committee faulted Babcock mainly for his administrative style, or lack thereof. The superintendent did not keep regular office hours. He kept his own schedule and could be hard to find. He had no system for maintaining records. He had no system for filing copies of letters sent out, letters received, and reports.[45] He had given up his former practice of meeting daily with the staff physicians. He received no regular reports on the conditions of individual patients. He had been out of touch with the "white male department"—Thompson's department—for many years and did not know the general conditions of those wards, just as Thompson had said. Thompson was not lauded, however, as "an atmosphere of disorganization" pervaded the white male department along with "want of cooperation with those in authority" and "a feeling of apathy and helplessness." In essence, the superintendent did not supervise.[46]

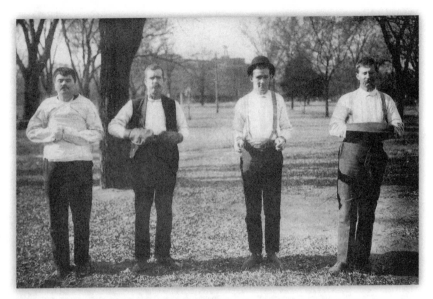

Forms of restraint used at the South Carolina State Hospital for the Insane included, from left to right, camisoles, mitts and wristers, wristers, and muffs and wristers. "Each day about 105 men and women are in restraint of this kind or some combination . . . . Modern hospitals use less than 1% under strict regulations, we use 7% indiscriminately."
Courtesy: South Caroliniana Library, University of South Carolina, Columbia, S.C.

The committee found patient care poor from start to finish. The admissions process was seriously flawed. Babcock had abdicated responsibility for approving admissions on a case-by-case basis as required by law. There was no special room for receiving and examining patients. Patients were often brought to the asylum "in iron shackles by deputies who have no training in the handling of the insane" with the result that "patients are often in an excited or despondent condition upon arrival . . . their ailment is thereby aggravated and their treatment begins unfavorably." They were admitted directly to the ward, often bringing "vermin and disease" that could spread to other patients. Medical records were essentially nonexistent: "We find that no clinical records whatever are kept at our Hospital."[47] There was little attempt to classify patients according to their disease or mental condition. There was little attempt to separate patients with infectious diseases, who often mingled "freely with the other patients, in some cases sleeping in the same room." There was little attempt to separate patients inclined to disturb other patients: "Reference to the testimony will show that disturbed

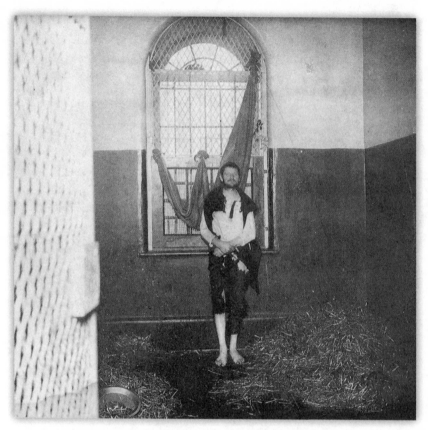

Inmate in restraint, New Building, seventh ward. "This violent patient is kept locked in this room, sleeps on straw and eats out of the tin dish. Door was opened and flash light of room and patient were taken just as they were. He receives no treatment worthy of the name. Each time hospital was visited several were found on this ward in this or worse condition."
Courtesy: South Caroliniana Library, University of South Carolina, Columbia, S.C.

and dangerous cases, suicidal cases, epileptics, chronic insane, inebriates, criminally insane, idiots, dipsomaniacs, and the feeble minded of all ages, are mixed together through the wards. Under these conditions, any effective treatment is difficult." Although white female patients were "fairly well clothed and kept, considering the lack of nurses," the same could not be said for the white men. Bed bugs, body lice, and head lice were common in the men's departments and were sometimes seen in the women's wards.[48] Conditions for blacks were abysmal irrespective of gender.

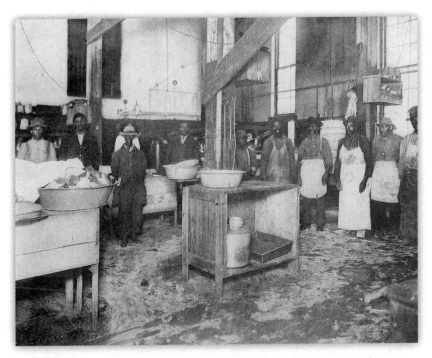

Main kitchen, cooks and patient helpers. "Man in light felt hat is one of a
number of patients who wander in and out of the kitchen at will."
Courtesy: South Caroliniana Library, University of South Carolina, Columbia, S.C.

The staff was deficient in both quantity and quality. The ratio of nurses to
patients was one to thirty-six on the wards for black men and one to eighteen
on the other services. Many of the attendants, especially on the male wards,
were incompetent. Some were illiterate, leading to medication errors as they
could not read the labels. Poor discipline sometimes led to brutality.[49]

Physical restraints of various types were in wide use. The committee
heard that on average about 1 percent of asylum inmates in the United
States were mechanically restrained on a given day. At the South Carolina
asylum, mechanical restraint was applied to about 10 percent of white men,
9 percent of black men, 7 percent of white women, and 1 percent of black
women. Nurses were given discretion to use mechanical restraint or seclusion
for difficult patients. A survey of thirty-six asylums revealed that records of
restraint were kept at all but one. No such records were kept at the Columbia
asylum. Moreover, all but one of the respondents indicated that mechanical
restraint required a doctor's order, as was not the case in Columbia. Committee members had "seen screaming white women strapped down to beds in

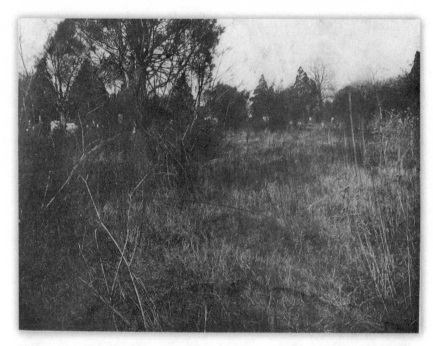

Hospital lot, Elmwood Cemetery. "After it had been filled new graves were dug
into old ones and the bones scattered over the ground. This went on about a year.
Nearly all the rough wooden head-boards are gone, graves are sunken and the lot
overgrown with weeds and brush."
Courtesy: South Caroliniana Library, University of South Carolina, Columbia, S.C.

locked rooms, and in other departments patients, in restraint, lying in defiled
beds." Thus, "our institution employs a maximum of restraint and allows
it to be used indiscriminately," and this was "largely the fault of management." Neither the superintendent nor the regents had addressed the issue
of restraint "as far back as we have examined the records."[50]

Babcock admitted that "we use a great deal of restraint, but I am not
theorist enough to say through this Commission to the people of South
Carolina that no person should ever, under any circumstances, be restrained."
The committee, however, obtained letters to the contrary from other asylums.
Dr. Henry A. Cotton, medical director of the New Jersey State Hospital
at Trenton, advised the committee: "Restraint in insane hospitals is largely
a matter of tradition, but the experience in such hospitals as the Danvers
Hospital, the Trenton State Hospital and others . . . will overcome all arguments against the method of no restraint." The committee concluded that "an
institution's attitude toward the use of 'mechanical restraint' is an index that

shows quite accurately whether its administration is abreast of the times." Although more and better attendants were needed, also needed was "a radical change in the attitude of the administration."[51] Medicinal restraint with powerful sedatives, on the other hand, was not abused at Babcock's asylum.

Treatment was minimal. There was little or no attempt at "moral therapy." Hydrotherapy—a new vogue involving the application of water at various temperatures and by various methods—was not used at the Columbia asylum in contrast to many hospitals. Drugs were at that time thought to play a minor role in the treatment of mental illness.[52] James Thompson testified that the major treatment modalities for mental illness were "diet and exercise," both clearly deficient at the Columbia asylum.

Diets were monotonous at best. The surveyors found no diet tables. After consulting with the steward they managed to construct a menu from which they concluded that there was "practically no variety, this menu being unchanged except as noted." Food was likely to be unclean since the three kitchens were small, poorly lighted, and unsanitary. Patients' opportunities for employment, exercise, and amusements were limited. The rules stipulated: "The Superintendent shall, as far as practicable, furnish employment to the patients, especially such employment as is accompanied with healthy exercise; and he shall establish such modes of sedentary or active amusement as may suit the various circumstances of the patients."[53] Little was done along these lines. At other hospitals, about 50 percent of patients were employed in farming and gardening, kitchen work, laundering, care of cattle and barns, road work, shoe repairing, printing, and other gainful tasks.[54] Employment rates at the Columbia asylum were 40 percent for black men and women, 24 percent for white women, and 16 percent for white men. There was little or no provision for systematic exercise. The exercise rooms were enclosed with high wooden fences. Those for white men and black women looked "more like pens than yards, and others not much better."[55] There were no amusements for blacks, and amusements for whites consisted mainly of a weekly dance during the fall, winter, and spring months.[56] The committee concluded:

> The lives of most of the patients at this Hospital are spent in the rooms, and the corridors, and the small yards where they are usually allowed to spend a few hours a day when the weather is good. The enforced idleness, even in sanitary surroundings, and the lack of exercise would be injurious to the mental and bodily health of a sane person. Members of your Committee have been deeply moved at the sight of these patients crowded in dismal, unsanitary, ill-smelling corridors and rooms or walking about in the cramped, pen-like enclosures surrounded by high board fences. In

other institutions visited by us the buildings have been fresh and clean, and the grounds have been unenclosed, the whole having the appearance of a hospital rather than a prison.

Overcrowding was horrific. Most toilets were unsanitary. The buildings were "virtually fire traps." There were no instructions on what to do in case of fire, and "in fact, no one knows what to do except to turn on the alarm for the Columbia fire department." The storage room was "in a state of disorder, no attempt being made to properly classify or arrange the goods it contained and keep them in a neat and orderly condition." The South Carolina State Hospital for the Insane was, just as Gibbes had charged, a grim place to be.[57]

Death may or may not have been a welcome relief, but was certainly more common than in other asylums. Death rates for blacks were twice those of whites, but in each instance were much higher than those of other states. Tuberculosis was by far the most common cause of death. The committee confirmed that while Babcock had written a major article on controlling tuberculosis in asylums, he had done little about it: "Patients suffering from this disease are on most of the wards, mingling freely with other patients, eating with them, drinking out of the same vessels and sometimes sleeping in the same rooms . . . . The State is now maintaining in its Hospital a breeding-place for this disease." The committee verified that the Old Building had become a death trap. The mortality rate for black women in the Old Building was 34 percent in 1908 and had averaged 28 percent over the previous five years. Reckoning that the death rate for black women should not exceed 10 percent, the committee calculated that the administration had been responsible for the deaths of 259 black women over the previous five years. Nor did the dead always rest in peace. The seldom-marked graves were often disturbed to make room for new corpses. A new burial ground had been established for whites but "on a steep hillside on a corner of one of the lots in which the Hospital's hogs are kept."[58]

The Majority Report was thus comprehensive and damning. The investigators charged: "Merely as a place of detention our Hospital is unfit. Not only does the State fail to provide proper or adequate treatment for the insanity for the patients there held, but its custodianship is a menace to the health and life of these afflicted citizens." The main positive observation was absence of fiscal dishonesty, graft, or corruption. Babcock insisted on scrupulous honesty for himself and everyone else. The Majority Report hinted but did not declare outright the need for a new administration. Its recommendations would increase state appropriations to $150 per capita for white patients and $125 per capita for black patients. Bonds amounting to one million dollars would be issued to buy land and build two new hospitals, "one for the white and one for the colored insane." When these were up and running the existing asylum and its land in downtown Columbia would be turned over to the state's Sinking Fund Commission for disposal. State law would "be amended so that idiots, inebriates, the weak-minded, and non-insane epileptics, who are not dangerous to life or property will be ineligible to admission to the Hospital." There were twenty-two specific charges, of which the most unflattering was that the superintendent and the regents had not been diligent about keeping the patient census at a more reasonable level. Persons who were not insane should not be admitted, and patients who had substantially improved should be discharged.[59]

The Minority Report

The three signers of the Minority Report disagreed with those of the Majority Report and perhaps among themselves as to the proper scope of the report, the root causes of the deficiencies, and the appropriate remedies. They asserted that legislators including themselves should not "manage or tell others to manage the Hospital for the Insane." They expressed "feelings of sympathy and love for the unfortunate inmates of the institution." They were poetic in their defense of Babcock: "Think of the tremendous effort of caring for fifteen hundred human beings with deranged intellects, many with reason dethroned and more with that bright light entirely gone. Our Saviour could by a simple command cause the reason of such unfortunate beings to resume her throne . . . . But how is mere man to minister to the needs of those whose bodies are diseased and whose minds are either gone or tottering in the balances? Warm must be the heart, and broad the sympathy and clear the intellect of him who is willing to undertake it. No calling could be higher, no work grander, and he who does it honestly, faithfully and efficiently is indeed a public benefactor." Although it was not their "purpose to unduly praise Dr. Babcock nor to unjustly censure him," still:

> The estimate we have formed of him is that he is high, scholarly, honest, sympathetic, kind, and has medical attainments of the highest order and is devoting his life to the State's most unfortunate class. We do not say that he has not made mistakes nor that he is faultless, nor that he has always carried out the strict letter of the law relating to the subject of insanity. He has for many years been doing the work of about three men, and the testimony shows it, executive head of the institution and until three months ago sole

physician to all the colored women and a large number of white women in addition to aiding the other physicians under him. Always at his post of duty and taking but one vacation in twenty years, and then for the purpose of studying the causes and treatment of that dread disease pellagra, which is puzzling the medical mind more than any other disease and on which he is recognized as high authority by all physicians, even those representing the United States Government. Shall a Legislative Committee undertake to strike down such a man or cripple his usefulness? We decline to do so.

In denying the state's abdication of responsibility to the mentally ill they were almost maudlin: "We know that South Carolina loves her insane . . . . We are unwilling to publish to the world that South Carolina is negligent in providing for these unfortunate people. We do not think the facts show it . . . . Our great aim has been to hold up to the members of the Legislature a photograph of the institution dedicated to the care and treatment of God's most unfortunate creatures and to be of some help to each one of them in answering the question: 'Canst thou minister to a mind deceased?'"[60]

They largely dismissed the Majority Report's twenty-two charges. They gave three options for overhauling the facilities: (1) the purchase of two farms "at some distance" from each other on which to build separate facilities for white and black patients; (2) transfer of black patients to a new facility while retaining the downtown facility for whites; and (3) construction of a new facility in the countryside where "epileptics, harmless inebriates and imbeciles could be colonized or to which the colored insane could be gradually transferred" while retaining the existing facility."[61]

Showdown

Division within the Committee to Investigate the State Hospital for the Insane left the legislature with two problems. What should be done with the competing Majority and Minority Reports? What should be done with Babcock and the regents? The legislators forged a compromise. New facilities would be built to relieve overcrowding. Babcock stayed on, although the hearings, outside consultants, and publicity undermined his long-term political viability.[62]

Babcock's supporters saw the Majority Report as a serious affront to his honor. Francis Hopkins Weston, a lawyer and farmer from lower Richland County, rose to praise his friend in the Senate: "I have been attracted to him by his high sense of honor, by the great humanity of the man, that he can never look upon suffering, whether it is from a white man or from a negro, without his whole heart giving out to him, a man consecrated soul and mind to this great problem of the insane in South Carolina .... Physician after physician in South Carolina can tell you and will tell you that Dr. Babcock among physicians in South Carolina has no peer and few superiors, that he is perhaps the leading alienist in the Southern States, that he is a man with as kind and gentle disposition as God ever bestowed on any human."[63] The issue came down to the Majority Committee's report versus Babcock's personal popularity.

Christensen proposed in the Senate a resolution that Babcock and the regents be asked to resign. The resolution was referred to the Judiciary Committee, which endorsed it for consideration by the legislature.[64] When it came his turn to speak, Christensen acknowledged that "the corridors and galleries have been crowded with the friends and relatives of the officers and physicians of this institution," and that he had been approached by them all. He spoke for about two hours, making "a plain, business presentation without any oratory." The question as he saw it was "not whether we shall or shall not condemn the six men [Babcock and the regents], but whether we shall or shall not inaugurate a new policy, a new system, new standards, and new methods at the South Carolina Hospital for the Insane." He continued: "It is quite possible that the gentleman at the head of this institution as superintendent is an excellent gentleman and at the same time it is quite possible that the superintendent is inefficient. It is quite possible that the board of regents are honest men and of good standing in their community, and yet, at the same time, it is quite possible that their administration of the Hospital for the Insane has been incompetent." As a result, "the South Carolina State Hospital for the Insane practically has had no head, it has no general director, each department has been running itself ... without system of administration or control." Christensen recited some of the major shortcomings uncovered by the Legislative Committee. The real issue was not Babcock but "the welfare of the insane of the State." Christensen had been getting letters "for a year imploring me to go to the bottom of this matter, and gentlemen, they need champions, too, on this floor; yes, they need a champion with the fearlessness of a Mart Gary to speak the truth boldly; they need a champion with the courage and cool judgment of a Wade Hampton, that they might listen to him and heed him above the clamor, one with the gift of a Calhoun to hammer forth the logic of their position." Christensen's directive was clear: "However lovable this man may be, whatever fine traits he may have, we must not, we can not, in considering this question, take that into consideration." Babcock must go.

Christensen had given it his best shot. By alluding to the memories of
Martin Witherspoon Gary, Wade Hampton III, and John C. Calhoun—
champions of white supremacy during previous eras—he had done all he
could to appeal to the conservative Democratic majority in the State Senate.
It did not suffice. It is doubtful that most senators took the young progressive
seriously. "The chairs of many senators were vacant," the *State* reported. "They
had decided how they would vote and didn't care to hear the argument."[65]

To Babcock's defense came Senator Thomas Irby Rogers, an attorney
from Marlboro County who seems to have been a personal friend.[66] Rogers
pointed out that nowhere in the two volumes before the Senate (that is, the
testimony from the hearings and the legislative committee's report) was
there any finding of incompetence or criminal neglect of duty by Babcock.
The conditions at the asylum, however unfortunate, were caused by underfunding and were common public knowledge, yesterday's news. Members
of the Senate were not competent to judge a doctor's treatment of patients.
Babcock's advocacy for patients was shown, for example, by the occasion
when he found a subordinate "treating one of the patients wrongfully, and
his indignation was so aroused that he broke his cane over the attendant's
head." Babcock deserved credit, not blame, for denying admission to no more
than three persons during his tenure at the asylum. He deserved credit for
declining an offer to have his salary raised, for having stated: "No gentlemen, in proportion to the meager appropriation for these unfortunates here
whom I have learned to love, whom I have so long tenderly cherished in
my soul, I have not the heart to ask the State of South Carolina to give me
more than the average salary paid others in public life." Rogers appealed to
the Code of Honor, suggested that many (including the legislature) were to
blame for the asylum's shortcomings. Rogers even likened Babcock to Jesus
of Nazareth: "Mr. President, I have seen a picture painted like this: On the
canvas was a man bleeding, footsore, staggering under a heavy burden; the
man was represented as staggering up a rocky slope; by his side marched
those with scourges and spears; when he tottered he was scourged, when he
fell he was speared; when I looked again I saw the burden that he bore, it
was a cross. In Heaven's name are you going to spear and scourge this man
who has so long borne his cross in patient suffering and honest endurance?
The Senate of South Carolina will not do it." Babcock should not be forced
to shoulder the cross alone.[67]

Babcock's defenders prevailed. The Senate by vote of twenty-seven to
nine killed the resolution asking Babcock and the regents to resign. The press
applauded. The *News and Courier* crowed that it had been a "battle between
the kindness and humaneness of the superintendent of the Hospital and

the crying needs of that institution on the one hand against those officials attacking methods in vogue at that asylum on the other hand."[68]

There remained the problem of overcrowding. The House of Representatives rejected the Majority Report by a vote of eighty-nine to twenty-nine, adopting instead the Minority Report. It also killed the proposition to issue $1,000,000 in bonds to build two new asylums, one for whites and one for blacks, which would have been along the lines of the cottage plan.[69] A compromise resolution created a five-member State Hospital Commission to buy land, make plans, and erect buildings "which will relieve the congested conditions now existing in said hospital."[70] This eventually led to a new campus for blacks on a property northeast of Columbia that became known as State Park.

Aftermath

On the same day that the legislature vindicated Babcock at the Capitol of South Carolina, Tillman collapsed on the steps of the Capitol of the United States. This time it was his right side that was paralyzed and he lost his speech entirely. Babcock left for Washington at once. Tillman made a "near-miraculous recovery"[71] but his health and therefore his ability to protect Babcock politically was clearly declining.

The investigation had brought out that first assistant physician James Thompson, while not overtly hostile, was willing and able to "tell it like it is" at Babcock's expense. Babcock now knew that Julius Taylor among the regents and Eleanora Saunders among the staff physicians were his only reliable supporters at the asylum. His outside support system was also dwindling. His closest friends among fellow asylum superintendents, Patrick Murphy of North Carolina and Theophilus Powell of Georgia, had both died in 1907, and George Searcy of Alabama was no longer a superintendent.[72] Things returned to a semblance of normal at the asylum. The new State Hospital Commission began its work toward a rural campus for black patients. Yet cards were in place for another legislative showdown less than four years later. There had been no change in the asylum's governance, which was in many ways the root cause of the deficiencies.[73]

Babcock took it personally. He was unable to acknowledge, at least publicly, that there was much truth in the charge that as an administrator he had many shortcomings—a reservation he had himself expressed before accepting the job. He never forgave Hunter Gibbes, and his coolness extended to Gibbes's brother, a physician.[77] Babcock's opinion, supported in

recent years by historian Gerald Grob, was that the investigating committee merely confirmed what he had been telling the legislature for years.[75]
Moreover, the committee and its outside consultants had not acknowledged
that overcrowding and underfunding plagued public asylums throughout
the nation, and that southern states, and especially South Carolina, suffered
more than most because of poverty.[76]

Years later, James Thompson related, a member of the investigating
committee came to the asylum and Babcock ordered him to leave, told
him to never set foot on the campus again, and followed him to the gate
with "a heavy walking stick in his hand."[77] The legislator in question was
probably Christensen, for in 1914 Tillman wrote Babcock: "I notice that
even Christensen has been civilized and humanized enough to become your
advocate, attributable no doubt to your escorting him from the asylum that
night."[78] Whether Babcock ever forgave Christensen—or, better, acknowledged that there was "nothing to forgive" since Christensen had been well
intentioned from the beginning and had treated Babcock with utmost
respect—is unknown. As an ally for improving the plight of the mentally
ill, Christensen with his progressivism might have served Babcock better
than did the largely conservative Board of Regents, which concluded early
in the investigation that while numerous improvements were needed, the
costs "might impose unjustifiable hardship and burdens" on the taxpayers of
South Carolina.[79] But Babcock was never one to break rank with the chain
of command.

CHAPTER 5

Sambon's Obsession

Pellagrins, Pellagrologists, and Pellagraphobia

Between the first (1909) and second (1912) national conferences at the South Carolina State Hospital, pellagra became epidemic in the Southeast and a concern throughout the nation. American physicians established a competence in the disease. Louis Sambon's version of the infection hypothesis replaced Cesare Lombroso's version of the spoiled-corn hypothesis as the most popular explanation.

Babcock and Claude Lavinder of the U.S. Public Health and Marine Hospital Service tracked the epidemiology and brought out the first comprehensive English language treatise on pellagra. Numerous Americans taught their colleagues through journal articles, meetings, and conferences. Two well-funded groups of American investigators—the Illinois Pellagra Commission and the Thompson-McFadden Pellagra Commission—claimed their data largely eliminated diet as the cause. Both groups favored an infectious cause despite the paucity of hard evidence. Lavinder with Babcock's assistance tracked the epidemiology of pellagra, tried to transmit the disease to animals, and became progressively discouraged.

Marie's Pellagra

William Osler, having written in the sixth edition (1907) of his bestselling textbook that pellagra did not occur in the United States, revised the seventh edition (1910) to read: "Searcy, Babcock, Wood, and Bellamy have shown (1907–1908) that it is not an uncommon disease in the southern parts of the United States; many of the cases are acute." Osler embraced Lombroso's version of the spoiled-corn hypothesis; the "measures to be employed are change in diet, removal from the infected district, and, as a prophylaxis, proper ripening and preservation of the corn, the toxic changes in which are apparently due to the action of a special organism."[1]

The medical literature on pellagra in English consisted mainly of papers by Fleming Sandwith. Babcock and Lavinder hesitated to write a textbook from scratch, since their "comparatively limited experience" posed the problem of credibility.[2] They decided to translate a then-new French text, *La Pellagre* (1908) by Armand Marie, which was in turn an abridgement and translation of Lombroso's massive *Trattato Profilattico e Clinico della Pellagra* (1892). Lavinder expressed doubts "whether we could get it published."[3] Who would buy a book about pellagra?

The project became more than a translation. They added numerous observations by themselves, other Americans, and Sandwith. They included twenty full-page photographs.[4] They prepared an English language bibliography.[5] Lavinder, who had tried unsuccessfully to find a national publisher, told Babcock: "We could have made a better book with less work, and it makes me angry to think that Marie's name must be put on what he deserves no credit for whatever."[6]

Babcock's family complained when Lavinder's name went first on the title page. They felt Babcock had done most of the work. Babcock answered that he "did not need the recognition the book would bring but the other man [Lavinder] did."[7] He had overcome whatever reservations he may have had about a government agency's stealing his thunder, and he wanted to promote Lavinder as the best-qualified American pellagra researcher. Babcock told Surgeon General Walter Wyman that Lavinder "has a better insight into the whole pellagra problem than anyone else in America" and urged that "plans now under consideration for Dr. Lavinder's further investigation of pellagra at home and abroad be carried out."[8]

Babcock may have had another reason for not insisting on first authorship: a patient at the asylum did most of the actual translating.[9] George W. Manly came from a prominent South Carolina family, was an accomplished linguist, had a doctorate from the University of Leipzig, and was still studying abroad when he developed "signs of intense nervous strain." His family brought him home and consulted Babcock. Manly became devoted to Babcock and his family and even lived with them for a while in the superintendent's house. Eventually he acquired his own quarters in the Main Building (or New Building; now the Babcock Building). According to one of Babcock's daughters, Manly did "literally <u>mounds</u> of translations from

French, German & especially Italian for Daddy."[10] Manly helped prepare the manuscript and oversee its publication in 1910 by The State Company in Columbia, South Carolina.[11]

Babcock and Lavinder reviewed the various hypotheses. They recounted how in 1810 Marzari "believed that corn caused the disease by reason of its deficiency in certain nutritive qualities," leading to "the great corn theory of pellagra" and, eventually, "the ultimate creation of the so-called 'Zeist' (from *Zea Mays*) and 'Antizeist' schools of thought." Although this division led to a "wordy war," still "the corn idea, in one form or another, has held the dominant place in the etiology of pellagra."[12] They added a six-page discussion of Louis Sambon's new hypothesis, fortified by details "kindly provided by Doctor Sambon." Sambon gave five reasons why pellagra was not due to corn, five reasons why pellagra was a parasitic disease, five reasons why pellagra was an insect-borne disease, and eight reasons why pellagra was transmitted by a specific insect, *Simulium reptans* (a black fly or sand fly). Babcock and Lavinder commended the "judicial mental attitude which American investigators have so far shown with regard to the etiology of pellagra" but felt Sambon's elaborate hypothesis was "well worthy of serious attention at the hands of American students and investigators."[13] Babcock refrained from zealous advocacy for any hypothesis but, when pressed, remained a Zeist—pellagra was somehow linked to corn.[14]

Babcock and Lavinder invited the aging Lombroso to write a preface. He happily obliged. Marie's book already included "experimental researches" by Lombroso and others. An alcoholic extract of corn meal infected with a microorganism named *Bacterium maidis* killed white mice. Dogs given mold-spoiled corn developed anemia, muscle spasms, and diarrhea. Chickens developed convulsions and lost their feathers. Previously-tame chickens became "very wild at the end of five or six months on the regimen of corn." An "alcoholic extract of pellagrosine" caused convulsions in frogs, rats, and dogs, and killed the only cat that got it. Human experiments included repeated injections of a "tincture of spoiled corn" to "twelve sound and healthy individuals, soldiers and laborers at work in the city." Nine subjects vomited, eight lost weight, and six got diarrhea. Only two of the twelve subjects stayed symptom free.[15] Lombroso told Babcock and Lavinder that he would use their invitation to announce "the more recent observations made this year, in my laboratory, upon the cause and prophylaxis of pellagra."[16] Lombroso defended sound corn and blamed "the fraudulent methods of millers" for much of the pellagra in Italy.[17] Babcock and Lavinder cautioned readers that it was "only fair to say . . . that the experimental work of Lombroso and others has not escaped criticism at the hands of many earnest and capable men."[18]

Supporters of one or another hypothesis prized bits and pieces of epidemiologic data. Lombroso pointed to the Mediterranean island of Corfu,
where the rural poor lived mainly on corn but never grew quite enough for
their own tables. They habitually bought corn from neighboring Albania and
the Epirus region of Greece. Then they discovered that grapes paid better
than corn. Vineyards replaced cornfields. The Corfu residents began import-
ing corn from afar and it often arrived in "very bad condition" after the long
sea voyages. Pellagra, according to a researcher named Pretenderis Thypaldos, appeared in one community on Corfu only after the residents stopped
growing most of their own corn.[19] The Corfu experience, while anecdotal,
resonated with Lombroso and his followers. Meanwhile, Louis Sambon in
London contemplated his 1905 observation that pellagra in northern Italy
seemed to occur mainly along the banks of fast-flowing streams teeming
with *Simulium* flies and their larvae.

Babcock and Lavinder stressed the difficulty of making an accurate
diagnosis of pellagra in its early stages. The manifestations could be "very
contradictory." There could be loss of appetite *or* voracity; constipation *or*
diarrhea; somnolence *or* insomnia; stupor *or* mental excitement; sensation
of burning *or* sensation of cold; mutism *or* loquacity; dilated pupils *or* con-
stricted pupils; salaciousness *or* impotence.[20] They agreed with Sandwith
that the rash from which the disease took its name was actually the least
important feature. And the rash could be confusing. The initial sunburn-like
redness evolved into a chronic dermatitis that could assume a wide variety
of appearances. Babcock and Lavinder observed that in African American
women it was "not unusual for the dermatitis upon the face and nose to
assume the 'butterfly' appearance common in lupus erythematosus."[21] Other
observations that may have been new, at least in the literature in English,
included spots on the palms and soles.[22] Babcock and Lavinder gave long
accounts of the effects of pellagra on the nervous system, the gastrointestinal tract, the eyes, the blood, and the urine. And there were of course the
changes found at autopsy.

They added an appendix with practical advice by the Italian Giuseppe
Antonini. "Instead of SPENDING YOUR MONEY IN WINES AND LIQUORS,
buy wheat bread . . . . If you have milk, eggs, cheese, limit the sale of these
articles to others, and use at least a part of such products for your own home
food." "REDUCE the cultivation of corn." "DO NOT BE ASHAMED to go
to the doctor if you are a pellagrin . . . . Get cured in time and so avoid the
HOSPITAL or the INSANE ASYLUM." "PROFIT BY YOUR INSTRUCTION
IN AGRICULTURE, and better your crops." Such advice became a mantra
for pellagra prevention in the United States.

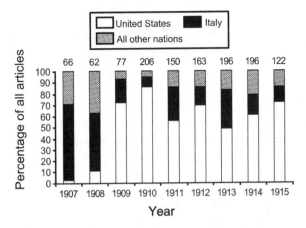

Percentage of all articles on pellagra by nation, 1907 through 1915, as referenced by the *Index Medicus* (the numbers of articles for the respective years are shown above each bar). The United States rapidly surpassed Italy and other nations in this regard.

Their last appendix summarized world corn production by nation and region. For the year 1907 the United States produced 79 percent of the world's 3.3 million bushels. The U.S. Department of Agriculture had already assigned Carl L. Alsberg, one of its top scientists, to pellagra, which by threatening corn consumption held huge economic implications.[23] They prepared two bibliographies, one of which presented for the first time a compendium of the literature on pellagra written in English. The second bibliography was a less-complete list of references in Italian, French, and other languages.

Marie's *Pellagra* was well-received. Sandwith probably wrote the review that appeared in the *Lancet*, still the world's most prestigious English language medical journal, concluding that "this book ought to be in every medical library."[24] All of the reviews were favorable, with the reservation by some that there was too much reliance on Lombroso, whose "moldy corn" hypothesis was fading in popularity.

An American Competence in Pellagra

Physicians throughout the U.S. and especially in the Southeast took notice. Americans quickly surpassed Italians in the number of papers on pellagra catalogued in the *Index Medicus*. Between 1907 (the year Searcy reported epidemic pellagra in the United States) and 1915 (the year Goldberger reported experiments confirming that a good diet prevented pellagra), 409 Americans wrote 746 articles on pellagra. Many of these were isolated case reports, but 118 of these 409 Americans (29 percent) wrote at least two articles and some were prolific.[25] American doctors who made even half-hearted attempts to stay abreast of new knowledge could now identify the salient features of pellagra. Even those who seldom read journals were likely to hear about pellagra one way or another. The more diligent physicians could trace the history of the disease, recite competing hypotheses and discuss treatment and prevention. The collective effort of so many American doctors in so many places focusing on a new disease had no precedent.

Whether Zeists or anti-Zeists, most American doctors recommended a better diet. Dr. James Nevins Hyde of Chicago, for example, wrote in 1910 of "the imperative demand for improved nutrition.[26] Dr. J. G. Wilkinson of New Orleans warned, "By all means nourish your patient."[27] Corn still got the most attention. One physician suggested that pellagra was uncommon among Jews because of "the comparative absence of corn from the Jewish dietary."[28]

Babcock, while praised for sounding the alarm, made little or no effort to consolidate a reputation as a national expert. He turned down most invitations for out-of-state speaking engagements.[29] He did not attempt a

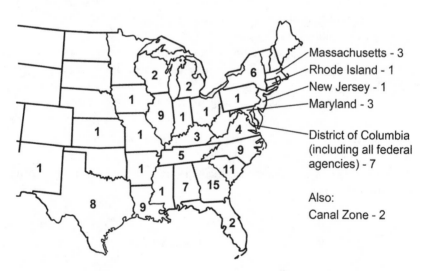

Between 1907 and 1915, 118 Americans—shown here by state (or, for federal employees, the District of Columbia)—wrote two or more articles on pellagra according to the *Index Medicus*.

review article for a major journal such as the *Journal of the American Medical Association*, the *Southern Medical Journal*, the *American Journal of the Medical Sciences*, or the *Boston Medical and Surgical Journal* (forerunner to the *New England Journal of Medicine*). He did not approach a national publisher to bring out a new edition of the locally published but well-reviewed Marie's *Pellagra*. Others were less reluctant. In 1912 Dr. Edward Jenner Wood of Wilmington, North Carolina, and Dr. George M. Niles of Atlanta brought out books on pellagra, and in 1913 Dr. Stewart R. Roberts, also of Atlanta, followed their example.[30] Wood was lavish in his praise for Babcock. Niles thanked Babcock and Lavinder "for both their encouragement and consideration." Roberts, who sketched an outline for his book in the back cover of his copy of Marie's *Pellagra*, barely praised or thanked anybody.[31] None of these monographs added substantively to basic or clinical science. Lavinder complained that Niles's was merely "the first paraphrase of Marie" and that Roberts was backed by "the corn crowd."[32] Babcock, true to form, refrained from criticizing anybody. He no doubt agreed with Wood's confession that "none of us are at best more than amateur pellagrologers."[33]

Babcock never took it as his responsibility to solve pellagra. He helped more-qualified researchers whenever and however he could. His twelve eventual publications on pellagra, while exceeded in number only by those of Joseph Siler, Lavinder, Charles C. Bass of New Orleans, and Herbert P. Cole of Mobile, Alabama,[34] reflect his own spheres of competence. These include the epidemiology of the disease (in collaboration with Lavinder), its history, its psychiatric and psychological manifestations, and its medicolegal implications. When he wasn't managing the asylum he stayed busy seeing patients with known or suspected pellagra (for which he did not charge fees), conducting teaching clinics, discussing pellagra with colleagues, corresponding with authorities, and reading everything he could find about the new red plague.

Historian of the Movement

Physicians of Babcock's era often took into account the observations and ideas of their predecessors. William Osler, for example, advised colleagues: "By the historical method alone can many problems in medicine be approached profitably."[35] Babcock applied the historical method to two problems. Was pellagra a new disease in the United States, and if so, to what extent? What did the early European students write that might be useful? He became the movement's unofficial historian-archivist.[36]

He poured over old case records at his asylum. He told the regents: "Carefully written records by Dr. James Davis, in 1834, undoubtedly prove that he had a case of the disease—the 118th admitted here under his observation, although he considered it purpura or a scorbutic habit." Previous superintendents—Trezevant, Parker, Ensor, and Griffin—had "all left records indicating quite clearly that pellagra has probably been with us since the opening of the institution." However, "even if this be true, it does not explain the great prevalence and increase of the disease."[37] Babcock suggested that he, too, had sometimes missed the diagnosis, and that James Thompson and some of "the old attendants" now felt they had seen the disease in the early 1880s.[38] Babcock sent his historical note to William Osler in Oxford, who wrote back that "Davis's notes are a great credit to him" and that he was now "on the watch" for pellagra in England.[39]

Babcock thus concluded that pellagra had long existed in the United States as a sporadic, seldom-diagnosed disease, but that epidemic pellagra was a new phenomenon.[40] As a sidelight he examined the possibility that pellagra might have explained in part the high mortality at the notorious Andersonville prison during the Civil War, a possibility raised by the former chief surgeon at the prison. Babcock asked Tillman to get him two volumes of the *Official Records of the War of the Rebellion.* "Of course," he wrote the senator, "I shall go at the problem with such discretion as I possess."[41]

He translated, or had translated for him by George Manly, just about everything he could find in the European literature.[42] Of special interest were the observations of Francisco Frapolli, the Italian who popularized the name "pellagra" although he spelled it with a single "l," which had not been previously translated into English.[43]

In 1771 Frapolli, unaware that the Spaniard Don Gaspar Casál and the Frenchman François Thiéry had described the same disease, reported that "the country people" of Lombardy knew a malady they called "pellagra." During the spring, as farmers began to work in the sun, their skin "changes suddenly to red" and "parts of the body exposed to the sun become repulsively disfigured." Victims developed mental and neurologic disturbances and refractory diarrhea. Frappolli asked the right questions. Was it a new disease? Was it contagious? What was the cause? Were the manifestations always the same? How could it be prevented, and how could it be cured?

Frapolli reasoned that pellagra was due to sun exposure and was clearly not contagious. Defining "contagion" as "that power or activity by which any disposition residing in one body excites one similar to itself," Frapolli cited "overwhelming experience that Pellagra, however produced, not only is not communicated at a distance, but likewise never by contact . . . . It ought to be justly and deservedly established that pellagra is free from all contagion."[44] Diet was the treatment of choice. A 30-year-old mother of four named Martha Bonfanti did not benefit from baths, cupping, leeching, or other regimens. Frapolli gave her a more generous diet and wine, whereupon she became happy, "nourished" and with "a healthy color," got out of bed, walked, and, being "better in all respects," went home. A 50-year-old woman named Francesca Cajellina failed to respond to bathing, cupping, or leeches but was "allowed [a] more generous diet and at length she went home well."

Paper after paper in the older literature supported two conclusions: pellagra was not contagious and could be cured, if caught early, by better diet.

In one notebook, for example, Babcock wrote that around the year 1845 a Frenchman observed: "Wherever pellagra is observed, you find a class of persons subsisting, nearly exclusively for a part of the year at least, on Indian corn, either alone or associated with some analogous cereal." Another European wrote: "A change in the diet, the interdicting of maize altogether and the providing of other kinds of food instead of it, has in many cases effected a complete cure where the malady was in its early stage." Babcock generalized from the earlier European writers that the "view held by some of the first observers of pellagra, that the disease spreads by way of <u>contagion</u>, is opposed in the most decided manner by all the later investigators both on positive and on negative grounds."[45] Babcock devoted a section of another notebook to "Of improper & insufficient food."[46]

The observations by Frapolli and other early Europeans—namely, the noncontagious nature of the disease and the curative effect of a more generous diet—were of course the salient features of Joseph Goldberger's 1914 hypothesis and 1915 demonstration. What went wrong? Why were pellagra researchers so seriously sidetracked first by Lombroso's "spoiled corn" or "toxin" hypothesis and then by Sambon's version of the infection hypothesis?

Marzari's 1810 suggestion that pellagra might be due to corn's "deficiency in certain nutritive qualities" was prescient, but it would take nearly 130 years to overcome the devil in the details: the chemical identity of such "nutritive qualities." Meanwhile, conflicting observations abounded.

Why, Frapolli asked, did many paupers who got the very worst food not get pellagra? Why did some people with access to the very best food sometimes get pellagra? In 1910, for example, it was reported to the Board of Regents of the Columbia asylum that one of their own members—J. Perry Glenn of Anderson, South Carolina, who owned and managed a large estate—had died of pellagra.[47] In 1911 an Italian physician named Attilio Caccini who had moved to New York City concluded that pellagra "is

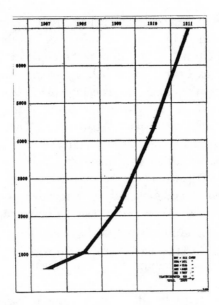

This illustration from Lavinder's 1912 paper, "The Prevalence and Geographic Distribution of Pellagra in the United States," shows the number of new cases in the U.S. (vertical axis; the scale is from zero to 7,000 cases) by year (horizontal axis) between 1907 and 1911.

relatively frequent among the well-to-do class in America, while in Europe it is essentially limited to the poor farming population."[48] Pellagra researchers of that era missed the forest for the trees partly because the forest contained so many "accidentals"—observations that defied any clear-cut pattern or generalization.

Epidemiologist, Clinician, and Teacher

Accurate epidemiologic data on pellagra in the United States before 1915 are unavailable. There was no standardized case definition, no legal requirement for reporting, and no well-coordinated effort to gather data.[49] Before 1912 Lavinder, assisted by Babcock and the South Carolina State Board of Health, was the main data compiler.[50] Lavinder showed that pellagra was spreading exponentially. In 1910 Babcock reported to the regents that there were in the U.S. more than 1,000 cases of pellagra, more than half of which were in the asylums of thirteen states. This indicated "the importance of this disease and justifies the early steps by our Board in seeking more information about this mysterious malady."[51] In 1911 Babcock wrote in a notebook that pellagra was "much more prevalent than ever before in VA, the Carolinas, GA, AL, MS, LA, TX, TN, and Kentucky and probably Fl [Florida]. In fact it may be claimed that in these states there have probably been 10,000 cases of pellagra in the year 1911 . . . and from 15,000 to 20,000 since the year 1906." On a page marked "private" he wrote for Lavinder's benefit: "This method of gathering and publishing estimated statistics will soon put us on the level with the Italian statisticians whose methods we are so prone to decry. I hope you will be able to evolve a method by which you can get accurate figures."[52] In 1912 Lavinder observed that through 1911 there were 25,545 known cases of pellagra in the United States. He estimated at least 30,000 victims with a case-fatality rate over 39 percent. "It may be safely said," Lavinder concluded, "that this matter has reached the dignity of a public-health question of national importance."[53]

Babcock's immediate concern was his own asylum. In May 1910 he told the regents: "Next in importance to tuberculosis as a cause of death among our patients we recognize the newly identified disease."[54] Three months later he told them "that pellagra even more than tuberculosis" explained "the high death rate that has prevailed here many years."[55] In August 1911 he elaborated: "Fifty percent of our mortality was due to pellagra, and the

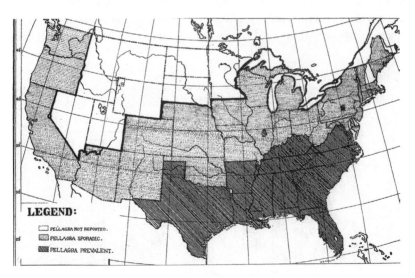

This illustration from Lavinder's 1912 paper on "The Prevalence and Geographic Distribution of Pellagra in the United States" shows the disease to be epidemic (or "highly prevalent," darkly shaded areas) in the Southeast but present ("sporadic," lightly shaded areas) in most other states. Note the "highly prevalent" foci in south central Illinois and eastern Pennsylvania.

applications for the admission of pellagrins continue unabated .... Several
times a week I receive inquiries as to whether pellagra is catching or not.
Upon the whole subject there seems to be a widespread pellagraphobia.
Other asylums notably those of Louisiana and Kentucky have stopped all
corn rations for insane patients .... If you do not wish to stop corn for the
other departments it certainly should be stopped for the Old Building where
the disease is most prevalent."[56] The Board ordered that corn should no
longer be shucked in the fields and left the "matter of corn and corn products
as articles of diet, especially at the Old Building ... to the discretion of Dr.
Babcock and Dr. Taylor."[57] Babcock promptly substituted rice for corn for
all patients. There was no immediate effect.

Pellagra replaced tuberculosis as the leading cause of death at Babcock's asylum. Between 1907 and 1915 there were 1,478 deaths attributed to
pellagra at the South Carolina State Hospital for the Insane, with substantial
racial and gender disparities. Blacks constituted 41 percent of the patient
population but 68 percent of the pellagra deaths. Babcock was apparently the
first to suggest that pellagra hit blacks harder than whites. Others disputed
this conclusion.[58] Females of both races constituted 53 percent of the patient
population but 61 percent of the pellagra deaths. Black females constituted
19 percent of the population but 42 percent of the pellagra deaths between
1907 and 1915. However—and this does not seem to have been previously
appreciated—substitution of rice for corn in late 1911 reduced black females'

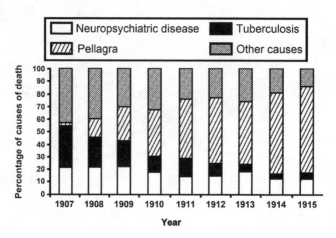

Pellagra, tuberculosis, neuropsychiatric diseases, and other conditions as
percentages of all causes of death, South Carolina State Hospital for the Insane,
1907 through 1915. Pellagra replaced tuberculosis as the leading cause of death.

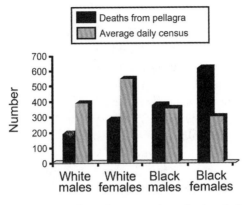

Percentages of deaths due to pellagra by race and gender in relation to the average daily census, South Carolina State Hospital for the Insane, 1908 through 1915, based on the author's tabulations of the original data.

percentage of all pellagra deaths from 53 percent for 1907 through 1911 to 39 percent for 1912 and 1913.[59]

Pellagra in the asylum could not be separated from pellagra in the community. By 1911 pellagrins had joined inebriates and epileptics as a class of patients sent routinely to the State Hospital for the Insane, the "convenient place for inconvenient people." Babcock complained that "this class of patients is being forced upon us whether insane or sane."[60] In 1912 he reported to the regents that "recovered or convalescent pellagrous women" became homesick whereupon their families demanded release. "If we yield to these demands," Babcock noted, "the patients on returning home soon suffer relapses and are then brought back to the institution either to die or to pass through long months of severe illness." There were also "frequent appeals … for the admission of pellagrous patients who are not yet strictly insane, but who are just developing nervous and mental symptoms. These doubtful cases I have tried to refuse, but I should like your opinion and advice on the matter."[61] Pellagra, at first a fascination, became a burden. But if Babcock ever complained about seeing so many pellagrins he left no record of it. He carved out pellagra as his "special disease."

He set Sundays aside for consultations.[62] He saw it as his duty to the doctors and patients of South Carolina. Where else could they turn? A doctor in Sumter, South Carolina, for example, wrote of "a patient who is depressed mentally. Suspect pellagra. If I send her to Columbia for a few days with her nurse, could you see her at the hotel and examine her for me?"[63] A doctor in Florence, South Carolina, wrote of a patient with "a very marked

case . . . . [her] husband is a poor man & [has] no one to assist him in caring
for his wife & requests me to write & ask if she might be sent to you for treatment . . . . This is a case, that . . . should have and deserves consideration at
the hands of the State. Let me hear from you at your earliest convenience."[64]
Pellagra became another strain on Babcock's limited discretionary time and
the asylum's limited resources. He soldiered on, filling at least four notebooks
with clinical observations. He devised a system that took into account the
competing hypotheses. One note, for example, reads in part: "Corn eater—l.
1 m. fr. [lives one mile from] stream—no mosquitoes—few gnats."[65] By thus
documenting how far the patient lived from a stream and whether she had
been exposed to mosquitoes or gnats, Babcock gave Sambon's hypothesis
at least a hearing.

Physicians and hospitals used denial as their defense against the
unwanted disease. In 1910 Babcock told fellow psychiatrists that pellagra
seemed a source of shame and embarrassment: "It is my impression that the
discovery of the existence of pellagra in their institutions is not welcomed
by some asylum officers. Recently while visiting such a hospital in which the
disease had not yet been recognized, I saw and called attention to an unmis-
takable case, but I was not invited to extend my observations."[66] He quoted
an article in the *Baltimore Sun* "that information regarding pellagra has
been suppressed at a number of institutions and that at the Johns Hopkins
Hospital the physicians and nurses have been forbidden to discuss pellagra
cases which they may have."[67] Such overt denials reflected, in part, the
growing belief that pellagra was contagious despite overwhelming evidence

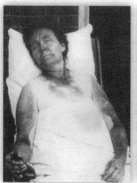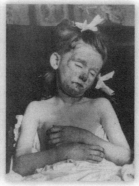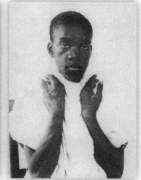

Illustrations of pellagra from Babcock's collection of photographs. The rash of
pellagra involves especially the face, neck (Casál's necklace), upper extremities, and
back surfaces of the hands—or, more generally, sun-exposed areas.
Courtesy: Waring Historical Library, Charleston, S.C.

to the contrary. Many hospitals refused to admit pellagrins. Some doctors blamed public panic on the newspapers.[68]

Babcock subscribed, presumably at his own expense, to a press-clipping service to keep up with what reporters were saying.[69] Pellagra was big news. Thus, "Pellagra is spreading at a rapid rate," "400 have pellagra," "Practically every mountain county in this state has scores of cases," and "Miss Denton victim of pellagra."[70] The *Baltimore Sun* reported that a man "had gone to Alabama several months ago to shuck oysters" only to come home "suffering from a well-developed case of pellagra."[71] Reporters played up hypotheses. "Illinois corn has been tried and acquitted of the charge of causing pellagra," trumpeted the *Rock Island News*. "Says Birds Carry Pellagra," headlined the *New York Times* of a speaker at the American Medical Association meeting who "claimed that germs carried by robins and other migrating birds contain the dread pellagra which is devastating the poor districts of the Southern states." "Corn liquor will cause pellagra," announced the *New Bern Sun* of a rumor in North Carolina, but: "We do not believe this, for if such is the case the population of North Carolina would be greatly on the decrease instead of increase."[72] Babcock wrote that some physicians considered pellagra an expression of leprosy, syphilis, tuberculosis, or other diseases.[73]

He kept up with unorthodox therapies. Dr. Herbert Cole of Mobile, Alabama, wrote fourteen papers between 1909 and 1914 about blood transfusion for treatment of pellagra. A few doctors followed his lead. A physician in Houston made national news by binding together the wrists of a pellagrin and a healthy person. He opened arteries in the two wrists and held them firmly together. When the donor "showed no signs of weakness, their blood was allowed to mix for 30 minutes."[74] A physician in Spartanburg, South Carolina, found a "sure cure" that involved opening the abdomen and exposing the appendix. The appendix was clipped off at the end in such a way as to admit the nozzle of a syringe, through which a germicide was infused into the bowels.[75] Some doctors experimented with drugs marketed for other indications. Many tried Salvarsan, the "wonder drug" introduced in 1910 by the German chemist Paul Ehrlich and his team for the treatment of syphilis.[76]

Fraudulent nostrums abounded. Of an estimated 200 "cures," the best-known story belongs to "Ez-X-Ba" or "Pellagracide," also known as "Dedmond's Remedy." Ezxba Dedmond was a millworker from Belton, South Carolina. He sold his remedy as a liquid or as tablets at $5.00 per bottle. According to the label it was "guaranteed . . . under the National Pure Food and Drug Act, June 30th, 1906." Dedmond claimed he had cured himself and was in partnership with God. He convinced some businessmen to help him manufacture and market the product, first through the Dedmond Remedy Company of Belton, South Carolina, and later through the National Pellagra Remedy Company of Spartanburg. Dedmond's mistake was to ask Babcock to try his remedy at the asylum. Babcock referred it to Lavinder, who sent samples to the Hygienic Laboratory in Washington. The main ingredients were various ferric, aluminum, and magnesium sulfates. "How long," asked the *Journal of the American Medical Association*, "will the United States Government ... actually aid the nostrum manufacturers by permitting the use of 'Guaranteed ... under the National Food and Drug Act' ... for the exploiters of nostrums to deceive the public?" Babcock wrote of Dedmond that "it would appear that his mind is weakened, and that he has become, or is, a religious crank."[77] Babcock nonetheless tried to accommodate physicians with reasonable credentials who wished to try something new. When a Philadelphia physician wanted to study the effect of radium on pellagra, Babcock agreed to do what he could for him.

In May 1910 Babcock addressed fellow psychiatrists at a national meeting on "The Prevalence and Psychology of Pellagra." He told them that, in the South at least, pellagra had become a leading cause of insanity. He catalogued the many ways pellagra could affect the nervous system. Symptoms included "a sense of heat in the head and spinal cord," tingling and darting pains, trembling, and weakness. Depression (melancholy) was the most common psychiatric manifestation, but patients could also be manic-depressive, delirious, catatonic, or in a stupor. They were often frightened and suspicious. For some "a slight insult, the threatening of some trivial danger completely carries them away." Some patients felt "persecuted, or possessed by the devil," while others had "exalted religious notions." Some were suicidal. Dementia in the late stages sometimes resulted in "an almost complete disappearance of mental activity." Although many of the late manifestations resembled "general paralysis of the insane" (an end-result of syphilis) pellagrous insanity differed from general paralysis in that it was usually "of a misty, ill-defined, contradictory character, like that produced by old age, or by anemia." The bottom line was that psychiatrists should consider pellagra in the differential diagnosis of just about everything. Babcock told his colleagues that "in the language of Dr. Zeller, when we understand what pellagra is—'root and all and all in all'—shall we not better understand what insanity is?" Babcock's review was published in the *American Journal of Insanity*.[78] He remained fascinated the rest of his life on the finer points of pellagra's effects on the nervous system. He believed, for example, that one should distinguish between "insane pellagrins" and "the pellagrous insane."[79]

Lavinder and Siler Stake Out Positions

Of the Americans who wrote about pellagra for medical journals between 1907 and 1915, by far the most prolific were Lavinder of the U.S. Public Health and Marine Hospital Service and Joseph Siler of the U.S. Army (twenty-four and twenty-one articles, respectively). Their opposite approaches largely defined American views on pellagra before 1914, when Goldberger joined the battle. Lavinder became a frustrated agnostic. He did not think corn held the answer, but neither did he think pellagra was an infectious disease. Siler felt the tug of Sambon's version of the infection hypothesis. Sambon's influence on Siler, it will be argued here, seriously harmed the American pellagra effort.

Joseph Siler was three classes behind Lavinder at the University of Virginia School of Medicine. There is no evidence they became close friends, but neither is there the slightest hint of animosity. Still, interagency rivalry

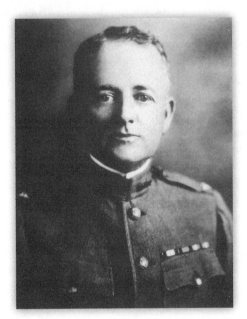

Dr. Joseph Franklin Siler (1875–1960) of the U.S. Army belonged to both major commissions that investigated pellagra in the United States during the pre-Goldberger era (that is, before 1914).
Courtesy: National Library of Medicine.

to "get there first" was inevitable. Lavinder, after visiting the Peoria State Hospital in Illinois in September 1909, wrote his superior: "I thought it might interest you to know that Dr. Siler of the Army went to the Asylum at Peoria shortly after my departure and is still there."[80]

The Army had the stronger track record in medical research. Army doctors took pride in William Beaumont, who changed for all time the way we think about digestion, and in Walter Reed, whose commission proved that mosquitoes transmit yellow fever. Beaumont and Reed remain visible if only because of the big Army medical centers that bear their names. The Public Health and Marine Hospital Service with its smaller medical corps had a less conspicuous but still substantial heritage. Joseph Kinyoun, working in a one-room laboratory at the Staten Island, New York, Marine Hospital, found a way to stain the tubercle bacillus. Henry Rose Carter, investigating yellow fever outbreaks in two small towns in southern Mississippi, described an "extrinsic incubation period" that helped pave the way for the Reed Commission.[81] Now these agencies pinned their hopes on Lavinder and Siler. As events unfolded, an expedition to Italy led by Louis Sambon in the spring of 1910, and in which both Siler and Lavinder participated, had momentous consequences.

Having speculated in 1905 that pellagra was transmitted by a fly of the genus *Simulium*, Sambon needed more data.[82] Supported by Sir Patrick Manson, he influenced the British Medical Association to convene a Pellagra Investigation Committee. The blue-ribbon committee was chaired by Sir Thomas Lauder Brunton, London's most eminent doctor, and its thirty-nine members included the editors of the *Lancet* and the *British Medical Journal*, the regius professors of medicine at Oxford and Cambridge (Sir William Osler and Sir Thomas Clifford Allbutt), Sir William Leishman, Sir Ronald Ross, Manson, Fleming Sandwith, and the Italian ambassador. Committee members heard that pellagra was spreading in the British Empire and therefore had to be solved. They agreed to raise 1,000 pounds to send Sambon back to Italy.[83]

On March 20, 1910, although only about one-fifth of the funds had been raised, Sambon left for Italy to get more data for his hypothesis that pellagra concentrated along fast-flowing streams teeming with *Simulium* flies and their larvae. He had invited Siler to join him. Fortuitously, Lavinder was also in Italy, sent by Surgeon General Walter Wyman with Babcock's support. Sambon invited Lavinder to join his party. Sambon already knew that most Italian physicians did not think pellagra was an infectious disease. He did not want to hear their opinions. He concluded that corn had nothing to do with pellagra, and that, sure enough, pellagra tended to occur during the spring and autumn in those who lived near fast-flowing streams.[84] Siler, being a specially invited guest, stayed with Sambon's entourage to the end.

Lavinder left Sambon's party. Although he enjoyed his time with the group he had been skeptical from the beginning. Six months earlier he told a reporter that "those physicians who have announced that they have discovered the specific germ of pellagra must be mistaken."[85] He now considered Sambon's obsession "hypothetical, and lacking scientific demonstration."[86] He wanted to hear what the Italians thought. In Bologna he visited Professor Guido Tizzoni but was unimpressed by Tizzoni's claims for an infectious agent he'd named *Streptobacillus pellagrae*. In Rome he listened to Professor Angelo Celli's opinion that "any etiologic relation between corn and pellagra" could "no longer be entertained." Professor Bartolomeo Gosio told him that "the subject of pellagra . . . [is] . . . so full of perplexities and difficulties that one might find apparent facts in almost any theory."[87]

Lavinder also went to several *pellagrosari*, the hospitals devoted exclusively to pellagrins. The diets, while simple, were abundant, varied, and corn-free. Northern Italy's poor took notice. Whereas previously "many pellagrins concealed themselves with shame," some now feigned symptoms in order to benefit from the free and varied food dispensed in the special hospitals for pellagra.

Lavinder returned from the two-month trip believing he'd learned nothing new except that the Italians were turning away from the spoiled-corn hypothesis since it didn't account for all the facts. Like Babcock he preferred not to side with one or another hypothesis and, in a paper prepared for *Public Health Reports*, wrote: "The judicial mental attitude which American investigators have so far shown with regard to the etiology of pellagra is certainly to be commended in the present unsatisfactory status of this question."[88] But he'd also confirmed—if indeed it needed further confirmation—that "diet is considered a matter of great importance in the treatment of the disease."[89]

Sambon returned to London a conquering hero. The British journal *Nature* called the three-month expedition "eminently successful."[90] "GNAT CAUSES PELLAGRA," announced the *New York Times*, citing Sambon's telegraphs from Rome that the British investigators had "definitely proved that maize or Indian corn is not the cause of pellagra," and that "the parasitic conveyer of the disease is the 'simulium repans', a species of biting gnat."[91] The *Journal of the American Medical Association* was more cautious, calling Sambon's evidence "strong, but more will be required to satisfy the profession that this covers the whole case."[92] Other Americans were more enthusiastic. Dr. Stewart Roberts of Atlanta reported that "the same conditions exist in Georgia to produce the disease that exist in Italy."[93] And Sambon reported soon after his return to London that "Captain Siler writes me that in the United States Simulium is being found wherever there is pellagra."[94] Siler had, unwittingly, been recruited to Louis Sambon's quest for personal glory.

Babcock encouraged both Siler and Lavinder, as he did anyone with a credible idea. He encouraged Tillman to support funding for pellagra research. He also asked Tillman to support pay increases for the medical officers of the Public Health and Marine Hospital Service, adding that if there were any questions Tillman could "call on my friend Lavinder."[95]

Joseph Siler and the Two Commissions

Of the various American groups and commissions that sprang up to examine pellagra, two were reasonably well funded and produced comprehensive reports. These were the Illinois Pellagra Commission and the Thompson-McFadden Pellagra Commission. Drs. Joseph Siler and Ward MacNeal belonged to both.

The Illinois Pellagra Commission convened in November 1909 and dissolved in November 1911 after issuing a 250-page report. The Thompson-McFadden Commission convened in 1912 and remained active through 1917, issuing three reports amounting to 771 pages with 20 maps, 88 photographs, 205 figures, and 312 tables. The reports of both of these commissions demonstrate diligence and competence by the standards of that era. Still, one senses the invisible guiding hand of Louis Sambon in the researchers' improbable conclusions, unsupported by solid data, that pellagra was in all likelihood an infectious disease.

THE ILLINOIS PELLAGRA COMMISSION

The Illinois State Board of Health took up pellagra after Lavinder confirmed the disease in Cook County and George Zeller showed its high prevalence at the Peoria asylum. Its members gleaned some evidence for "deficient animal protein in the diet" as a predisposing factor, but concluded that pellagra was probably "due to infection of the body with some micro-organism."[96]

The commission suffered a setback in May 1910 when Howard Taylor Ricketts died of typhus while studying that disease in Mexico. Ricketts had been one of that era's most accomplished infectious diseases researchers. He had proved tick transmission of Rocky Mountain spotted fever and had isolated the causative organism, later named *Rickettsia rickettsiae* in his honor. The commissioners "had counted greatly upon his knowledge and investigative skill."[97] However, the commission still had infectious diseases talent: Siler and Henry J. Nichols, both on loan from the U.S. Army, and Ward MacNeal, then at the University of Illinois.

Dr. H. Douglas Singer, a young psychiatrist from Chicago,[98] wrote the final report's introductory chapters. He leaned heavily on Sambon's hypothesis while, perhaps unknowingly, citing two observations against it. First, "none of the employés suffered from the disease in spite of the fact that they were exposed fully as much to the bites of insects and drew their food and water supply from exactly the same source as the patients." Second, pellagra in Illinois concentrated in the two largest cities, Chicago and Peoria, neither situated on the banks of a fast-flowing stream teeming with *Simulium* flies and their larvae.

The Illinois researchers tried to prove the case for infection. They inoculated forty rhesus monkeys, two guinea pigs, and a kitten with blood, spinal fluid, spleen emulsions, and other materials from pellagrins. Nothing much happened and the results had to be "regarded as entirely negative."[99] They painstakingly analyzed the intestinal bacterial flora of persons with and without pellagra. This, too, led nowhere.[100] They confirmed Siler's observation that stools of pellagrins often had increased numbers of amebic parasites, but "the majority" of the amebae were nonpathogenic.[101] Subcutaneous injections of corn extracts to patients with pellagra gave little or no evidence of hypersensitivity.[102] The state entomologist reported that Illinois contained at least nine of the sixty-five known species of *Simulium*, and that these insects frequently inflicted "a bite much more severe than that of a mosquito," yet could not be more definite.[103]

They did not overlook the possibility of dietary deficiency. Dr. Rachel Watkins, a staff physician at Peoria State Hospital, supervised a feeding experiment at two cottages. All of the patients were initially free of pellagra. Patients at one cottage were given "a generous corn diet," with about 16 ounces of corn per day. Patients at the other cottage were given a corn-free diet in which corn was replaced by rice, rice pudding, or tapioca pudding. The diets were otherwise kept the same. At the end of one year there was no difference between the groups. Five of fifty-nine patients on the corn-containing diet and ten of fifty-eight patients on the corn-free diet acquired definite or suspected pellagra. In retrospect, all of the patients received beef on a daily basis, either as boiled beef (five days per week) or as beef and gravy (two days per week). The authors concluded that the diet should contain adequate protein and should "at all times possess variety," yet could not be more specific, recognizing that their data might be inadequate to rule out a dietary cause of pellagra.[104]

The Illinois Pellagra Commission ultimately concluded that deficient diet *contributed* to pellagra but did not *cause* it. Poor nutrition was "an important factor in predisposing to the disease," since "a diet deficient in animal protein may so alter the body that the infecting organism has a better chance to grow."[105] This conclusion—*monotonous diet predisposes to pellagra but is not the actual cause*—reverberates in the previous and subsequent pellagra literature. The commissioners thus resigned themselves to an unknown infectious agent as the best explanation.

THE THOMPSON-MCFADDEN
PELLAGRA COMMISSION

The most elaborate American effort to solve pellagra during the pre-Goldberger era became known as the "Thompson-McFadden Commission of the New York Post-Graduate Medical School," or "Thompson-McFadden Commission." This commission although well intentioned ultimately proved extremely counterproductive. The last article in the final report, published in 1917 (two years after Goldberger's breakthrough and without mentioning Goldberger), concludes: "Pellagra is probably communicable, but how the communicated 'germ of the disease' shall progress in the body depends, in part, upon constitutional factors."[106]

Evidence strongly suggests the Thompson-McFadden Commission resulted from the following sequence of events.

During late 1910 or early 1911, when Joseph Siler and Ward MacNeal both worked with the Illinois Pellagra Commission, Siler almost surely told MacNeal about his trip to Italy and Sambon's thesis that an insect, probably a *Simulium* fly, transmitted a pellagra-causing infectious agent, probably a trypanosome parasite. This excited MacNeal. At the University of Michigan MacNeal had worked extensively on trypanosomes with the eminent microbiologist Frederick Novy, with whom he had written a monograph "On the Trypanosomes of Birds."[107] In 1911 MacNeal moved from the University of Illinois to the New York Post-Graduate Medical School and Hospital. He invited Siler to lecture on tropical diseases and made sure his new boss, Dr. George N. Miller, attended. Miller had connections. He got two philanthropists, Colonel Robert Means Thompson of New York and John Howard McFadden of Philadelphia, to donate the then-large sum of $15,000 for a systematic research program.[108]

The commission's headquarters were in New York, with MacNeal as coordinator. MacNeal asked the Army, the Navy, and the Public Health and Marine Hospital Service to loan physician-researchers. The Army loaned Siler and the Navy loaned Philip E. Garrison. The surgeon general of the Public Health and Marine Hospital Service turned him down, being too short-staffed himself.[109] Siler, Garrison, and MacNeal coauthored the commission's major publications. Siler headed up the field studies, assisted by Garrison. MacNeal stayed in New York and analyzed the data, using methods developed by the English mathematician Karl Pearson and the American biologist Charles Benedict Davenport.

When plans were being drawn up for the Thompson-McFadden Commission, Babcock sought the regents' permission to go to New York to lobby for bringing a proposed "pellagra hospital" to Columbia. Subsequent consultations in which Babcock participated led to the conclusion that Spartanburg would be a better choice, since pellagra in South Carolina concentrated in the state's northwestern Piedmont region, with its thriving textile industry.[110] In June 1912 the commission set up headquarters in Spartanburg County, where much of the subsequent research on pellagra would take place.

The researchers chose to study pellagra mainly by descriptive epidemiology. They would try to resolve *what* caused pellagra, and *how* and *why* people got pellagra, by painstaking analysis of *who* got pellagra, and *when* and *where* the cases occurred. Siler and Garrison, under MacNeal's supervision, thus marched in the footsteps of the English physician John Snow, who in 1854 pinpointed a London cholera epidemic to contaminated water at the Broad Street pump—a classic precedent for labor-intensive "shoe-leather" epidemiology.[111] Unfortunately, as it turned out, this was not the best approach. To assess the role of diet, they relied on dietary histories, asking people what they ate. We now realize that dietary histories are fraught with potential pitfalls.[112] To crack the riddle, Goldberger would later use the experimental method rather than descriptive epidemiology.

Having decided that "an intensive study of the disease as it occurred among the population of a limited area" would be more useful than "a more superficial investigation over an extended area," Siler and Garrison analyzed the habits and circumstances of 282 pellagrins in Spartanburg County between June 1, and October 15, 1912.[113] They, like the Illinois Pellagra Commission, concluded that diet was not the main problem. They wrote that while "the most striking defect in the general dietary of the working classes … appears to be the limited use of fresh meats … the thesis that deficiency in the quality and quantity of food can be regarded as the essential cause of pellagra seems not to be supported by our studies." On the other hand, they found little evidence for Sambon's *Simulium* flies. But instead of looking for a different disease paradigm, they turned to other insects, notably the stable fly.[114]

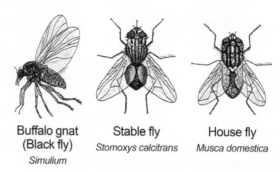

Buffalo gnat   Stable fly   House fly
(Black fly)   Stomoxys calcitrans   Musca domestica
Simulium

When American researchers influenced by Louis Sambon concluded that flies of the genus *Simulium* (such as the sand fly, buffalo gnat, and black fly) were unlikely to explain pellagra, at least in the United States, they turned to other insects such as the stable fly and house fly.
Courtesy: Florida Center for Instructional Technology, College of Education, University of South Florida.

The Thompson-McFadden Commission's reports offer vivid photographic documentation of living conditions in early-twentieth century mill villages in the South Carolina upstate. The first report contains seven photographs of houses, six of wells, and six of privies. Using the Rockefeller Sanitary Commission's classification of privy types and sanitary indices, the researchers determined that 63 percent of the privies were of the "ordinary open-in-back surface" type and that 72 percent of the privies had a sanitary index of 25 percent or less. Such poor sanitary conditions promoted "the contamination of food with the excretions of pellagrins"[115] and swarms of stable flies.

It would take enormous effort by Goldberger, his colleagues, and other researchers to show the world that the privies and stable flies were merely surrogate markers of poverty. Poverty might condemn a family to an "ordinary open-in-back surface type privy" with swarming stable flies, but it also condemned that family to a monotonous, niacin-deficient diet.

Claude Lavinder and the U.S. Public Health Service

Most accounts of pellagra in the United States pay relatively little attention to the contributions of the U.S. Public Health Service between 1907 and 1914 except for Lavinder's epidemiologic studies. However, Public Health Service researchers produced additional data against the infection hypothesis. These data helped Goldberger conclude that infection was not the cause.

The June 30, 1911, issue of *Public Health Reports* begins with an article that seems to have been neglected by most historians of pellagra. John F. Anderson, director of the Hygienic Laboratory in Washington (precursor to the National Institutes of Health), and a slightly younger assistant named Joseph Goldberger reported their inability to transmit pellagra to rhesus monkeys.[116] Historians and also Goldberger's bibliographer seem to have overlooked his role in this study, possibly because the editors of the *Index Medicus* inadvertently listed Anderson as the paper's sole author.[117]

Anderson and Goldberger had previously used rhesus monkeys to study typhus, Rocky Mountain spotted fever, and measles. They had shown that typhus and Rocky Mountain spotted fever were separate diseases despite some common features. They had shown that a condition known as Brill's disease is merely another manifestation of typhus. Now they used their

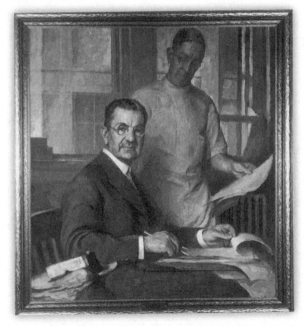

In 1911 John F. Anderson (1873–1958) (seated), the third director of the Hygienic Laboratory in Washington, D.C. (now the National Institutes of Health), reported with Joseph Goldberger an unsuccessful attempt to transmit pellagra from humans to rhesus monkeys. (The assistant behind Anderson is not Goldberger.)

Courtesy: National Library of Medicine.

animal facility to investigate pellagra. Unaware of previous attempts to infect higher animals such as monkeys "with the blood or tissues from pellagrins," they drew blood from two cases of well-marked pellagra and spinal fluid from one of them and injected the material into five rhesus monkeys. One monkey developed "bronzing of the face and a pinkish tint of the neck and upper chest" but otherwise nothing much happened.

Anderson and Goldberger were conservative in their conclusions. It was possible that rhesus monkeys were not susceptible to pellagra. It was possible that "the infective agent was not present in the blood nor in the spinal fluid" when the patients were sampled. Therefore: "A final conclusion . . . is not justified." This article matters to the historian not so much because of the methods, data, and conclusions but rather because it implies that Goldberger surely discussed with Anderson the competing hypotheses on pellagra. Hence, statements to the effect that Goldberger had no experience with pellagra before February 1914—that he went south behind a "veil of ignorance"—are incorrect.

The June 30, 1911, issue of *Public Health Reports* also contains an article by Lavinder entitled "A Note on the Inoculation of the Rhesus Monkey with Blood, Spinal Fluid, and Nervous Tissue from Pellagrins."[118] Lavinder's article was published back to back with the paper by Anderson and Goldberger. On October 20, 1910, Anderson proposed that Lavinder go to Columbia, take some monkeys with him, and inoculate the monkeys with blood and spinal fluid from cases of pellagra in the *acute* stage of the disease.[119] Anderson knew that if the cause was an infectious agent, such an agent might be present in blood, body fluids, or tissues during the *acute* stage but not in the advanced or "well-marked" stage. It is unclear where Lavinder's study was carried out, but the paper hints that Lavinder may have taken monkeys in their "small wire cages" to Columbia since he thanked "Dr. J. W. Babcock for permission to make use of material and for generous assistance, and . . . Dr. E. B. Saunders also for valuable assistance." He may then have taken them back to Washington, as the monkeys were "kept under observation for about six months" and there were no animal facilities in Columbia. Lavinder inoculated nine monkeys with various combinations of blood, spinal fluid, and portions of spinal cord (obtained at autopsy) from patients with pellagra. None of the monkeys showed "any change of note."

These experiments—his own with Goldberger and Lavinder's separate studies—did not fully answer Anderson's question whether pellagra might be an infectious disease. Although the patients from whom blood and spinal fluid were obtained displayed "the acute phenomena of the disease, including marked erythemas of both the 'wet' and 'dry' forms," all of them "were alienated and had probably suffered from the disease for some months or longer." Thus, none were in the "incubation" stage—that is, after the introduction of an infectious agent but before the appearance of diagnostic features— which as everyone knew might be the only time that blood, body fluids, or tissues contained infectious material, as had recently been shown to be the case with yellow fever.[120]

Anderson assembled a committee and outlined a plan.[121] He told the surgeon general that "some decided changes are necessary." There should be a Pellagra Commission, chaired by Lavinder. Work should proceed along three lines: gathering of statistics, epidemiologic studies, and clinical studies on patients with the disease, with "the relegation of corn purely to a secondary place." Field studies could help determine whether the disease was infectious, but there should also be a research laboratory. The Hygienic Laboratory in Washington had good facilities by the standards of that time, but patients would be hard to come by. "On the other hand," Anderson noted, "if it is attempted to take a laboratory to Columbia, S.C., or other place, where material exists for the work . . . little of worth can be accomplished" without an adequate and fully-staffed laboratory. Even if adequately equipped, such a laboratory would "have to be established with some other institution, and this institution would not be under our control." Another drawback to sending Lavinder to Columbia was that the patients would be mainly asylum inmates, "a class of cases which are probably not the most desirable for research use."

The committee decided to make use of existing marine hospitals. Patients otherwise not eligible for treatment in a marine hospital could be admitted "wholly for scientific and research purposes."[122] Congress passed the necessary legislation and the Marine Hospital in Savannah, Georgia, was selected.

There were no patients with pellagra at the Savannah Marine Hospital when Lavinder arrived in June 1911, and it would take nearly a year before fourteen patients were recruited by advertising in newspapers and medical journals.[123] Lavinder became bogged down in administration and patient care. Anderson assigned Dr. Randolph M. Grimm, a recent Johns Hopkins medical graduate, to assist Lavinder. Grimm, on Lavinder's recommendation, went to Columbia to learn pellagra from Babcock.[124] Lavinder and Grimm then agreed to divide up the work. Lavinder would stay in Savannah, do animal experiments, and coordinate field surveillance. Grimm would go out into the towns and cities where pellagra occurred in the Southeast.

Grimm began his studies in Spartanburg, Chester, and York counties in South Carolina. "The local physicians," he reported, "have everywhere received me with kindness and have been of greater assistance to me in seeing cases of pellagra."[125] He recorded on index cards details from 380 cases, more than half of them from Spartanburg and its vicinity. Some of the data supported Sambon's hypothesis: "Running streams are abundant in these counties . . . . None of the pellagrous homes that I visited were located more than a half mile from a stream, and in the majority of cases there was a stream 200 or 300 yards from the house." Other data supported the dietary-deficiency hypothesis. Textile workers and their families relied heavily on refined corn stripped of its germ: "Each of the 83 pellagrins whom I saw gave a history of having used corn products more or less regularly as an article of diet . . . . On account of passing of the old gristmill, to which the farmer took his corn and had it ground, the meal now used is chiefly that which has been ground at some of the large mills of the country and shipped out in large quantities. This kind of meal has been used by all of the 83 pellagrins excepting one. The exception was a farmer's wife, who stated positively that for years she had used only corn raised on her husband's farm. Her husband, however, kept a little "crossroads" store . . . . [and therefore it was] needless to say that the store was drawn upon to furnish the family larder." Grimm's field studies thus complemented to some extent the work in Spartanburg by the Thompson-McFadden Commission.[126] However, unlike certain members of the Thompson-McFadden Commission, neither Grimm nor Lavinder was willing to concede that pellagra was in all likelihood an infectious disease.

On November 2, 1911, the fourth annual one-day conference and clinic on pellagra took place at the State Hospital for the Insane in Columbia. (These conferences were in addition to the triennial meetings of the National Association for the Study of Pellagra.) There were about 150 attendees.[127] Rather than preside himself, Babcock turned the meeting over to James Adams Hayne, South Carolina's newly elected state health officer.[128] Babcock's deference to Adams Hayne created problems in the long run, for, after Goldberger became involved in 1914, the bombastic and highly opinionated state health officer did much to destroy the goodwill that had previously characterized the American effort against pellagra.

Another newcomer at the November 1911 conference was Philip E. Garrison, the Navy physician assigned to the Thompson-McFadden Commission. Garrison spoke on *Simulium* flies. After the conference he told his superiors that some attendees liked the spoiled-corn hypothesis and a few liked Sambon's ideas, but that the "prevailing attitude" was "of suspended judgment regarding the cause of pellagra and at the same time the determination to attack the disease along all possible lines until a satisfactory demonstration of its causation makes plain the true prophylaxis." What impressed Garrison most were the attendees' earnestness, thoroughness, and sense of urgency. He also wrote: "The treatment of pellagra does not appear to be so fruitless a task as it was considered a year ago. This applies particularly to cases recognized early—and much stress is laid upon early diagnosis. In the absence of specific drug treatment, undoubtedly the two most important measures are rest and a full nutritious diet."[129]

Meanwhile, Lavinder in Savannah became increasingly discouraged. He was bogged down in administration and patient care, leaving little time for research.[130] He asked for a third man but was turned down.[131] In January 1912 he told the surgeon general that his hospital service always included about thirty-five to forty acutely-ill patients, that it was difficult to do his job and work on pellagra at the same time, and that it was "almost useless for me to say that pellagra is a very large subject, much larger indeed than is fully appreciated."[132] In April he wrote John W. Kerr in Washington that "I have never worked harder in my life, and yet I do not seem to get anywhere very much. It is discouraging at times."[133] To Babcock he was even more vivid: "I think I dream pellagra these days, but no inspiration comes to help me get a clue. The whole thing gets worse and worse to me. I can see no light anywhere." He described his going back and forth between and among hypotheses as "mental gymnastics with a vengeance."[134]

Lavinder was nevertheless on the right track. In August 1911 the *Savannah Morning News* reported that "Dr. Lavinder quite agrees with the general idea that the disease is not contagious or infectious, and that the discovery of its origin will show it to be caused by some such agencies as have been claimed in theories already announced."[135] Within a year such an "already announced" theory would resurface in the form of Casimir Funk's refinement of Marzari's 1810 suggestion that pellagra might be caused by deficiency of an unknown dietary constituent.

CHAPTER 6

So Near, So Far

Funk Was Right but Few Listened

IN 1912 CASIMIR FUNK, a 28-year-old Polish-born chemist working in London, proposed the vitamin-deficiency hypothesis for pellagra. Among those who took him seriously were Surgeon General Rupert Blue of the U.S. Public Health Service, and Fleming Sandwith of London. On the evening of October 3, 1912, at Babcock's invitation, Blue and Sandwith separately brought up Funk's hypothesis at the second triennial meeting of the National Association for the Study of Pellagra held at the South Carolina asylum. Babcock and Carl Alsberg of the U.S. Department of Agriculture commented on its reasonableness. However, Claude Lavinder and Joseph Siler, their respective agencies' point men for pellagra, missed or dismissed the significance of Funk's hypothesis. Louis Sambon's version of the infection hypothesis appealed to many but not most participants at the 1912 meeting. Nicotinic acid and also tryptophan were well known in 1912, but it would be another quarter of a century before researchers established that niacin deficiency causes pellagra. Thousands died before Funk's ideas and observations were put to practical use.

Casimir Funk and the "Vitamine" Hypothesis

No discrete historical event explains "the discovery of the vitamins." Each of the now clinically important vitamins—vitamin A, the B vitamin complex, and vitamins C, D, E, and K—has its unique history.[1] The idea of vitamins as substances that must be present in the diet because the body cannot make them in sufficient quantities began to take shape during the late nineteenth century when researchers experimented with measured quantities of proteins, sugars, and fats. They found that something else was necessary for health;

hence, the idea of "accessory food factors."[2] Precise chemical identification of the vitamins was a twentieth-century development.

It began with beriberi, known mainly for its effects on the nervous system.[3] Asian physicians had long suspected monotonous diet. During the late nineteenth century the germ theory prompted enthusiasm for an infectious cause of beriberi. Among the researchers was a young Dutch military physician named Christiaan Eijkman, who attempted to cause beriberi in rabbits by injecting them with a recently discovered bacterium. He decided to try chickens since they were cheaper to buy and keep. In 1890 the chickens in one batch staggered, couldn't perch, lost weight, and died. Autopsies showed degenerative changes in the nerves of the legs similar to those of human beriberi.

Eijkman suspected bacterial or toxin contamination of his chickens. By chance he learned that the chickens' keeper had been skimping on their feed to save money. He had given them leftover cooked rice instead of feed-grade unpolished rice. Eijkman's scientific impulse led him to prove that the substitution of polished for unpolished rice caused "fowl polyneuritis." Caught up in the germ theory, he concluded that beriberi was "linked" to the substitution of polished for unpolished rice but not necessarily "caused" by it.[4] He missed the full significance of his discovery: an animal model for beriberi.

Japanese physicians and two Americans—Drs. Edward B. Vedder and Robert R. Williams—used every means at their disposal to identify the key substance(s) in "extract of rice polishing." In 1912 Vedder and Williams returned to the United States only to learn that Casimir Funk had beaten them to the punch.[5]

Casimir Funk was born in Warsaw, the son of a dermatologist. At age 16 his father sent him to college in Geneva to study biology. He transferred to Berne, got a doctorate in chemistry at age 20, worked for a while at the Pasteur Institute in Paris, and in 1906 moved to Berlin with a letter of introduction to the Nobel laureate Emil Fischer.[6] In 1910 the young chemist's wanderlust took him to London and a job at the Lister Institute of Preventative Medicine. One day a middle-aged man showed up in the laboratory and suggested that he and the ill-at-ease newcomer stroll along the Thames Embankment. The man, who did not introduce himself at first, was the institute's director, Dr. (later Sir) Charles James Martin. Martin made Funk a Scholar of the Lister Institute and told him of some work being done on beriberi in the British colonies. Martin suspected beriberi might be caused by deficiency of an amino acid contained in rice polishings.

In 1911 Funk published "On the Chemical Nature of the Substance Which Cures Polyneuritis in Birds Induced by a Diet of Polished Rice."

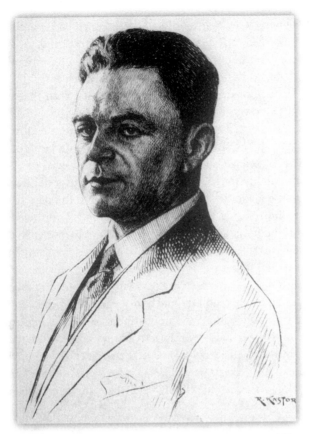

In 1912 Dr. Casimir Funk (1884–1967), born Kazimierz Funk in Warsaw, proposed the "vitamine hypothesis." He suggested that beriberi, scurvy, rickets, and pellagra were all caused by specific deficiencies.
Courtesy: Photo Researchers/ScienceSource.

Other technical papers followed. Funk was invited to write a review article, for which he did not need his supervisor's approval. He proposed that beriberi, scurvy, rickets, and pellagra were all deficiency disorders. He called the missing substances "vitamines"—*vita* for "life" and *amine* for a type of nitrogen-containing substance derived from ammonia. As it turned out, the term "vitamine" (later shortened to "vitamin") was not technically accurate, since not all vitamins are amines, but the name stuck despite opposition. The paper, published in the *Journal of State Medicine*, is now considered a classic. Funk's proposal became "the vitamin hypothesis."[7]

Funk explained in his paper that "deficiency diseases break out in countries where a certain unvarying diet is partaken of for long periods. When this food happens to be deficient in a substance which is necessary for the metabolism, we have the real conditions for the outbreak of this type of disease." Beriberi and scurvy had already been shown to respond to adding something back to the diet, even though the "something" had not been identified: "It is now known that all these diseases, with the exception of pellagra, can be prevented and cured by the addition of certain preventive substances; the deficiency substances, which are of the nature of organic bases, we will call "vitamines"; and we will speak of a beri-beri or scurvy vitamine, which means a substance preventing the special disease." He did not claim originality for suggesting that pellagra was a deficiency disease: "The idea that pellagra is due to some deficiency in the diet was expressed by several authors, but at the present time there is no positive evidence in favour of this theory, as against any other theory. A glance at all the existing theories suggests that an investigation of this disease on the lines mentioned above for beri-beri might yield valuable results. Up to now the only evidence in favour of this view is its close analogy with beri-beri, and especially with scurvy. Research on this subject, which in the past has been very one-sided, is rendered more difficult by the impossibility of producing experimental pellagra in animals, and also by the lack of knowledge on the prevention of this disease by means of a change in diet." Funk perceived correctly that "the present state of the pellagra investigation is the same as that of beri-beri ten years ago." Pellagra researchers badly needed an animal model analogous to Eijkman's chickens.

The 1912 Triennial Conference—
Sandwith Comes Close

While Funk tried to publicize his vitamin-deficiency hypothesis, Babcock prepared for the upcoming conference of the National Association for the Study of Pellagra, of which he was outgoing president. The venue would again be his underfunded asylum. He wanted to do all he could to make the meeting a success. In May 1912 he asked Tillman to get support from the surgeon generals of the Public Health and Marine Hospital Service, the Army, and the Navy, and also from the Secretary of Agriculture. "All of these Departments," Babcock told Tillman, "now have specialists engaged in the study of Pellagra and we wish to enlist their cooperation very early as to contribute to making our meeting a success."[8] Babcock encouraged pellagra researchers in other countries to submit papers, which could be read if they were unable to attend. These included Sandwith and Sambon in London, Victor Babes in Rumania, Giuseppe Antonini and Eugenio Bravetta in Milan, Bartolomeo Gosio in Rome, and Jean Nicolaidi in Paris, to name a few. He asked the regents' permission to go to Washington to drum up interest.[9] He encouraged the regents to attend, and also the state's probate judges since they kept sending people with pellagra to Columbia.[10]

Babcock's efforts to beef up the meeting's scientific content were hugely successful. Only 19 percent of the papers were from South Carolina, compared with nearly 39 percent at the 1909 conference.[11] Many of the papers came from abroad, including eight from Italy. The meeting's eventual product was a 409-page book summarizing essential knowledge on pellagra.

Less successful were his efforts to promote attendance. There were only 152 registrants (versus 394 at the 1909 meeting), and a majority (63 percent) were from South Carolina. Pellagra was no longer a novelty. The press was less interested. Hosting a major conference on pellagra no longer engendered civic pride; rather, it was a bit embarrassing. The conference organizers and presenters were to some extent preaching to the choir.

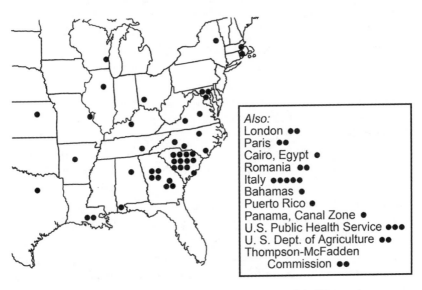

Also:
London ●●
Paris ●●
Cairo, Egypt ●
Romania ●●
Italy ●●●●●
Bahamas ●
Puerto Rico ●
Panama, Canal Zone ●
U.S. Public Health Service ●●●
U. S. Dept. of Agriculture ●●
Thompson-McFadden Commission ●●

The papers presented at the second triennial conference of the National Association for the Study of Pellagra, held October 3–4, 1912, at the South Carolina State Hospital for the Insane, reflected greater geographic diversity than those at the 1909 meeting (see page 106). (Each dot represents the hometown of one speaker.)

Less than a third of the papers at the two-day conference, held October 3 and 4, 1912, in the asylum's assembly hall, dealt mainly with causation. Most papers were descriptive of one or another aspect: epidemiology, clinical and laboratory observations, or response to different treatments. The latter included an update on blood transfusion by Herbert Cole of Mobile, whose series now included thirty-four cases without "ill effect"; two trials of the new chemotherapeutic drug Salvarsan; and use of an "organo-mineralized radio-activated serum" concocted by Dr. Jean Nicolaidi of Paris.[12] As to possible causes, as Etheridge summarizes, "the emphasis shifted to the germ theory" or "strongly toward the anti-Zeists."[13] Yet the conference was by no means a coronation of the germ theory or, more specifically, of Louis Sambon's version of it.

Lombroso's spoiled-corn hypothesis was down but not yet out. Gosio and Antonini reported from Italy that while "weak points in the doctrine of Lombroso have been noted all along" there were still reasons to support it. A plant pathologist from the Virginia Agricultural Station claimed he'd found a fungus-produced toxin "similar or identical with Lombroso's *pellagrozein*." Two researchers from the U.S. Department of Agriculture reported on the metabolism of molds belonging to the genus *Penicillium* (the genus that later gave the world penicillin).[14] Novel ideas included Dr. George Mizell's oil hypothesis. The Atlanta gastroenterologist claimed that pellagra in Georgia farmers was "entirely limited to those who are using cottonseed oil." Dr. Herman Adler of the Boston Psychopathic Hospital described lesions in rabbits resembling those of human pellagra after feeding the animals large quantities of oils.[15] But despite the plethora of opinions an undercurrent of the germ theory tugged at most if not all attendees.

Setting the stage for Sambon's hypothesis on the first morning were two entomologists, Allan H. Jennings and William Van Orsdel King, on loan from the U.S. Department of Agriculture to the Thompson-McFadden Commission. They doubted that Sambon's insect of choice—flies of the genus *Simulium*—had much to do with pellagra in upper South Carolina. *Simulium* larvae could be found in streams but local residents seldom reported bites from adult flies. *Simulium* flies did not abound in the mill villages. Jennings and King favored the more cosmopolitan stable fly if the pathogen turned out to be a protozoan parasite, as Sambon thought.[16] They felt the house fly was the more likely vector if the pathogen turned out to be an intestinal bacterium. Dr. Stewart Roberts of Atlanta favored mosquitoes.[17] *Simulium* did not, however, lack supporters. Samuel J. Hunter, the state entomologist for Kansas, correlated pellagra with the distribution of sand flies (a *Simulium* species).[18] Edward Jenner Wood of North Carolina felt the concentration of pellagra cases along fast-flowing streams in his state supported Sambon and *Simulium*.[19] On the other hand, a Texas doctor suggested that "had Sambon's expedition gone out to Texas instead of to Italy, especially during the last three years of drought, we should now be little concerned with the distribution of *Simulium*."[20] Dr. Victor Babes of Bucharest expressed dissatisfaction with all of the recent hypotheses. He thought pellagra had something to do with corn: "I think I can close this interesting discussion by saying that we are all in accord on the maidic origin of the disease."[21]

Poor timing—a late-evening session at the end of the long first day—may have limited the impact of Funk's new vitamin-deficiency hypothesis. The "Symposium on Pellagra" began at 8:30 P.M. with an introductory address by Surgeon General Blue, followed by eight papers from London, Italy, Rumania, France, and Egypt. It was an ambitious, jam-packed program but whether the assembly hall was jam-packed with attentive listeners is another question. One suspects it was not. The registrants sat through a morning session on "Etiology, Epidemiology, and Statistics" and what must have been a tiresome afternoon session on "Local History and Diagnosis of Pellagra" during which one after another speaker gave statistics from this or that state or country. The attendees had dined and likely had access to alcoholic beverages. Most if not all of the papers from abroad were read that evening *in absentia*, enhancing the soporific effect of passive listening.[22] Thus, it is unknown whether attendees paid close attention to what turned out to be a conceptual breakthrough: the vitamin-deficiency hypothesis. Blue mentioned it briefly; Sandwith provided more detail.

Surgeon General Blue gave Babcock credit for recognizing pellagra and bringing it "to the attention of the medical profession, thereby performing a praiseworthy labor which has proven of great value not only to the people of his own State and our nation, but to all the world."[23] Blue outlined four "well-defined" theories of etiology: infection, intoxication, auto-intoxication, and food "deficiency." He intended to focus on the first (and specifically on Sambon's hypothesis) and fourth (and specifically on Funk's hypothesis) because these seemed the most promising. He like others found Sambon's hypothesis intriguing but lacking data. Blue continued: "A second promising line of investigation as regards the causation of the disease is to be found in the deficiency theory as advanced by Casimir Funk. He states that 'it is beyond any doubt that pellagra has some close association with maize diet.' Pellagra is thus placed in the same category with scurvy and beri-beri. It is only in the case of an exclusive or one-sided diet of corn: and, if the corn is

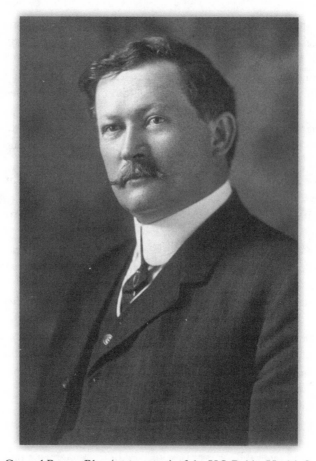

Surgeon General Rupert Blue (1868–1948) of the U.S. Public Health Service
gave a keynote address at the 1912 pellagra conference in Columbia. He
mentioned Funk's "vitamine hypothesis" as one of two promising lines of
investigation, the other being Sambon's version of the infection hypothesis.
Courtesy: National Library of Medicine.

spoiled, it is all the more deficient in nutritive values." Blue had little more
to say about Funk's hypothesis, but the next speaker, Sandwith, said a lot in
his compact paper, "Can Pellagra be due to Deficiency of Nutrition?"

Babcock had written Sandwith on May 2, inviting him to attend and
submit a paper for the conference. Sandwith wrote back that he could not
attend because he was overwhelmed with routine work. Sir Patrick Manson
was about to retire, and Sandwith had to take over Manson's wards. He
promised Babcock a short paper, "though I have really nothing fresh to say

on the subject."[24] Earlier that year Sandwith had published a comprehensive review of "Pellagra in the Thirty-Five States of America."[25] Sometime between May and October 1912 he learned of Funk's hypothesis, and, as they were both in London, they possibly met.[26]

Sandwith through his submitted paper told the conference attendees that "some of my valued correspondents in the Southern States" had been impressed with the discovery that beriberi was caused by "too continuous use of polished rice" and that "now a young chemist, Dr. Casimir Funk," had closed in on the key substance in rice polishings. Pointing out that scurvy, beriberi, and rickets were "all diseases due to some deficiency of nutrition, but capable of cure if that deficiency be banished from the diet," Sandwith asked: "Is pellagra, too, a deficiency disease, waiting for a 'Vitamine' to be discovered?" He mentioned Gowland Hopkins's demonstration that young mice needed tryptophan, and proposed that "tryptophan might be directly utilized as the normal precursor of some specific 'hormone,' or other substance essential to the processes of the body." Sandwith closed with a prophecy: "Some day soon the mist will clear before our eyes and we shall all be wondering how we came to be floundering near the goal so long without actually reaching it."[27]

Many attendees probably forgot about Sandwith's paper while listening (if they were still awake) to the windy paper that followed, submitted by Louis Sambon and like Sandwith's read by a stand-in. Sandwith's paper was pithy—just four pages in the eventually-published *Transactions*—but Sambon's stand-in droned on for 15-pages-worth of musings on *Simulium* flies, fast-flowing streams, and the like. Sambon was gratified that various doctors had "already confirmed my topographic findings" in the United States, and that evidently "in Georgia and the Carolinas pellagra is limited to the Piedmont section of the Appalachian system." Once again, he conveniently overlooked the glaring fact that pellagra was epidemic in asylums—and especially in the asylum where his paper was now being read!

Sandwith polished his paper for publication the next year in the *Transactions of the Society of Tropical Medicine and Hygiene*, again posing the question in his title: "Is Pellagra a Disease due to Deficiency of Nutrition?"[28] He extolled the benefits of balanced diet as reported by the early Europeans and confirmed in spades by others, including his own studies in Egypt. He again discussed tryptophan. He acknowledged that the feeding experiments sponsored by the Illinois Pellagra Commission pointed away from diet, but hinted that the experimental design might have been flawed.

Sandwith's 1913 paper in the *Transactions of the Society of Tropical Medicine and Hygiene* constitutes the clearest statement of the vitamin-deficiency hypothesis before the Goldberger era, which began the next year. Sandwith had taken Funk's hypothesis and brought it to the United States in the form of his paper read late in the evening of October 3, 1912, in the assembly hall of the South Carolina State Hospital for the Insane. Among those who obviously knew about the hypothesis and took it seriously was Rupert Blue, who in 1914 sent Joseph Goldberger south to study pellagra.[29]

Did Babcock and Carl Alsberg Almost Get It Right?

Babcock's published remarks in the 1912 conference transactions give little insight into what he really thought about the competing hypotheses. His presidential address consisted of his studies of the origins of pellagra in the United States.[30] He also presented on the medicolegal aspects of pellagra, reflecting his growing interest in forensic psychiatry.[31] He later told the regents: "The pellagra conference held here last week seems to have been a success scientifically, even if no report was made that would settle finally any of the long disputed points regarding the cause of the disease."[32] The state medical journal described the program as a "distinct advance over those of the previous meetings" and "the spirit of the meeting" as "broad, scientific, and tolerant," but likewise gave no hint of a conceptual breakthrough.[33] What Babcock thought about Sambon's version of the infection hypothesis had, however, come out less than two weeks before the conference. At the annual meeting of the state and provincial boards of health held in Washington, D.C., Babcock had sounded a strong cautionary note: "This question of the communicability of the disease forced itself upon the very early students certainly a hundred to a hundred and twenty-five years ago: those who advocated the non-communicability of the disease, I believe . . . subjected themselves to inoculation and none of them contracted it. Of course the Sambonian theory that pellagra is of parasitic origin is a very fascinating one but I believe the most ardent have not yet claimed that the disease is communicable . . . . I think it is very much better to take the attitude borne out by the one hundred and twenty-five years of human experience, that the disease is not communicable."[34] Sandwith had written Babcock the previous year that "Sambon may eventually prove to be partly right, but I do not think any of us in this country [Great Britain], except Manson, are his converts yet."[35] Babcock would therefore have been receptive to a new version of the dietary-deficiency hypothesis.

Less than three weeks after the pellagra conference in Columbia, Dr. Beverley Randolph Tucker, professor of neurology and psychiatry at the

Medical College of Virginia in Richmond, indicated that Babcock had done just that—he had suggested that pellagra might be caused by deficiency of an essential nutrient. Tucker reported on the Columbia conference to members of the Medical Society of Virginia. He related that "the maize theory seems to have lost ground," that the insect-transmission hypothesis "had many followers" with advocates for one or another pest such as "the sand fly, the stable fly, the flea, the mosquito, the bedbug and the louse," and that "various bacteria and toxins" and "foodstuffs, especially carbohydrates" each had their champions. He then credited Babcock for summarizing the vitamin-deficiency hypothesis: "After reviewing them all, probably the strongest and most logical suggestion of the cause of pellagra was that expressed by Dr. Babcock in a discussion. He made an analogy between beri-beri, sprue, scurvy and pellagra, and advanced the idea that pellagra was due to a monotonous diet, in which there was a deficiency of some food element, and that this diet with the deficiency affected the debilitated, whether their disability was caused by tuberculosis, insanity, alcohol, syphilis, or what not." Tucker continued: "The longer one thinks of this suggestion the stronger is its appeal. This could account for the non-febrile character of the disease, for its occurrence in institutions and in rural districts among the poverty-stricken, for its occasional occurrence among the better class who have through fear of dyspepsia or some other cause reduced their diet to only a few articles, for its apparent seasonal recurrence, as there is much less variety of diet during the winter, and for its widespread [distribution] over the country." He hoped that "Dr. Babcock will push his investigations to a definite conclusion, for, if this is true, pellagra will become a preventable disease."[36]

Carl Alsberg, the chief biologist with the Bureau of Plant Industry at the U.S. Department of Agriculture, had the same thought. Apparently, Babcock had sent Alsberg a clipping of Tucker's comments on Babcock's discussion of the deficiency hypothesis, for on October 23, 1912, Alsberg wrote Babcock:

> I certainly do not recall that your remarks at all warrant any one in quoting you as fathering a new theory of pellagra. However, what you said at the time impressed me very strongly as I had been thinking along the same lines, largely because I had been working upon a disease of cattle known as loco weed disease, and because I had been looking into the recent work on the etiology of scurvy. It seems to me that there is a possibility of there being more than a grain of truth in your remark concerning the monotonous diet. In fact I have been asking myself whether or not it would be worth while to see whether pellagra may be cured in the same way that beri-beri had been cured. As you are no doubt aware, Dr. Casimir

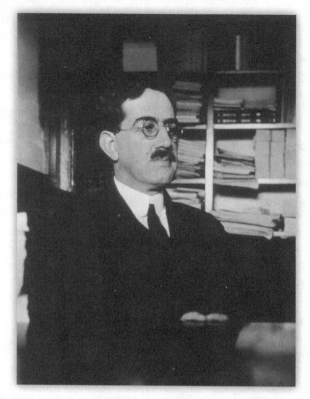

Dr. Carl L. Alsberg (1877–1940) of the U.S. Department of Agriculture wrote
Babcock after the 1912 pellagra conference about Babcock's discussing the idea
that pellagra "might, after all, be a deficiency disease."
Courtesy: National Library of Medicine.

Funk, of the Lister Institute of London, England, has recently published
an article in the Journal of Physiology, in which he reports that he has
succeeded in isolating and crystallizing the chemical substances in rice
polishings, to which the curative action of the rice polishings is due. He
has also proved that the same substance is present in yeast, in milk and
in ox-brain, all substances which have been recommended as a cure for
beri-beri. Funk has called this substance vitamine and has proved that it is
probably related to some of the substances which occur in nucleic acid. I
have been wondering whether it would be worth my while to prepare some
of the substance according to the procedure utilized by Funk, and to feed
it to pellagrins. I certainly mean to examine maize to determine whether
it contains any of this substance. If your suggestion concerning diets is a

factor it is conceivable that one might get interesting results. How does this whole matter strike you?[37]

How close they came!

There is little evidence that anyone at the 1912 conference seriously followed up on this idea—which would have required a strategic plan for a systematic research program—leaving it to Goldberger to discover the preventative and curative value of brewer's yeast more than a decade later.

The careers of both Babcock and Alsberg had assumed new directions. Babcock was not a researcher, and he was now spending much of his time developing the new State Park campus of the asylum (see Chapter 7). Alsberg had just been promoted to chief of the Bureau of Chemistry at the U.S. Department of Agriculture, a job that evolved under his leadership into the now-powerful position of director of the U.S. Food and Drug Administration. His focus turned toward drug regulation, research, and enforcement policy and philosophy. He like Babcock had little time for another exhausting project on pellagra.[38]

Had Babcock been interested in feeding some of the substances mentioned by Alsberg to pellagrins, a logical collaborator would have been Claude Lavinder, still in Savannah and the new president of the National Association for the Study of Pellagra. However, Lavinder did not even mention the vitamin-deficiency hypothesis in a three-page article he wrote about the Columbia conference for *Public Health Reports*. "The general tone of the meeting," he reported, "was encouraging, and it was abundantly evident that American students of the disease had come to recognize the need of less speculation and more work if important results are to be achieved." Those who wished to speculate, he went on, fell mainly into two camps. Some felt strongly that the disease might be "due to some profound metabolic disturbance in which spoiled corn might be very largely concerned." Others had "a feeling, almost a conviction, that the disease is of an infectious nature, and probably insect-borne."[39]

Lavinder became involved in yet another major effort to transmit pellagra to nonhuman primates. At least three attempts to transmit pellagra from humans to monkeys—his own, Anderson's (with Goldberger), and the Illinois Pellagra Commission's—had failed. However in 1913 Dr. William H. Harris of New Orleans reported that two of three monkeys injected with material from pellagrins developed skin changes suggestive of pellagra.[40] Beginning in August 1913 Lavinder and three colleagues—including Dr. Edward Francis, for whom the causative organism of tularemia is now named—tried to transmit pellagra from humans to twenty-seven rhesus monkeys, two Java monkeys, and three female baboons. The results were again essentially negative.[41] These data did, however, help Joseph Goldberger conclude that pellagra was not an infectious disease.

Sambon's Spash in Spartanburg

While Lavinder and his U.S. Public Health Service colleagues injected monkeys in Savannah, Joseph Siler and his fellow members of the Thompson-McFadden Commission planned the public announcement of the commission's first progress report, scheduled for September 3, 1913, in Spartanburg, South Carolina. Louis Sambon sailed from England to attend, notifying Babcock by telegram.[42] When Sambon reached New York in late August he called a press conference. He told reporters all about *Simulium* flies and fast-flowing streams. He told them that "food had absolutely nothing to do with the spread of pellagra," and that American doctors had given up on the spoiled-corn idea.[43] Ward MacNeal showed him the sites of New York. Sambon then went to Spartanburg for the much-anticipated event, sponsored by the Spartanburg County Medical Society. The *Spartanburg Herald* billed "the distinguished pellagra expert connected with the London School of Tropical Medicine" as "the leading, dominant figure in the great meeting."[44] The *State* hailed Sambon as "the world's greatest authority on pellagra."[45]

About 225 people, including 185 physicians, more than half of whom were from out of town, crowded into a conference hall above the Merchants & Farmers Bank. The president of the medical society called the meeting to order, then turned the gavel over to Babcock "as an honor to ... the one man who has done so much to promote the study of pellagra in South Carolina."[46] Babcock introduced Sambon, who apparently did most of the talking during the largely-unstructured, four-hour daytime meeting. The other papers, including the Thompson-McFadden progress report, were given that evening at an "informal smoker" at the Spartanburg Country Club.[47] When Sambon returned to New York nine days later he called another press conference. He told reporters at the Hotel Astor that it had been agreed in Spartanburg "that pellagra was an infectious disease, the germ carried by an insect." On September 13 the *New York Times* ran the story under the headline, "INSECT CARRIES PELLAGRA. ENGLISH SCIENTIST SAYS SPARTANBURG CONFERENCE ESTABLISHED THIS."[48] It was a classic example of science by consensus.

It was also a classic example of Sambon's misleading ebullience. Local newspapers, archival sources, and a comment made during a medical meeting nineteen years later strongly suggest that Louis Sambon's North American adventure seriously weakened his swaggering self-confidence in the insect-vector hypothesis.

Most if not all of those who heard Sambon in Spartanburg no doubt came away impressed and took his ideas seriously.[49] Yet the local newspapers gave a rather different story than did the *New York Times*. The *Spartanburg Herald* reported the morning after the conference that "no decision was reached as to the cause of pellagra and no definite course of treatment was arrived at." Although Sambon was praised for who he was—"a man world-famed as an epidemiologist and a scientific investigator of international repute"; the president of Wofford College described Sambon as "a great power, and the medical profession will not be same because he is in it"—it was Claude Lavinder, not Sambon, who grabbed the local headlines: "PELLAGRA IS NOT TRANSMISSIBLE BY DIRECT CONTACT. This is the Theory Advanced Yesterday by Dr. C. H. Lavinder, And Was Concurred in By Other Physicians."[50] The *Greenville Daily News* headlined: "PELLAGRA DISCUSSED BY EMINENT DOCTORS; ITS CAUSE A MYSTERY. Famous English Scientist Believes Pellagra is Caused by Insect, but has Not Yet Succeeded in Finding What the Insect Is." The Greenville newspaper noted that among the discussants was "Dr. J. W. Babcock [who] . . . expressed the view that there were . . . striking points of resemblance between pellagra and scurvy or beriberi."[51]

After leaving Spartanburg, Sambon went to Columbia with Siler and the entomologist Allan Jennings. Babcock later told the regents that Sambon wanted to stage an international pellagra conference in the District of Columbia.[52] It was probably from Columbia that Sambon went to Charleston to study pellagra in the neighboring barrier islands, where pellagra was endemic among African Americans. Nineteen years later Dr. Robert Wilson Jr. related, "Sambon came to Charleston to study pellagra, confidently expecting that he would find a verification of his hypothesis. We took him to Johns Island and other places where pellagra existed in abundance, and I recall clearly his eagerness in looking for Simuliae."[53] He did not find them.

Later, and probably after returning to New York, Sambon with Siler and Jennings sailed to the British West Indies for more studies of pellagra and *Simulium* flies. As in Spartanburg County and on Johns Island, they found pellagra but no evidence for transmission by *Simulium* flies.[54] Siler returned to South Carolina and announced that *Simulium* had been falsely accused.[55] Sambon went back to England. Six months later Siler wrote Babcock: "Have heard nothing directly from Sambon since his return to England. I have heard, however, from his wife and she informs me that immediately after his return to England he proceeded to Italy for further investigations. It is my opinion that his trip over here, and more particularly his observations in the West Indies, have given him some further light on the disease called pellagra and that he has returned to Italy for the purpose of looking at things in a somewhat different light."[56]

Although we don't know when Sambon "gave up on the theory," as Robert Wilson Jr. reported nineteen years later, Sambon apparently never published on pellagra again. He left pellagra for other pursuits. However, he apparently failed to disclose his new doubts to Americans. Ward MacNeal and the Thompson-McFadden Commission clung to the insect-transmission hypothesis. Sambon *in absentia*, as the intellectual force behind the creation of the Thompson-McFadden Commission, thus became the champion of those who refused to accept Joseph Goldberger's premise that pellagra was caused by monotonous diet, caused in turn by poverty.

Paradigms, Personalities, and the Tragedy of Casimir Funk

In summary, although by February 1914 (when Surgeon General Blue assigned Goldberger to pellagra) there were many hypotheses on pellagra causation, the field had been basically narrowed down to two. Sambon's version of the germ theory represented the infectious diseases paradigm. Funk's vitamin-deficiency hypothesis posed a new paradigm. Funk's hypothesis had now been aired by Sandwith, Blue, Babcock, Tucker, Alsberg, and other physicians and scientists who correctly saw an analogy between pellagra and beriberi.[57] The tragedy of Casimir Funk is that nobody acted on his reasonable proposal. As Virgil Sydenstricker puts it, "a little more armchair research involving thoughtful perusal of Funk's early work might have saved years of effort and a great many lives."[58]

Funk concluded in 1913 that one of the three substances he had isolated from the vitamin fraction of yeast "appears to be nicotinic acid." He had demonstrated that nicotinic acid was present in rice polishing.[59] He examined the effect of milling on the nutritive value of corn and concluded that the "distribution of the vitamines in the grain of maize resembles closely that of rice," and that it would therefore "be advisable to abandon the present mode of milling since only the whole grain including the skin can be regarded as a complete food."[60]

Scholars through the years have studied the resistance to Joseph Goldberger's 1914 conclusion and 1915 demonstration that diet explained pellagra. Few have addressed why the vitamin-deficiency hypothesis got so little attention before Goldberger went south. An obvious explanation is that ideas behave as epidemics. Paradigm shifts usually spread glacially, if at all, and the vitamin-deficiency hypothesis had yet to assume a critical mass of advocates.[61] Another, and complementary, explanation can be found in the personalities of the leading proponents. Funk and Sandwith had little chance against the flamboyant, charismatic Sambon.

Fleming Sandwith, who in 1914 at age 61 was approaching the end of a strenuous life, had qualities most people would treasure in their physicians. One colleague called him a "great gentleman, an invaluable friend, a tower of strength in time of trouble" who "never spared himself if in any way he

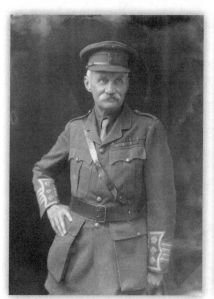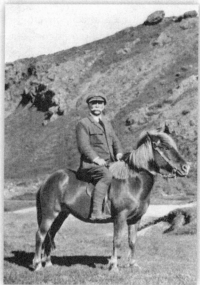

The body languages of Drs. Fleming Sandwith (left) and Louis Sambon in these photographs suggest the forcefulness of their respective personalities, which may in turn have affected the influence of their ideas about the cause of pellagra.
Courtesy: National Portrait Gallery, London (Sandwith); PhotoResearchers/Science Source (Sambon).

could alleviate the sufferings and sorrows of those around him."[62] Another wrote: "He had the real divine gift of simplicity . . . . He had in his life, and it was visible in the look of his face, a touch of the ascetic spirit . . . . There was about him an air of great refinement. He hated self-assertion, advertisement, gossip against other men, and all conceited or irresponsible talk. He lived for what he could do to help the world, not for what the world might do to help him. Quietness—that was one of the many graces of his character: a quiet voice, a quiet manner, a quiet mind. One cannot for a moment imagine him anything but the master of his fate and the captain of his soul."[63] A third colleague described "a charm about his personality which greatly endeared him to his friends," adding: "Very quiet, almost reserved in manner, with a half-cynical pose which was much more assumed than real and which was greatly relieved by a most delightful sense of humour he was one of the kindest of men, always ready to help, saying little or nothing about it, and never grudging trouble in doing it."[64] There was not in Sandwith the faintest hint of self-aggrandizement or showmanship.

Louis Sambon, who in 1914 was 49 years of age and at the height of his power and influence, was as extroverted and self-asserting as Sandwith was introverted and self-effacing. He was a "romantic and colorful figure" with an "electric temperament" who came across as "grandiloquent in style," "assured in judgment and pugnacious in tone," and nearly always "exuberant." He could charm an audience not only as a scientist but also as a *cordon bleu* cook, an accomplished amateur archeologist, a naturalist, a mountaineer, a linguist, and a connoisseur of the arts.[65] As a lecturer, "Sambon was brilliant and entertaining and his histrionic performances were always a great draw. He strutted and gesticulated on the stage, using the arts and actions of a great actor. It did not matter if his facts were drawn on a too generous scale from the realms of mythology or were based upon his fertile imagination. It was sensational; it was stimulating, and invariably invoked applause."[66]

Among the charmed was Julius Taylor, Babcock's friend and supporter. Taylor, who had been attracted to Sambon's hypothesis from the beginning, delivered at the 1912 pellagra conference a paper on "Sambon, the Man, and his Later Investigations on Pellagra." Taylor effusively praised Sambon as a man who had grown up "in a charming atmosphere of culture," as a man of "splendid ability and linguistic accomplishments," as a man of "amazing scientific versatility," and as a man with "true genius of intuition" who had no equal in tropical medicine "with the possible exception of Sir Patrick Manson himself."[67] But it seems that nobody praised Sambon as a good listener.

A vignette told by Casimir Funk's biographer strongly suggests that Sambon heard Funk present his hypothesis and immediately dismissed it: "Casimir had difficulties getting the word 'vitamine' accepted. But he had worse difficulties with the many medical men who refused to accept his theory of deficiency diseases and their relations to vitamins. To many of the medical fraternity, pellagra, beri-beri, etc., were in some way connected with an infiltration of certain pathogenic bacteria. As an illustration of this attitude, at a meeting in London during these days [1911–12], a lecturer at the School for Tropical Diseases maintained that pellagra was transmitted by some kind of fly and was particularly prevalent in localities near swift streams! Casimir's rebuttal was received with scant attention."[68] Almost certainly the "lecturer" was Louis Sambon.[69] Funk, a small, shy man, had little or no chance to prevail in a verbal showdown with Sambon.

Funk is a difficult study. Born in Poland at a time when Russian domination threatened Polish culture and even the Polish language, Funk was encouraged by his father to make his mark elsewhere and spent the rest of his life as a peripatetic scientist. He seems never to have felt at home anywhere with the possible exception of his last years in the United States as head of the Funk Foundation for Medical Research.[70] In 1915 Funk left the Lister Institute in London to take a higher-paying job as a cancer researcher at Cornell Medical College in New York. It is unclear whether Funk ever saw a patient with pellagra. Pellagra never became a cause célèbre for Funk as it did for Goldberger. We are left wondering "what might have been" had some combination of Funk and Sandwith in London (or Funk later in New York), Alsberg and Blue in Washington, and Babcock, Lavinder, Siler, and members of the other pellagra research groups tested nicotinic acid, yeast, or even unprocessed corn for the treatment and prevention of pellagra.

Data from the South Carolina State Hospital for the Insane might have strengthened the case for nutritional deficiency had they been duly appreciated. As noted in the previous chapter, the Board of Regents in August 1911 authorized Babcock and Julius Taylor to discontinue "corn and corn products as articles of diet."[71] Between 1912 and 1913—after a full year in which rice had been substituted for corn—the number of deaths due to pellagra fell by 28 percent even though the number of admissions rose by 10 percent. In March 1914 Babcock was sharply criticized for the extravagance of buying rice, since "Dr. Sambon had expressed an opinion that use of corn was not responsible for the new disease."[72] The administration that replaced Babcock's that month went back to corn, which might explain at least in part why deaths due to pellagra in 1914 exceeded by 116 percent those of

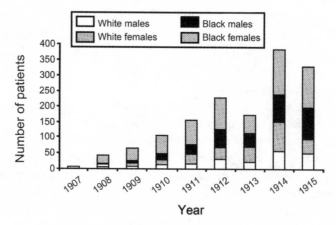

Pellagra deaths at the South Carolina State Hospital for the Insane, 1907–15. In August 1911 rice was substituted for corn. In March 1914 corn was resumed.

the previous year.[73] To the present author's knowledge, nobody put these observations together, perhaps because Babcock and his incredibly bright, energetic, and idealistic young protégée, Dr. Eleanora Bennette Saunders, were gone.

CHAPTER 7

A Plain Farmer's Daughter

"The War against the Woman"

IN MARCH 1914 BABCOCK RESIGNED UNDER PRESSURE from Coleman Livingston Blease, possibly the most controversial governor in South Carolina history. As the story is usually told, Blease had at least two reasons to get rid of the superintendent. First, he wanted to get even with Ben Tillman, Babcock's friend and sponsor but Blease's mentor-turned-enemy who had contended during the 1912 gubernatorial election that Blease was morally unfit for office.[1] Second, Blease begrudged Babcock for testifying in the murder trial of James Tillman, Ben Tillman's nephew but Blease's ally. Blease stacked the Board of Regents in his favor and struck when staff physicians complained that Dr. Eleanora Bennette Saunders, Babcock's favorite protégé, "interfered" with their work. The showdown, the state's major legislative news story for 1914, resulted in complete vindication for Babcock and Saunders. The press portrayed Blease, the other staff physicians, and most of the regents as epitomes of pettiness. Yet Babcock and Saunders found their state-salaried positions no longer viable. They left the asylum and started a private practice.

The evidence, which includes a 542-page legislative report, much of which reads like a good screenplay, suggests a more nuanced narrative than the standard account summarized above. The conclusion presented here is that Babcock could easily have survived Blease's governorship had it not been for resentment harbored by first assistant physician James Thompson toward him, and even more toward Saunders. Thompson drew the other physicians and most of the regents into a conspiracy. When pressured to sacrifice an incredibly capable and dedicated young colleague—indeed, the best "asylum doctor" with whom he had ever worked and who happened to be a woman—Babcock fell on his sword.

State Park

Babcock during his last two years as superintendent focused mainly on developing a new campus for African Americans at a suburban location known as State Park. He delegated daily operations to assistant physicians even more than he had done before, setting the stage for accusations against Eleanora Saunders.

Overcrowding got worse during Babcock's tenure as the patient census outpaced the building program. Blacks suffered more than whites. Between 1900 and 1913 death rates at the asylum, expressed as percentages of admissions, were 33 percent for whites versus 58 percent for blacks. Incredibly, more black women died at the hospital during 1912 than were admitted to it. Only a small fraction of the patients—20 percent of whites, 14 percent of blacks—made full recoveries.[2] Nearly everyone familiar with the situation agreed something had to be done, if only to patch an eyesore to the state's reputation.

The most positive outcome of the 1909–10 investigation of the asylum was the creation of a five-member State Hospital Commission to develop a new campus somewhere in the countryside. Babcock was made chairman. Other members included Dr. Robert Wilson Jr. of Charleston, dean of

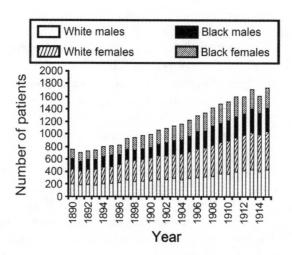

Year-end census at the South Carolina State Hospital for the Insane (formerly, the Lunatic Asylum) by race and gender, 1890-15. During Babcock's tenure (September 1891 to March 1914) the census nearly doubled and outpaced the building program.

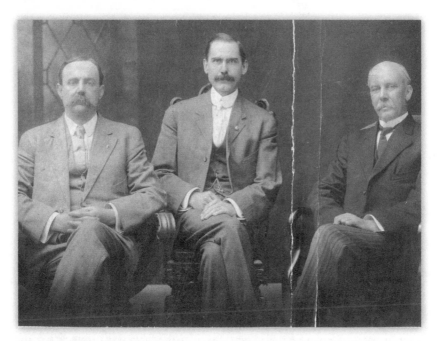

Members of the State Hospital Commission who planned the new facility at State Park, photographed in 1912, included Babcock (left; chairman), Colonel Elbert H. Aull of Newberry (right; secretary), and Dr. Robert Wilson Jr. of Charleston (center), dean of the Medical College of the State of South Carolina and chairman of the State Board of Health.
Courtesy: South Caroliniana Library, University of South Carolina, Columbia, S.C.

the state's medical school and, unofficially, of the state's medical profession. Babcock, Wilson, and several others toured asylums in northern and western states.[3] Babcock found them all "greatly overcrowded," but none, with the possible exception of an asylum in St. Louis, more crowded than his own.[4] The commissioners located suitable land about ten miles northeast of Columbia, near a railway depot known as Dent's Station, in a sparsely-settled community later named Dentsville. With support from the legislature they pieced separate parcels into a 2,582-acre tract that became known as State Park.[5] Payments began in November 1910.[6]

The State Park project promised fulfillment of a dream: a new asylum based on the "cottage plan."[7] It had become increasingly apparent that the massive Kirkbride buildings dominating that era's campuses were poorly suited for care of the mentally ill. In 1899, for example, Walter Taylor urged "separate cottages rather than ... [adding to] the already too large central structures." Babcock and other members of the State Hospital Commission recognized the prohibitive cost of relocating all patients to the suburban location, at least in the near term. They wrote in their first report: "It is, however, planned to remove the colored insane as rapidly as practicable."[8] Humanitarian considerations trumped concerns some had expressed about a separate, potentially better facility for blacks. A 1910 resolution stipulated that blacks would receive priority for transfer to State Park.[9] In 1912 Babcock recommended that black women go first.[10]

Babcock assumed the tasks of a real estate developer. The land at State Park, much of it "very sandy and poor" but with patches of soil suitable for truck farming and with stands of timber, had to be surveyed. Landscape architects, building architects, agricultural consultants, forestry consultants, and engineering consultants had to be brought in; arrangements made for water, electricity, and sewage; and spurs added to the railway and trolley lines from Columbia. The first building foundations were laid in the spring of 1912, by which time plans called for an amusement hall with a seating capacity of 1,000, an athletic field, a power plant, a laundry, fire houses, and further development of the farming operations.[11] In 1911 Babcock suggested that "more vegetables be raised" and by 1912 the farm was producing corn, peas, potatoes, and cotton.[12] Babcock rejoiced that in the State Park campus

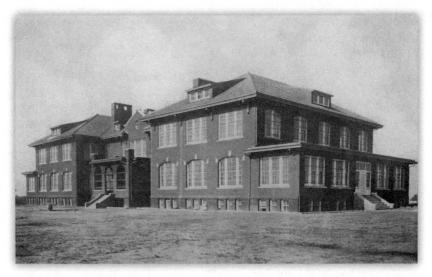

Building 1 at the State Park campus of the South Carolina State Hospital for the Insane, photographed on January 10, 1914, at which time plans for its occupation were being debated.
Courtesy: South Caroliniana Library, University of South Carolina, Columbia, S.C.

"we finally have seen materialize the hopes and aspirations of several generations of Regents and physicians" whereby "each of us has been the feeble instrument in the hands of an unseen Power."[13]

Ecstasy gave way to agony, caused, as usual, by the legislature's reluctance to commit funds for the mentally ill, especially the black mentally ill. In 1912 Babcock asserted that "the most urgent question" was securing "from the General Assembly a definite policy in connection with the development of State Park."[14] In 1913 state appropriations were sharply reduced, although special committees were appointed by both the Senate and the House of Representatives to "determine, so far as possible" policies for the new campus.[15] Despite these obstacles the first building on the State Park campus was essentially complete by January 1914.[16]

While Babcock worked to develop State Park, his extraordinarily capable second assistant physician, Eleanora Saunders, worked overtime to lead the asylum into the mainstream of American psychiatry. The other staff physicians admired but resented her, claiming that Babcock in his absence had made the energetic young woman *de facto* superintendent. Their resentment put Babcock and Saunders on a collision course with the regents and, as a consequence, with Blease, the stormy governor.

Nora Saunders and Cole Blease

"Sometime between 1910 and 1912 in this country," Harvard physiologist Lawrence J. Henderson famously remarked, "a random patient, with a random disease, consulting a doctor chosen at random had, for the first time in the history of mankind, a better than fifty-fifty chance of profiting from the encounter."[17] It is unlikely that institutionalized mental patients had a better than fifty-fifty chance of profiting, but psychiatrists like other doctors saw the promise of a new, science-based medicine. Thus, in 1913 Dr. Henry M. Hurd of Johns Hopkins proclaimed an "era of scientific care" for the mentally ill.[18] Although therapeutic options were still limited—the most widely used methods were hydrotherapy and purgatives—there were at least three grounds for optimism. Efforts to arrange and catalogue the symptoms and signs of mental illnesses that would lead to a uniform classification were well underway, holding the promise that psychiatry, like other branches of medicine, would have a sophisticated nosology—a logical system for classifying diseases.[19] Analytic psychiatry pioneered in Europe by Sigmund Freud promised a new diagnostic and therapeutic approach.[20] And the discoveries that "general paresis (or paralysis) of the insane" was a late manifestation of syphilis, could be diagnosed with the newly developed Wassermann test, and could be treated with the new drug Salvarsan promised that for the first time a relatively common mental illness could be diagnosed in the laboratory and treated with a specific drug.[21]

The quiet crusader for science-based progress at the South Carolina State Hospital for the Insane was Eleanora Bennette Saunders, "Nora" to her friends. She was born near York, South Carolina, grew up in McConnells-ville, attended Winthrop College, and received a scholarship to the Medical College of the State of South Carolina where her graduation, according to the *State*, marked "the first time in the history of the venerable institution and probably the history of any medical college in this country that the first honor of the graduating class goes to a woman."[22] Soon after she arrived at the asylum in May 1907, Babcock knew he'd found a star, indeed a superstar. He put her in charge of the white women's department and gave her free rein to develop it.[23] She lived on the second floor of the central administration building (now the Babcock Building), and aside from voice lessons—music was her sole outside interest and she had virtually no social life—she was nearly always at the asylum. Described as "a small package of incredible intelligence and energy,"[24] Nora Saunders by the standards of any time and place was an exceptionally capable and dedicated doctor.

She was extremely conscientious. Each of her patients received a thorough history and physical examination on admission followed by a mental examination that usually extended over several months. Picking up one of her patient charts at random, Dr. Julius Taylor found it "better work than some I get paid for." She looked hard for treatable conditions. She kept up with the medical literature and sought opportunities to expand her knowledge. When outside experts visited Babcock—for example, Dr. Charles W. Stiles (an authority on hookworm), Dr. Howard Fox (syphilis and the Wassermann test), and Dr. John Rogers (thyroid diseases)—she invited them to her wards to "give some criticism." She often asked Babcock to see her patients and she consulted with town physicians. Patients loved her.[25]

She combined continuing education with efforts to improve conditions throughout the asylum. At her own expense she took courses in New York and Philadelphia to learn new approaches.[26] She introduced hydrotherapy, mechanotherapy (exercise prescriptions and massage), and, for selected cases, electrotherapy.[27] She standardized the record-keeping system in the central office, established a central supply room, and improved the dining facilities. She went through the wards preaching cleanliness and neatness. She developed amusements for the patients such as dances, motion picture shows, and automobile rides. The nurses loved her and considered her "the soul of our undertakings here," adding: "Without her our inspiration would be gone."[28]

Nearly every year she set a specific goal for improving patient care. One year she worked on making smallpox vaccination routine; another year she worked on making typhoid immunization routine; another year she worked on identifying all patients with hookworm. For lasting scientific value her observations on pellagra probably surpass those of all of the other asylum doctors, including Babcock's. At the 1909 conference her presentation on the gynecological, obstetrical, and surgical aspects established her as the American authority on pellagra as it specifically affected women. Her plea that "care should be exercised to avoid needless surgical or other treatment" also drew notice.[29] She confirmed that pellagra was more common in women than in men. She confirmed that pellagra often appeared during pregnancy—an early hint that women are predisposed to niacin and/or tryptophan deficiency.[30] Her observation at the 1912 conference that substituting rice for corn at the asylum led to the appearance of beriberi was, in retrospect, a hint that vitamin deficiency caused both disorders. She was apparently the only assistant physician during Babcock's tenure to ask the regents' permission to attend a national meeting to present a paper.[31]

Now, in 1913, she set as her goal the testing of all of her patients—the white women—for syphilis using the Wassermann test. Unforeseeably, this admirable goal led to open warfare with the other staff physicians, most of the regents, and Governor Coleman Livingston Blease.

Blease, "Coley" to his adoring constituents, was a native of Newberry, South Carolina, and a lawyer by profession. He has been described as charismatic, combative, confrontational, erratic, explosive, flamboyant, inconsistent, shrewd, temperamental, and unscrupulous—to list just a few of the adjectives he provoked. He is best remembered as a racist who endorsed lynching, as a populist demagogue who appealed to textile workers, and as a wholesale pardoner of convicted felons. During his two terms as governor between 1911 and 1915, he exercised executive clemency for an estimated 1,700 prisoners, undoing the work of some 21,000 jurors. Undercover agents investigated, but could not prove, charges that he took bribes for pardons. And despite his blatant racial rhetoric, an estimated two-thirds of his pardons were for blacks.[32] Like other Southern demagogues he championed white female virtue, family unity, and individual dignity. He vowed to pardon any man or mob who killed a doctor who had examined a young girl without parental consent.[33]

However, Blease, as historian Walter Edgar puts it, is "one of the most misunderstood figures in South Carolina history."[34] Blease was and remains

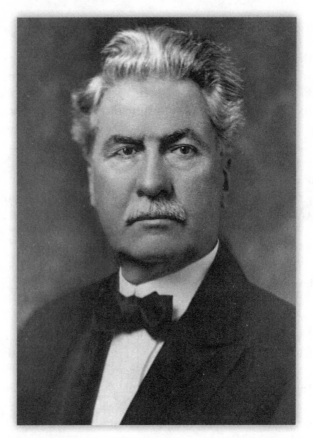

Governor Coleman Livingston Blease (1868–1942) pressured Babcock to dismiss
his talented and capable young assistant Dr. Eleanora Bennette Saunders, leading
to Babcock's resignation.
Courtesy: South Caroliniana Library, University of South Carolina, Columbia, S.C.

many things to many people, but there is little or no evidence that he was
an inveterate liar.[35] The weight of the evidence suggests he played a prominent role in the drama leading up to Babcock's resignation but was not the
primary instigator.

Blease became governor with "the full intention of removing Dr.
Babcock from the State Hospital for the Insane." He felt Babcock had been
"a traitor to my friend, Col. James H. Tillman." All that changed the day
Babcock invited him to ride out to State Park. Heading out of Columbia in a
buggy on a Sunday morning, Babcock disclosed circumstances that changed
Blease's perspective on Babcock's role in James Tillman's trial for the murder

of newspaper editor N. G. Gonzales. Babcock offered his resignation but Blease refused to accept it.[36] They established a working relationship, indeed a good working relationship. In November 1911, for example, Blease gave a welcoming address at one of Babcock's pellagra clinics, told how Babcock had given him statistics, and offered to help.[37] Babcock on several occasions consulted the governor about problems at the asylum. Each time Blease responded immediately. On one occasion Babcock learned the nurses were about to strike, went to the Executive Mansion, and found the governor at breakfast. Blease took one sip of coffee and headed to the asylum, reassured the nurses, and urged them to stay at their posts.[38]

Blease had reasons to keep the superintendent beyond their new personal relationship. Dismissing Babcock carried a political price. The superintendent was popular among the general public and with many legislators. Babcock supporters included Blease confidants, such as Colonel Elbert Aull from Newberry, Blease's lifelong friend and former schoolteacher,[39] and Dr. Robert Wilson Jr., who in 1913 saw the governor often during his successful campaign to transfer the endangered Medical College of the State of South Carolina to state ownership.[40] Finally, Babcock's performance by at least one Blease criterion—making do on a limited budget, thereby helping keep taxes low—was superb.

But Blease also had had reasons to rein in the superintendent. The governor like many public men prized power above nearly everything else. He sought power, used power, and retaliated against those who threatened his power. He wanted Babcock like others to feel the weight of his authority. Also, more than most governors in South Carolina history, Blease favored small government, minimal interference in people's lives, and little aid for the disadvantaged. In a later era he would probably be called a libertarian. He took a dim view of the financial burden that State Park would impose on taxpayers mainly for the benefit of blacks.

Although Blease's tours of State Park with Babcock were pleasant, the governor began to devise his own scheme—"plan" would perhaps be too generous—for the state's mentally ill. He would sell most of the "little sandy bottom land" with its scrub oaks and loblolly pines, which in his opinion had been bought at exorbitant price "under the pretense of benefiting poor insane people." He would keep the nearly finished first cottage at State Park, but would "take that place out there and make a pellagra hospital out of it . . . and let these fellows that drink corn liquor go out there in the sand hills and sweat it out." He would keep white patients at the downtown asylum campus, but would send all the black patients to the state penitentiary after the convicts had gone back to their counties of origin to work on chain gangs:

"Your State Penitentiary will soon be depopulated. The Representatives and the Senators are asking that these prisoners be sent back to the county chain gangs . . . . What are you going to do with your Penitentiary when all of these people are gone out? My idea is to take these insane colored people, spend a few dollars and put it in shape and put the colored people in there." Although he had reluctantly signed a bill authorizing a public vote on issuing bonds for the State Park project for black patients, he later vowed to "veto every dollar that this Legislature gives it in behalf of the people of South Carolina."[41]

Blease was accustomed to having his own way with the asylum, as with other state institutions. Thus in February 1911 he sent a rowdy man to the asylum, without any accompanying medical history, "to be held until arrangements could be made to send him to Ireland, his native country."[42] Babcock's problems with the governor possibly began in January 1912 when he declined to accept on Blease's recommendation a convicted felon named Richey. Babcock explained that he could not provide a private room staffed with adequate attendants to keep Richey from escaping.[43] This refusal almost surely did not sit well with the governor. Blease often used medical reasons to justify pardons and fumed when doctors didn't cooperate. A Blease supporter even tried to murder a beloved Columbia physician, Dr. James Higgins McIntosh, after McIntosh refused to supply a medical reason for a convict's release. (The assailant as he fled shouted, "Coley won't be bothered with you tomorrow." Fortunately for McIntosh, the bullet lodged in his ample abdominal fat pad.[44]) Just two months after Babcock's refusal to accept Richey, Blease began to fill the Board of Regents with loyal Bleasites.

In March 1912 Blease appointed to the Board of Regents Dr. Thomas E. Carothers and Iredell Jones, both of Rock Hill, and Fred H. Dominick of Newberry.[45] Iredell Jones, a Confederate veteran, had been a major Ku Klux Klan organizer.[46] Dominick was Blease's former law partner. Later that year Blease appointed State Senator John D. Bivens to replace a regent who had resigned, and in 1913 Blease appointed W. L Settlemeyer when Dominick resigned to become Blease's assistant attorney general. Dr. Julius Taylor, whose local prominence and family connections would complicate arbitrary dismissal, thus became the only holdover friendly to Babcock.

In January 1913 Carothers presented to the regents a resolution that appointments of all physicians, officers, and employees of the asylum would be for two years, the terms to end on the first of July. All employees would be "subject to removal by the Board at any time they [the regents] may deem for the best interests of the hospital." The resolution passed easily. It reduced the staff physicians' job security and the superintendent's already meager authority.

Further undermining Babcock's authority were the aftershocks of the 1909–10 investigation. In September 1911 Babcock told the regents that he "had been aware of a spirit of disloyalty . . . since the legislative investigation." The treasurer, John William Bunch, had chosen an assistant—his own son, David Sumter Bunch—without consulting Babcock. Babcock told the regents that 28-year-old Sumter Bunch had been "especially antagonistic" towards him. James Thompson had granted his assistant—who happened to be his daughter, May Thompson—a leave of absence without consulting Babcock. The regents promptly dismissed Sumter Bunch and May Thompson. Treasurer J. W. Bunch resigned immediately, necessitating an emergency meeting for "adjustment" of his terms of employment with the result that he withdrew his letter of resignation.[47] In 1912 Thompson took a three-month leave of absence, and when he returned Babcock accused him of usurping his authority by getting permission from the board rather than the superintendent for the leave, which Thompson denied. Thompson and also Dr. H. H. Griffin had given testimony damaging to Babcock during the 1909–10 investigation, and the superintendent now knew that Bunch, the treasurer, was a potential enemy.

Babcock lacked the Machiavellian instinct to never leave a wounded enemy in the field. Julius Taylor later testified that after the 1909–10 ordeal he had approached Babcock "four or five times" about Taylor's introducing a resolution to the board to remove those who opposed the superintendent. Babcock "objected to having these enemies resign from the institution."[48] Taylor was not alone in this regard. Two other regents—W. J. Gooding and W. W. Ray—sought Babcock's approval to remove Thompson and Griffin after the 1909-10 investigation; Babcock objected.[49] Babcock, it later came out, had been consistently gracious toward enemies and potential enemies. All of the regents except Julius Taylor were potential enemies when the trouble started for Nora Saunders.

Dr. Saunders, Dr. Cooper, and the Wassermann Test

Resentment toward Nora Saunders and, indirectly, toward Babcock surfaced during the spring of 1913 and became open war that summer. Her detractors found their *casus belli* when Dr. Ernest Cooper, defeated for reelection as pathologist on July 1, returned to the campus to teach Saunders how to do the technically difficult Wassermann test for syphilis.[50]

The minutes of the Board of Regents suggest the trouble began on April 11, 1913, when Babcock asked the regents to transfer the Patients' Personal

Fund from Treasurer J. W. Bunch to Saunders.[51] The fund consisted of contributions from family members or friends for patients' personal use. Administering the fund was no doubt a nuisance for Bunch. He told Babcock in early 1913 that he would not do it any longer. Saunders volunteered to oversee the fund contingent on the availability of an adding machine, a safe, and a trustworthy secretary. The regents granted Babcock's request. At the same meeting Dominick resigned as president of the Board of Regents to become Blease's assistant attorney general.[52] Dominick allegedly said in the presence of a secretary, "We will get rid of Babcock just as soon as we can find a suitable man to take his place."[53]

Dominick set out to make things difficult for Saunders and Babcock. Julius Taylor got wind of Dominick's intent and made several trips to his office only to be told the assistant attorney general was unavailable. In July Dominick ruled that the Patients' Personal Fund be transferred back to the treasurer's office.[54] The minutes and later events suggest that the other assistant physicians resented Saunders's frequent small favors for their patients, even when these favors were for the patients' benefit and did not adversely affect their care. Dominick's ruling that the fund should go back to Bunch's office seems incongruous—Bunch had previously "refused to keep ... the money [any] longer"—unless one postulates that Bunch saw an opportunity to avenge Babcock's role in the dismissal of Bunch's son, Sumter. Nobody ever complained that Saunders misused the funds or that her biweekly purchases hadn't helped the patients. Her final reconciliation showed an overdraft of only $2.22 in a single account. The assistant physicians (and possibly Bunch) influenced certain regents—probably Carothers and John D. Bivens—to persuade Dominick to punish Saunders and Babcock.[55]

Meanwhile, Nora Saunders set out to do Wassermann tests on her patients. The Columbia asylum like most hospitals of that era did not have a full-time pathologist. It was a part-time position then occupied by Dr. Ernest Cooper.[56] Cooper, a 1910 graduate of the Johns Hopkins University School of Medicine, spent several hours a day at the asylum and the rest of his time building up a private practice of general medicine. Cooper like Saunders had a zest for doing more than his job required. During 1911 he sometimes stayed up nights taking blood samples for the "possibility of a nocturnal parasite being discovered in the blood of pellagrins."[57] At the 1912 conference he presented on "Intestinal Parasites of Pellagrins and Nonpellagrins—A Comparative Study."[58] Cooper also studied the pathology of pellagra at autopsy. He shared specimens with members of the Thompson-McFadden Commission and with Lavinder.[59] In January 1912 he went back to Johns Hopkins to learn how to do the Wassermann test.

The Wassermann test was a complicated procedure for testing a patient's serum for antibodies against syphilis. It required a supply of fresh sheep red blood cells, a supply of rabbit antibodies, and basic laboratory equipment such as test tubes, graduated cylinders, a water bath, and a long thermometer. Months passed before Cooper had everything he needed. On June 6, 1913, he performed his first Wassermann test on one of Saunders's patients.

Babcock and possibly Saunders sensed trouble brewing with the upcoming election of assistant physicians, scheduled to take place on July 1 because of the new regulation requiring reappointment every two years. The incident over the Patients' Personal Fund had brought resentment out into the open. Fearing Saunders would not be reelected, Babcock appealed directly to Blease. The governor pledged to support Saunders.[60]

When Nora Saunders received notice that the staff physicians were required to reapply to the Board of Governors, she correctly deduced that "surely it must be for some purpose." She told Babcock she would "rather not reapply." Babcock reassured her of the governor's support. Saunders wanted to hear it directly from Blease. On the Saturday before the applications were due, she went to the governor's office accompanied by her head nurse. Blease told her "it was perfectly right for me to reapply."[61]

Saunders reapplied and was reelected to a two-year term. Thompson and Griffin were reelected. Ernest Cooper was not so fortunate. Although there had been no indication that anyone objected to Cooper, he was replaced as part-time pathologist by Dr. R. Golding Blackburn, who was scarcely known to the regents if at all. Blease, however, later testified that "Dr. Blackburn is my friend, personal and political, and I stand by my friends . . . . I have often said, and say yet, that I would rather be at the devil with my friends than anywhere else with my enemies." There were two other changes. Dr. W. E. Fulmer replaced Dr. D. Strother Pope as the fourth assistant physician, and Dr. L. L. Toole replaced Dr. S. F. Killingsworth as dentist. For the first time, the regents had elected a slate of officers without consulting the superintendent.[62]

To summarize, the medical staff as newly constituted on July 1, 1913, consisted of three full-time physicians—Babcock, Thompson (in charge of the white males), and Saunders (in charge of the white females) and three part-time physicians who combined their visits to the asylum with private practices in town—Griffin (in charge of the black males), Fulmer (in charge of the black females), and Blackburn (the part-time pathologist). Cooper and Pope were gone.

On July 2 Cooper took Blackburn, his replacement, through the laboratory and showed him the sheep and rabbits for the Wassermann test.

Blackburn did not know how to do the complicated procedure. It would take him a while to learn it, and he had a medical practice in town. Saunders, determined to test all of her patients for syphilis, decided to go off and learn how to do the test herself. Cooper then offered to teach her in his spare time. They set up a makeshift laboratory in the nurses' living room. Saunders and Cooper were never alone. Two nurses always accompanied them, and other nurses "were going in and out constantly." By November 15, at which time Blackburn was still not ready to do the Wassermann test, Saunders with Cooper's assistance had tested all of the white women for syphilis. Forty-three of her patients, or about 6 percent, tested positive. Saunders carefully examined these patients, found that most of them had structural brain lesions that might predispose to a reaction from Salvarsan, and then gave the drug to the ten or twelve patients who had no contraindication.[63] She concluded that syphilis involving the nervous system was present but not rampant among the white women patients. Babcock felt it was "the best piece of scientific work that has ever been done in connection with the State Hospital for the Insane."[64]

The trouble started when Blackburn, the new pathologist, discovered that equipment was missing from the laboratory. Blackburn complained to Babcock. Saunders returned the borrowed equipment at once. She bought some of the supplies she needed and received donations from Johns Hopkins and a physician in Boston. This did not satisfy Blackburn. He complained about Cooper's returning to the campus to teach Saunders how to do the Wassermann test. He felt Cooper had trespassed on his turf. No laws, rules, or regulations prevented any licensed physician in South Carolina from working at the asylum at a staff physician's invitation. No policy prohibited any physician to use the laboratory.[65] It had been Saunders's impression that the philosophy among the staff physicians had always been "to share and share alike," and indeed she'd given Blackburn some things he'd needed.

Thompson, the records suggest, added Blackburn to his list of conspirators. Thompson, Griffin, and Blackburn complained to Carothers, president of the Board of Regents. Babcock was not consulted.

One evening in early September, probably September 10, three of the regents—Carothers, Bivens, and Settlemeyer—met at the St. Johns Hotel in Columbia with Drs. Thompson, Griffin, and Blackburn to review complaints against Saunders and to hatch a strategy. Babcock, Saunders, and Taylor were not told of the meeting, making it a "conspiracy" by definition.[66] One or more of the conspirators told Governor Blease what was happening. Blease right away summoned Babcock to his office and, as Babcock recounted, told him: "Doctor, I feel it is my duty to inform you in the friendliest way possible that the Board of Regents, at least three of them, Dr. Carothers, Dr. Settlemeyer and Mr. Bivens had a meeting at a Columbia hotel this last week with all of your subordinates except Dr. Saunders." A purpose of the secret meeting, Blease told Babcock, was to secure the removal of Dr. Saunders on the grounds that she and Cooper had "interfered." Babcock replied: "Governor Blease, this is, as you have always been to me, a very friendly act; and I want to tell you that if that Board of Regents lays the weight of a feather upon that woman's head you have my resignation, and I will stand out in the open and I will proclaim them to the people of South Carolina, because they won't stand for that kind of thing. Dr. Saunders is the best officer that the institution has had since I have been there. Her work is constantly constructive; and because the Board of Regents is offended because Dr. Saunders is learning from Dr. Cooper, the former pathologist . . . if they are going to remove her you write my resignation and I will sign it, and, so help me God, I will proclaim this thing to the people of South Carolina." Blease responded: "I don't want your resignation; but it would possibly be better for Dr. Saunders to quietly leave the institution."[67]

The lines were drawn. Thompson, Griffin, Blackburn, Carothers, Bivens, and Settlemeyer opposed Saunders and Babcock. Blease was caught in the middle. The governor began to harden his heart toward Nora Saunders, who didn't measure up to his ideal of white southern womanhood. He felt that no decent white woman would concern herself with the diagnosis and treatment of syphilis.[68] He felt that Cooper's visits to the asylum smacked of impropriety. Babcock of course disagreed. He had made it clear that he would not go quietly into the still night of an asylum without Nora Saunders.

On November 10 Blease wrote Babcock asking him to "see that Dr. Saunders quietly retires from the Hospital for the Insane at as early date as you can make it convenient." The governor understood that "Dr. Cooper is still there hanging around . . . and that he and Dr. Saunders are frequently seen together, and that Dr. Blackburn is still deprived of the work which he was elected to do." He added: "I do not intend by this letter to impugn the motives of Dr. Saunders for a moment. From what I can learn of her there is no question that she is a good woman. But I think she has placed herself in a very unfortunate position, and you will please take the steps advised by me in this letter, as I do not longer propose to allow her to stand between the administration of the affairs of the institution and Dr. Cooper . . . . I have discussed this matter with you, and had hoped that you would see the propriety of acting. As you have not, I must." Babcock told Blease that many of the white women nurses threatened to resign if Saunders was dismissed. Blease answered that "if they knew the talk that is going on now, I think the decent women would withdraw, anyhow, if conditions were not changed."[69] Babcock shielded Saunders from the unpleasantness as best he could. She completed her study of syphilis and began to plan her project for 1914, which would be to examine every patient in the hospital for tuberculosis.

At about six o'clock on the evening of December 11, 1913, Nora Saunders went into the central office. Thompson drew her attention to a letter left for her by Bunch, the treasurer:

Columbia, S.C., Dec. 11, 1913

Dr. E. B. Saunders.

Dear Doctor: Acting under instructions of the Board of Regents in the meeting today this is to notify you to attend a meeting of the Board of Regents tomorrow morning at 11 o'clock, December 12th. The Governor, the Superintendent and the Medical Staff are requested to be present at this meeting.

Yours truly,

J. W. BUNCH, Secy.

Saunders asked Thompson what the letter meant. He said he did not know—which was almost certainly disingenuous. She walked over to Babcock's residence. Babcock "said he was sorry to tell me that there was to be a meeting tomorrow, [and] that the members of the staff had complained against me, that I had been complained against and that the whole meeting was to be held for my detriment." Saunders called her father, Olive Lee Saunders, who came down from York County. The three discussed the trouble well into the night.[70]

"Like Burnished Steel"

Friday, December 12, 1913, became for many South Carolinians a day of infamy because of the cauldron into which Nora Saunders was thrown at an evening's notice.

She and Babcock entered a room filled with all the regents except one (the elderly Iredell Jones, who had suffered a stroke), all the staff physicians, the dentist, and the governor. O. L. Saunders brought several attorneys. He and the attorneys were excluded on the grounds that it was to be an executive session. There was no stenographer to take minutes.

Thompson, Griffin, Fulmer, Blackburn, and Toole, the dentist, alleged that Saunders had "interfered with the professional work of the others of the medical staff in departments under their charge, and over which, in their opinion, she should exercise no control." Saunders denied "any intention to interfere with the other physicians . . . or to injure them in any way," that she "never hesitated to do any work that came to hand if in her opinion it would benefit Dr. Babcock, the institution or the patients," and that Dr. Cooper had only continued helping her with the special project.

Blease bellowed that the "institution was suffering because of the lack of harmony among the officers of the Hospital." Blease asked Griffin: "Dr. Griffin, Dr. Saunders is a single woman, is she not," to which Griffin, allegedly with a sneer, replied: "She is supposed to be."

Regent John D. Bivens took from his pocket a resolution with the charges against Saunders. He called for her dismissal.

Saunders, who later testified that the accusations had "burned into my whole being like burnished steel,"[71] began to cry and asked to leave the room. Julius Taylor moved to table Bivens's resolution. The other regents—Bivens, Carothers, and Settlemeyer—prevailed by a vote of three to one to keep the resolution on the floor. Blease reentered the fray. The governor ordered Bivens to withdraw the resolution.

Babcock made an impassioned plea in Saunders's behalf. He asked they blame him, not Saunders, for any "errors" and petitioned the board "to take into consideration the valuable services that have been rendered the Hospital by Dr. Saunders" and to exonerate her in full. The regents asked Babcock, the staff physicians, and the governor to retire. Taylor moved the board "take immediate action to exonerate Dr. Saunders." The other regents voted him down.

When the meeting was over, Babcock asked Blease what he should do. "By all means keep Dr. Saunders here," the governor replied. "It is clear to me that you and Dr. Thompson cannot stay in this institution, but you stay because if you leave the whole institution will be in a state of insurrection."[72]

They had not heard the last from James Thompson. The acrimonious meeting had not changed a thing. He was bitterly disappointed by Blease's demand that Bivens withdraw the motion to dismiss Saunders.

To that point, Thompson had left no paper trail implicating himself as the primary perpetrator of the conspiracy against Saunders and Babcock. He now dashed off a letter to the Board of Regents: "I have been connected with the State Hospital for the Insane for over thirty-two years . . . . During this time I have devoted my entire services to the institution, and have always been assured that I was giving entire satisfaction. Without any explanation

Dr. Saunders began to encroach on my duties. This was about two or three years ago. She now holds full control of them all but the 'title.'" Thompson continued: "This has been very unpleasant to me. But I have endured it rather than cause more friction than already existed in the management of the Hospital. I feel that Dr. Saunders has taken advantage of me in assuming the above stated duties."[73] He sent the letter to Carothers.

The next meeting of the regents took place on January 6, 1914, and the main agenda item was a petition by O. L. Saunders that began: "Charges of a grave nature have been preferred through the Board of Regents affecting the character of my daughter." Pointing out that he had come to the December meeting with counsel "to hear and answer these charges" only to be excluded, he demanded "that these charges be taken up and investigated and that I may be confronted by the party or parties who are responsible for these malicious and unwarranted accusations." On a motion by Settlemeyer, who earlier in the meeting objected to Julius Taylor even speaking, Mr. Saunders's petition was accepted as information.[74]

On January 16 Blease again summoned Babcock to his office. He read a letter he'd just written: "I have a very important matter, in reference to your personal and public life which I desire to read to you, and at the same time, to read to you a message which I have prepared to send to the General Assembly in regard thereto. Your Associates on the Hospital Commission have been requested to be here at the same time. I beg you to be sure to attend. Your personal character, as well as your public actions, have been seriously questioned, so much so that I feel it is absolutely necessary for me to call it to the attention to the General Assembly, and I want you to first know of it directly from me."[75] One can only conclude that a regent, probably Carothers, had told Blease about the charges and resolutions.

On January 19 the regents held another special meeting. Bivens and Settlemeyer brought resolutions. Bivens recited the "certain friction among the officials of this institution" and reports that Saunders had been "interfering, meddling, and thereby hampering" the other staff physicians, more specifically "taking lessons from Dr. Cooper." He asserted that "while the Board does not request, at present, the resignation of Dr. Saunders, that the same would be very acceptable to them, and that they think, from the friction that is evident in said institution, that it is her duty to resign, and that said resignation would do more to bring about peace and harmony in the Institution and among the employees thereof than any other action they could conceive of." He moved the board "place itself upon record as condemning the conduct of the Superintendent, Dr. J. W. Babcock, in upholding Dr. Saunders in her defiance of the rules and wishes of this Board."

Taylor moved to table Bivens's resolution. Opposition was unanimous, and the resolution passed by a vote of three to one. Settlemeyer then presented his prepared resolution "to the effect that Mr. O. L. Saunders's petition be dismissed, on the grounds that there had been no charges by the Board as to the moral character of Dr. Saunders, his daughter." This likewise passed.[76] Taylor complained about the secret meetings—the first was not the last—and about regents coming to board meetings with "resolutions already prepared." The other regents were unmoved.[77]

Babcock was admitted to the room. He "gave notice that he would refuse to submit to the dictation of the Board." He vowed to refer the matter to a higher tribunal.[78] He no doubt had in mind the state legislature, where Blease supporters were in the minority.[79] Nora Saunders's father, O. L. Saunders, belonged to the House of Representatives and had many friends and supporters.

On January 20 a concurrent resolution was introduced in the Senate and in the House of Representatives to conduct "a thorough investigation of the matters relating to the State Hospital for the Insane" and that "any party whose conduct is brought into question or whose character is affected shall have the right to be present" and be represented by counsel. Preceding the resolutions in both chambers was a lengthy message from Blease, the one he'd shared with Babcock four days earlier. Blease pointed out among other things that he had declined to accept Babcock's offer to resign the previous year.[80]

Six legislators—three from each chamber—were appointed to the Special Legislative Committee to Investigate the State Hospital for the Insane and State Park. This time Nora Saunders would have access to counsel and a stenographer would be present.

The Higher Tribunal

The hearings extended over ten days, from February 3 through February 20, and the witnesses included all the regents, all the staff physicians, the new dentist, Babcock, Cooper (the dismissed pathologist), Killingsworth (the dismissed dentist), and Colonel Elbert Aull. Blease cross-examined most of the witnesses, as did Babcock, Taylor, and Saunders, in that order. The *State* reported midway through the hearings that Babcock had just given most of his books pertaining to the history of Columbia to the library of the University of South Carolina.[81] He knew he would probably resign, but not before he and Saunders had their day in court. Tillman encouraged Babcock to "pull off the gloves and fight like a man" and to "let your motto be, 'Lay on McDuff [*sic*].'"[82]

The hearings established that the other staff physicians' complaints against Saunders were laughable, that three of the regents (Carothers, Bivens, and Settlemeyer) were less than evenhanded, and that Blease was a bully who reacted mainly to perceived threats to his power. The hearings also established that Nora Saunders would have made a superb trial lawyer.

She drew out of James Thompson that he had no legitimate case against her. Although he and Saunders, as the only full-time staff physicians living at the asylum, had worked closely for nearly seven years, he had no specific complaints. He could only whimper that she'd gradually usurped his authority:

Q (Saunders). Dr. Thompson, I believe you said that you and I worked together harmoniously?

A (Thompson). Never had a word.

Q. And each lent a helping hand?

A. Yes, ma'am.

Q. And you and I have worked more closely together than any other two?

A. Yes, ma'am.

Q. And spent more time together naturally from working in the office?

A. Yes, ma'am.

Q. We have exchanged more ideas?

A. Yes, more ideas than any others.

Q. And whenever you conceived a new plan for improvement didn't you give it to me?

A. Yes.

Q. And didn't I always give you mine?

A. You always did, cheerfully.

Q. And, after all, ours was a kind of a feeling of co-operation?

A. Certainly.

Q. When I first began to supersede you, as you say, did you object in any way?

A. Not at all. Not at all. I didn't object, because, as I stated, I said nothing on account of existing—

Q. Didn't you rather think it was helpful for the two us to work together?

A. Yes, ma'am. I admit that.

Thompson agreed that Saunders had implemented a new record system, devised a card index system for the central office, assisted the stenographer, provided amusements for the patients, improved the dining room for white males (among others), helped him improve his own wards, and helped him with specific patients. Indeed:

Q (Saunders). Have I ever failed to help you in any way that you asked me?

A (Thompson). I cannot remember a single time.

Moreover:

Q (Saunders). And you feel that you and I have worked very harmoniously?

A (Thompson). I think so.

Q. And decidedly so, more than any other two doctors?

A. Decidedly so. Our work has been for the twenty-four hours.

Q. And you didn't oppose any efforts for the general improvement?

A. Generally I did not; I have raised no objection.[83]

Thompson's only gripe was that Saunders was doing all these things on Babcock's authority, not his own. Julius Taylor later testified that Thompson was a conscientious physician who worked hard, but had not kept up with the medical literature and new developments in psychiatric care. In Nora Saunders the nurses recognized competence, energy, and enthusiasm. They began to look to her rather than Thompson for advice and leadership, eroding Thompson's self-esteem.

  Dr. H. H. Griffin, the part-time physician in charge of the black male patients, had three specific complaints against Saunders. All were petty. One concerned a patient with tonsillitis for whom Griffin had ordered a liquid diet. Saunders allowed a tray of solid food, presumably because the patient had improved and could now swallow normally. Another complaint concerned a patient's wife who wanted to visit her husband. Griffin had restricted visits; Saunders liberalized them.[84] The third incident occurred when Griffin began to dictate to a stenographer who was in the midst of taking a dictation from Saunders. Saunders asked Griffin to wait until she'd finished her own dictation.

Griffin's main grievance was that Saunders wasn't sufficiently friendly towards him:

Q (Saunders). So, our differences after all, have been personal?

A (Griffin). There have been no great things; no, ma'am.

Q. So our wards were separated so that we came in conflict very little?

A. There should have been no conflict at all.

Q. It has been but little?

A. Not a great deal. But enough to make things unpleasant for me.

Q. Did you feel from your daily visits to the Hospital that short time that you were embarrassed by my antagonism?

A. I must say that I felt rather bad that I should be treated that way.

Q. It didn't interfere with your efficiency in your duties, did it?

A. Well, if I asked the stenographer to take my letters and you tell her not to do it, it would have interfered with me.

Q. You are sure that that occurred?

A. That is what she said. She told me that.

Q. How often did that happen?

A. That happened only once in nine years, almost ten.

Q. The differences have been personal?

A. Doctor, there has never been any great thing, but enough to make it disagreeable and unpleasant.

Griffin acknowledged that his visits to the asylum averaged only an hour and a half, that he spent most of his time there doing paperwork, and that Saunders never hesitated to help out with his patients when asked to do so. Griffin apologized for his now-infamous insinuation that Saunders was "supposed" to be a single woman, claiming it was a mere figure of speech.[85] Babcock drew out of Thompson an acknowledgement that Griffin was hypersensitive. Julius Taylor said he was sorry to have to point out in a public forum how hateful Griffin had been toward Saunders, "because Dr. Griffin has been a life-long friend of mine … and he was probably, in my first school, my desk-mate."[86]

Dr. W. E. Fulmer, the part-time physician in charge of the black female patients, and Dr. L. L. Toole, the new dentist, had little to say against

Saunders. Fulmer claimed to have seen Cooper's automobile on the asylum grounds after Saunders had completed the Wassermann tests. Cooper produced evidence that the vehicle had been in a shop for repairs during the dates in question. Toole said that at first "Dr. Saunders was right horrible, but she has been recently very nice to me." Saunders interjected that the only disagreement she'd had with Toole came one morning when she'd asked him to come to a ward to see a patient who was too frail to go down to the dental clinic. Saunders gave the patient a small drink of whiskey after the procedure, as was her custom with "very feeble" patients. Then, "Dr. Toole, to my surprise, took a drink himself—a big one." She told Toole that his generous swig had no precedent at the asylum.[87]

Blackburn, the new pathologist, was not so benign. Even though the laboratory lay fallow much of the time—he spent only "a few hours a day" there—Saunders's borrowing equipment and doing Wassermann tests was somehow a violation of medical ethics. Blease backed him up:

Blease: Were you elected for that work, or Dr. Saunders?

Blackburn: I was.

Blease: Why did she have to do it?

Saunders (*interjecting*): May I say it was voluntary work?

Blease: Then I think you did wrong to volunteer this work. I think you made a
     mistake. I don't volunteer to try to go to the Attorney-General or Chief
     Justice to do their work.

Blackburn could not explain how Saunders had harmed him or given him less than "a square deal." Blackburn—like all of the witnesses except Babcock and Saunders—did not acknowledge the importance of testing mental patients for syphilis, which soon became routine at most if not all asylums.[88] Blackburn did, however, point out perceptively that "the fundamental cause of the entire trouble" was a dual government whereby "the Constitution of South Carolina gives the Superintendent and Board of Regents the same power over the same thing."[89]

Nora Saunders never backed down. Blease could not intimidate her. She insisted her name be cleared of any wrongdoing, and specifically from the insinuation that she and Cooper were having an affair. This had been absurd from the beginning. Nobody established that they were ever alone. Cooper, who as a youth had lost a leg in a railroad accident, was in 1913 newly-married and was later remembered as a "man of resolute character."[90] Saunders confronted Blease:

Saunders: I am perfectly willing to leave the institution, but I don't want to leave it with any darkness or any reflection on my name. My name is all I have.

Blease: So far as I am concerned, there has never been any reflection on your name.

Saunders: Excuse me; I read your two letters.

Blease: I think you made a mistake in having Dr. Cooper here after he was defeated for re-election, and I think Dr. Babcock ought to have asked for your resignation when I requested it, and only one thing kept me from asking for his, and he knows that.[91]

She stood up to the governor's accusation that she was running the asylum:

Blease: Whom do you consider Superintendent of the Asylum?

Saunders: Dr. Babcock; and I have always respected him as such.

Blease: Why did you proceed to run the institution?

Saunders: I do not. I told Dr. Babcock I wanted to do my tests [the Wassermann tests], and he did not object.[92]

Under her relentless questioning Blease disclosed his paranoid streak:

Blease: Has any other person who was defeated in July been hanging around here? Why should Dr. Cooper be singled out to be hanging around here? Because he was against me, and you are against me, and it was to flaunt a red flag in the face of my administration.

Saunders: Excuse me; I have yet to do anything against the Superintendent, the Board of Regents, or the Governor.

Blease: I would not think the Board of Regents would give you a chance to do anything else. I think this whole thing was done to hurt me politically—that Dr. Cooper was kept here for that purpose, and that people consented to it who pretended to be my friends who are not. It took me a long time to see it, but this array of counsel and stenographers here this morning absolutely verifies my judgment, and I am willing to take the political consequences.[93]

When on the ninth day of the hearings Saunders was at last called to testify and submit to cross-examination, Blease, who had sat through most of the testimony, was conspicuously absent. Perhaps he decided at the last minute not to come, after reading what the *State* had had to say that morning.

The newspaper ran an editorial on "The War Against the Woman." It described an orchestrated campaign against an "enemy" who happened to be "a country girl, a plain farmer's daughter" who had "fought her way" through medical school to render high-level, altruistic service to unfortunate patients only to "live and work in 'an atmosphere of insinuation'"—an embarrassment not only to the governor but to the entire state. The newspaper exhorted the "citizens and voters of South Carolina" to protest, for if "this is the kind of thing that we stand for, at least let us have sense enough not to talk about 'grand old South Carolina.' . . . Let us face the cold and common fact that in South Carolina a working woman has no chance when she blocks the way of the 'friends' of the political powers in the state." But, "Don't blame the government. It REPRESENTS THE PEOPLE."[94]

Nora Saunders's testimony that morning was straightforward and largely unchallenged. She had come to the asylum "willing to give generously of time and effort," and "though my time at the Hospital has not rippled along like a summer brook, it has not been unhappy." The revelations that began on December 12, 1913, had taken her by surprise, for she had every reason to think that Thompson and the regents "approved of my work." She was of course mistaken. They admired her work—Julius Taylor observed of the December 12 meeting that "I never heard any higher tributes paid to any one than they unconsciously paid to her"[95]—despite the hateful resolutions. When Saunders stepped down from the witness stand her friends and supporters rushed forward. The crowd had to touch her.

The 542-page *Report and Proceedings of the Special Legislative Committee to Investigate the State Hospital for the Insane and State Park* rewards the patient reader with a denouement worthy of a good whodunit. Blease had little or nothing to do with starting the war against Saunders and Babcock.[96] Thompson, Griffin, and Carothers had everything to do with it.

Before the elections of July 1, 1913—possibly about the same time as the controversy over the Patients' Personal Fund—Thompson had complained to Carothers about Nora Saunders's "running the asylum." Thompson threatened to resign if something were not done about Saunders. On the evening of June 30, 1913, Carothers drove from Rock Hill to Columbia convinced he'd located the "source" of friction among the medical staff. He came "with the full determination of not supporting Dr. Saunders."

On the morning of July 1, Carothers went to the governor's office. Blease told him of Babcock's insistence on keeping Saunders and that he supported Babcock in that regard. Carothers then decided to play chess with the medical staff positions.

Carothers had nothing against Cooper, whom he'd known for about ten years. However, "the strong personal friendship between Dr. Saunders and Dr. Cooper" called for Cooper's removal strictly because of the "want of harmony" voiced by Thompson and Griffin. Carothers reasoned that a new position—that of medical director—would soon become available at State Park. The salary would be more than Thompson was making as first assistant physician. Carothers reasoned that Thompson could take the new job at State Park, and that Griffin would also go there when the black males were relocated. Cooper could then take Thompson's place as first assistant physician. Cooper had actually run the white male wards during the three months in 1912 when Thompson took a vacation and, since he already knew the job, Carothers reasoned he would probably accept it. Cooper and Saunders could then work together as the two full-time staff physicians at the downtown campus.

Carothers admitted, when cross-examined by Babcock, that he'd deduced that Saunders "was the cause of the trouble" on the basis of Griffin's "one trivial misapprehension" and Thompson's complaints about "lack of harmony." Carothers had "no animosity against anybody," but decided Saunders had to go to keep the peace. Saunders, her father, and Cooper took him to task. Carothers finally acknowledged: "I have done the best, gentlemen, for peace and harmony, according to my judgment, and if I erred I am only human."[97]

Although Carothers despite his scheming may have ultimately held a benign view of Saunders and Babcock, his fellow regent John D. Bivens did not. He called Babcock "the present and chivalric defender of Dr. Saunders."[98] Bivens proposed a resolution calling for Saunders's removal, just as he'd done two months earlier. Before the motion could be seconded, Blease—just as he'd done two months earlier—intervened: "I think it would be best for you gentlemen to consider that matter among yourselves . . . . I think if you could get all parties together and just simply say to the public that you have had your investigation and that everything was satisfactory, it would be much better, than having a great newspaper story about a whole lot of friction at the Asylum . . . . Personally and officially I have absolutely nothing to conceal, here or anywhere else."[99] Blease squelched Bivens's resolution, but he was less successful with the press after the Investigating Committee reached its conclusions.

Vindication

The Investigating Committee attributed much of the "discord, trouble and friction leading up to and resulting in the investigation" to the State Constitution of 1895, which, among other things, denied the superintendent authority and control over his staff. The committee's exoneration of Eleanora Saunders was complete and effusive:

> She is not guilty of any wrong intention or wrong doing. There is no breath or even a suspicion as to her moral character . . . . The few and insignificant acts on which complaints were based were the direct result of requests from the Superintendent . . . and were executed in the discharge of duty to suffering humanity and are to be commended and praised rather than condemned.
>
> Her work and labors in the State Hospital for the Insane bear eloquent tribute to the remarkable initiative, aided by tireless energy and dominated by the womanly woman's overflowing love for unfortunate humanity, which

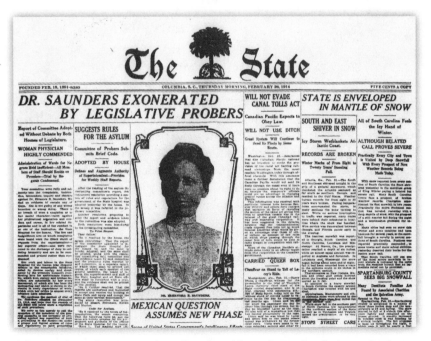

After ten days of testimony about her alleged "interference" with the work of other physicians at the asylum, Eleanora Saunders was completely exonerated and her critics humiliated by the press (*State*, February 26, 1914).

love and energy and tireless devotion is manifested by her every movement, of which she has been the mainspring and which is shown in the results of every department of work which she has touched and which her critics in almost every instance have admitted.

Babcock was also praised: "We commend the stand of the Superintendent ... in this acute exigency and throughout the subsequent aftermath, when he championed the right, not only of his loyal and true subordinate and staff officer, Dr. Eleanora B. Saunders, but of a woman, whose every instinct is shown to be for the right, the interests of the unfortunate patients under her care, and the best interests of the institution." The committee, without naming Blease, the regents, or the members of the medical staff, strongly recommended new rules and regulations to prevent such "irresponsible use of power," which it defined as "that power which is exercised without rule or reason and from which there is no recognized method of appeal."[100]

The press had another field day. A woman's successful defense of her honor made front-page headlines.[101] Public support for Babcock and Saunders was overwhelming. There were suggestions that Babcock run for governor and that Saunders would make a fine attorney general.

Resignation

Despite wide support from the legislature, press, and general public, Babcock and Saunders were expected to resign.[102] At the next meeting of the Board of Regents, on March 12, Blease again asked that the regents and Babcock "consult together and if possible settle their differences and agree to work together in harmony." Babcock expressed "a willingness to serve the institution provided matters are settled satisfactorily, but without harmony it would be impossible" to stay on. Newspapers even reported that the session resembled a love feast.[103]

Yet Babcock knew that reconciliation with the regents would not suffice. Neither he nor Saunders could continue to work with the other staff doctors, especially Thompson. Babcock had testified that all of them were hostile towards him. He had attacked Thompson's character. He tendered his resignation in writing to Blease that afternoon. Blease accepted it the next day.[104] Saunders submitted her resignation that afternoon. She offered to "hold on for a day or two" to persuade nurses to remain. The regents accepted her offer. The press continued to heap praise upon her, and "the women of Columbia" gave her a silver loving cup.[105]

The regents did not act on a set of resolutions proposed by Julius Taylor to commend Babcock for nearly twenty-three years of service to the institution.[106] Later that month Babcock asked the regents to purchase some 6,000 to 7,000 white duck suits of clothes, which he and Taylor had bought, at their own expense, as U.S. government surplus several years earlier at 50 cents per suit. Thompson advised the regents against the purchase, saying the hospital already had enough white duck suits.[107]

Friends, relatives, patients' families, and newspaper reporters rallied to Babcock's support, as did fellow asylum superintendents. John T. Searcy wrote from Tuscaloosa, Alabama: "I hardly know whether to express sympathy or congratulations to you, on your withdrawal from the State Hospital. It has been unpleasant to you no doubt to have been the center of so much political firing. I believe I have understood it all. I congratulate you, however, on your having removed yourself from such surroundings."[108] Joseph Siler of the Thompson-McFadden Commission joined the chorus: "Needless to say, we all admired you for the stand you took in this matter."[109] Saunders and Babcock had won a clear-cut moral victory.

CHAPTER 8

The Blind Men of Hindustan

"The Diet of the Well-to-Do"

B ABCOCK DID WELL IN PRACTICE. He set up a clinic and built a small private sanitarium in Columbia. He taught medical students at the Medical College in Charleston. Nora Saunders worked with him until 1919, when she went north to start a new career. Despite success in practice and at teaching, one of his daughters reminisced that "Doctor Babcock never concealed the fact that private practice brought him none of the satisfaction he had felt as a public servant."[1]

In February 1914, while Babcock and Saunders were enduring the legislative hearings, Joseph Goldberger replaced Claude Lavinder as the U.S. Public Health Service's chief pellagra researcher. Within four months Goldberger concluded that diet was the answer. During the 1915 meeting of the National Association for the Study of Pellagra, held at the Columbia asylum, news broke that Goldberger had prevented pellagra by wholesome diet. Ward MacNeal of the Thompson-McFadden Commission and Adams Hayne of the South Carolina State Board of Health emerged as Goldberger's most vocal opponents. They and others destroyed the goodwill and cooperation that had characterized the American pellagra effort. Goldberger, to win public support, had to disprove the Thompson-McFadden Commission's conviction that pellagra was in all likelihood an infectious disease. This necessity helped delay by at least several years the demonstration that brewer's yeast prevents pellagra at nominal cost. Thousands may have died as a result.

Babcock remained a diligent student of pellagra and psychiatry until shortly before his death in 1922 from complications of a heart attack. Newspapers and medical journals throughout the United States noted his death and the *Revista Pellagrologica Italiana* praised him as a "pioneer and humanitarian, whose fame will grow with time."[2]

A New Start

After resigning from the state hospital, according to family tradition, Babcock asked his wife, "What *shall* I do?" Private practice had always been a barely-viable option for alienists (psychiatrists). By 1914, however, a small niche had emerged for outpatient clinics and small private sanitariums.[3] Citizens in Greenville and elsewhere expressed a desire for his services. He chose to remain in Columbia. On March 17, 1914, he opened a practice at "the old H. P. Clark place," at 2315 Taylor Street. He borrowed money and built his own sanitarium. He and Saunders treated both races and genders as outpatients but limited their inpatients to white women.

In 1915 the Board of Trustees of the Medical College in Charleston voted him chair of psychiatry. He thoroughly enjoyed his weekly trips to Charleston by train, which he did without pay until 1918, when the trustees gave him a $500 honorarium to express "very great appreciation of your valuable services to the college."[4] His class usually consisted of no more than five medical students and often involved a case presentation. He also taught nurses at Charleston's Roper Hospital. Returning to Columbia he would take a trolley to its terminus at Taylor Street and Millwood Avenue and walk the remaining two miles deep in thought.[5] August Kohn wrote that it "was a tax for him to go there every week, but he frequently spoke of the happiness it gave him to meet such a group of fine young spirits. Nothing gave him more keen delight than to help young folks."[6] Through his relationships with lawmakers Babcock influenced constructive legislation related to mental health.[7]

Although no longer at the center of the American pellagra effort, he planned the 1915 triennial conference of the National Association for the Study of Pellagra, another turning point in the conquest of the disease.

Joseph Goldberger goes South

In early 1914 Claude Lavinder sought relief from pellagra work. He had helped sound the alarm, clarify the extent of the epidemic, and show that pellagra could not be transmitted from humans to rhesus monkeys and other animals, at least not easily. Now his research seemed to be heading nowhere.

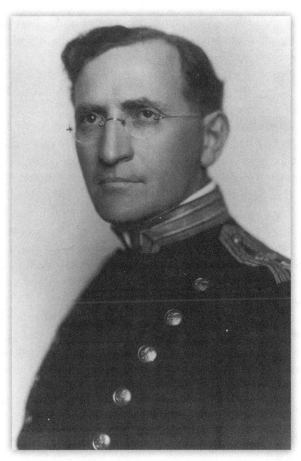

In February 1914 Dr. Joseph Goldberger (1874–1929) replaced Claude Lavinder as the chief pellagra investigator for the U.S. Public Health Service. He quickly concluded that faulty diet was the likely cause.
Courtesy: National Library of Medicine.

On February 7, 1914, Surgeon General Rupert Blue asked 39-year-old Joseph Goldberger to assume leadership of the U.S. Public Health Service's investigation of pellagra. Blue told Goldberger he was "preeminently fitted for this work and ... it could be placed in no better hand."[8] Goldberger accepted and received instructions to go to Savannah and Milledgeville, Georgia, and then to Spartanburg, South Carolina, to "inspect the operation of the Service in respect to pellagra investigations at those points."[9]

Goldberger's biography resembles a Horatio Alger story. He was born Josef Goldberger, the youngest child of a shepherd in a mountainous region of what was then the Austro-Hungarian Empire and is now Slovakia. A plague destroyed most of the sheep. His father took the family to New York where they scraped out a living on the Lower East Side and saved enough to start a grocery for which Joseph ran errands. Taking advantage of the free education at the College of the City of New York, the shy young man aspired to be a civil engineer until the day a friend, Patrick J. Murray, took him to hear a lecture by Dr. Austin Flint Jr. at the Bellevue Hospital Medical School. Joseph was hooked. He received his MD in 1895, did a two-year internship at Bellevue Hospital, and set up practice in Wilkes-Barre, Pennsylvania, which he found unfulfilling. In 1899, to his parents' disappointment, he joined the U.S. Marine Hospital Service.[10]

Goldberger's intelligence, drive, and focus brought invitations to join investigations of typhoid fever, yellow fever, and dengue. He contracted each of those diseases but survived. He was next assigned to work with Dr. John F. Anderson at the National Hygienic Laboratory in Washington, D.C., where he studied typhus, measles, and—usually overlooked but as previously noted in Chapter 5—pellagra. Goldberger went south in February 1914 and entered South Carolina in March, just as Babcock was leaving the state asylum.

Goldberger's conclusion that monotonous diet caused pellagra is often depicted as an "aha moment"—a sudden, brilliant flash of insight. Goldberger, the story goes, was expected to identify the causative germ. For example: "In 1914, the U.S. Public Health Service assigned Joseph Goldberger to study pellagra, presumably to help find its infectious agent."[11] And: "Goldberger was expected, by the USPHS and himself, to find an infectious cause of pellagra."[12] Goldberger, the story continues, observed monotonous diets in asylums and orphanages. At asylum after asylum, orphanage after orphanage, he learned that none of the staff ever got pellagra. As an experienced infectious diseases researcher he realized that an infectious cause was unlikely. The answer was in what people ate or did not eat. The root cause was poverty.[13]

Goldberger never told the story quite this way. The standard narrative oversimplifies in several key respects what he knew and thought about pellagra in February 1914 when he went south.

First, although the pendulum of opinion had swung toward the germ theory, the matter was far from closed. Most thoughtful physicians were reluctant to commit to any hypothesis. The programs of the triennial meetings of the National Association for the Study of Pellagra in Columbia—in 1909, 1912, and, later, in 1915—reflect considerable diversity of opinion. And new ideas were still coming.

TABLE 8.1   The Leading Hypotheses on Causation of Pellagra in February 1914

	Nutritional Deficiency Hypothesis	Infection Hypothesis
Essence	Pellagra is caused by a monotonous diet deficient in one or more key nutrients.	Pellagra is caused by an unidentified infectious agent possibly transmitted by an insect.
School of thought	Zeists (but open to the possibility that eating corn is not a prerequisite for pellagra)	Anti-Zeists (holding that pellagra has nothing to do with corn)
Historical context	Observations by Europeans, beginning with Gaspar Casál (between 1720–1735) that pellagra occurs almost exclusively in persons whose diet consists mainly of corn	Late nineteenth-century germ theory of disease, setting off a pursuit for infectious causes of most if not all diseases of then-unknown origin
Prime originator(s)	Giovanni Battista Marzari (1810)	Various Italians
Refinement	Pellagra is caused by a vitamin deficiency (Casimir Funk, 1912)	Pellagra is transmitted by an insect, possibly a fly of the genus *Simulium* (Louis Sambon, 1905)
Chief proponents	Casimir Funk and Fleming Sandwith in Great Britain; in the United States, no clear champion, although Rupert Blue, Babcock, Carl Alsberg, Edward Vedder, and others mentioned the idea and many saw an analogy with beriberi	Sambon and Sir Patrick Manson in Great Britain; in the United States, members of the Thompson-McFadden Commission (notably, Joseph Siler and Ward MacNeal) and others attracted by Sambon's force of argument
Supporting data	Pellagra is uncommon among persons with access to a diet varied with meat, milk, and leafy vegetables. If caught early, pellagra responds to treatment that includes a varied diet.	In Italy, according to Sambon, pellagra occurs mainly along the banks of fast-flowing streams teeming with *Simulium* larvae. A few Americans confirm this observation.
Opposing data	Pellagra sometimes occurs in persons with access to a varied diet; it also occurs in persons who never eat corn. Studies by the Illinois Pellagra Commission and the Thompson-McFadden Commission point away from dietary deficiency.	Pellagra in the United States often occurs in closed institutions and in places remote from fast-flowing streams. No causative organism has been convincingly demonstrated despite claims made for numerous bacteria, fungi, and parasites.

Second, while the competing hypotheses made up a crowded field, the smart money was betting on just two: the infection hypothesis and the dietary-deficiency hypothesis (Table 8.1; see also Chapter 6). Some still favored the spoiled-corn hypothesis but the odds against it mounted. People who never ate corn sometimes got pellagra. Rigorous enforcement of South Carolina's 1910 corn-inspection law failed to slow the epidemic.[14] Goldberger was in a position familiar to all student test-takers: a multiple-choice question essentially narrowed down to two.

Third, Rupert Blue, the man who sent Goldberger south, almost surely favored dietary deficiency. In 1909, two years before he became surgeon general, Blue told members of the San Francisco Medical Society that although "the communicability of the disease has ... received considerable attention .... I do not believe that the evidence thus far presented warrants us in the belief that pellagra is contagious or infectious, or in establishing quarantine against it."[15] (Previous accounts seem to make no mention of this paper.) At the 1912 conference in Columbia Blue identified the most promising hypotheses as those summarized in Table 8.1, and, based on his previous experience, had reason to think that what people ate held the answer. It is safe to assume that Blue shared his hunch with Goldberger before sending him south.

Finally, Goldberger had himself participated in unsuccessful experiments to transmit pellagra from humans to rhesus monkeys and therefore, as detailed in Chapter 5, did not head south knowing little or nothing about pellagra. Goldberger's first biographer's statement that he "had no previous experience with the disease, and knew nothing about it"[16] is incorrect.

To assert that Goldberger did not choose the dietary-deficiency hypothesis during an "aha moment" by no means belittles his accomplishments. Goldberger designed and carried out crucial experiments solidifying the case for diet beyond a reasonable doubt. He came close to identifying the essential dietary component. He made practical recommendations and, just before he died, identified in brewer's yeast a cost-effective therapeutic and preventative measure.[17] Goldberger, a steady and careful researcher, turned a hypothesis (a reasonable idea) into a theory (an idea that accounts for the known facts to a reasonable degree of certainty). Goldberger gave credit to others and did little or nothing to advance his own hero-myth.

The usual narrative that in February 1914 most people attributed pellagra to infection is, however, accurate to the extent that infection was getting the most publicity at that particular time. Driving the case for infection was the Thompson-McFadden Commission (which had been renamed the "Robert M. Thompson Commission," presumably because McFadden no longer contributed; the original name will be kept here for simplicity). In January 1914 the *Journal of the American Medical Association* published a summary of the Thompson-McFadden Commission's first progress report, concluding that pellagra was "in all probability a specific infectious disease communicable from person to person by means at present unknown."[18] The *State* ran the story on the front page: "PELLAGRA SPREAD BY BAD SEWERAGE. New Theory Advanced by Scientists. FOOD NOT THE CAUSE. No Definite Relation between the Disease and Any Particular Diet."[19] Pellagra correlated with poor sanitation and, more specifically, with outdoor privies around which stable flies swarmed.

In late January 1914 Joseph Siler, still on assignment from the U.S. Army to the Thompson-McFadden Commission, went to Columbia to lobby for state support. He wanted a pellagra hospital and a state-sponsored pellagra commission. Colonel Thompson had by then contributed about $40,000, and, Siler told legislators, "justly maintains that if no aid is received from the State the commission will discontinue."[20] The bill passed in the Senate but died in the House of Representatives.[21] However, Tillman, probably at Babcock's urging, successfully lobbied Congress to help fund a pellagra

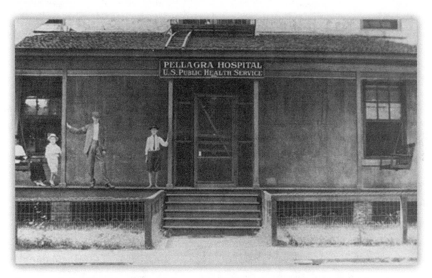

In 1914 federal legislation—supported by Tillman probably at Babcock's instigation—helped create a Pellagra Hospital in Spartanburg, South Carolina. In 1917 this hospital became Goldberger's base of operations for now-classic studies in mill villages that refuted the Thompson-McFadden Commission's conclusions about pellagra.
Courtesy: National Library of Medicine.

hospital of the U.S. Public Health Service in Spartanburg.[22] Citizens in the South Carolina upstate also contributed. Both the Thompson-McFadden Commission and the U.S. Public Health Service now had a presence in Spartanburg County, where much of the ensuing drama would occur.

In June 1914 Goldberger published his conviction that the problem was poor diet.[23] His short paper begins with six observations to the effect that in closed institutions where pellagra was common staff members never got it. He took his first three observations from the transactions of the 1909 national meeting at the State Hospital in Columbia. He took the fourth and fifth observations from Sambon and Lavinder, respectively, who had heard that in the *pellagrosari* of Italy the staff never got pellagra. He quoted Babcock for the last observation, namely that the staff in the South Carolina State Hospital for the Insane did not get pellagra, either.[24]

In June 1914 Goldberger was not the only member of the U.S. Public Health Service to make a case for dietary deficiency. Dr. Carl Voegtlin, a pharmacologist with the U.S. Public Health Service, read a paper on "The Treatment of Pellagra" that month at the American Medical Association's annual meeting in Atlantic City. Voegtlin said that "recent advances in the field of nutrition" suggested pellagra might be due to a vitamin deficiency, an amino acid deficiency, or toxic substances in the diet. In the audience was Ward MacNeal of the Thompson-McFadden Commission. MacNeal challenged Voegtlin. He cited his own conclusions from the Spartanburg County data that diet had nothing to do with it. Voegtlin shot back: "It is a great mistake to make such superficial dietary studies, which often lead to false conclusions, a fact well illustrated in the history of beriberi."[25]

This exchange between MacNeal and Voegtlin was the opening salvo to a war between the Thompson-McFadden Commission and the U.S. Public Health Service. MacNeal became increasingly defensive to the charge that he had made poor use of dearly-bought data. MacNeal became Goldberger's fiercest intellectual adversary.

On September 4, 1914, Goldberger strengthened the case for dietary deficiency in a second article. He pointed out that Lavinder and other researchers had taken "every kind of tissue, secretion, and excretion from a considerable number of grave and fatal cases . . . and inoculated [the material] in every conceivable way into over a hundred rhesus monkeys, [and] the results so far have been negative." Hence, the "inference may . . . be safely drawn that pellagra is not an infection, but that it is a disease essentially of dietary origin."[26]

On September 26 the Thompson-McFadden Commission issued its second progress report.[27] The commission had visited more than 5,000

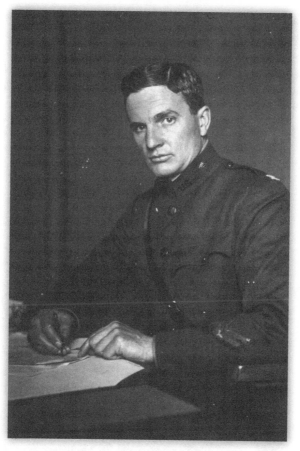

Dr. Ward J. MacNeal (1881–1946) directed the Thompson-McFadden Commission's work at the New York Post-Graduate Medical School and became Joseph Goldberger's fiercest intellectual opponent.
Courtesy: National Library of Medicine.

pellagrins—nearly every known case in six South Carolina mill villages—in their homes. There was no "definite relation of the disease to any element in the dietary." Most of these pellagrins had been in "close association with a preexisting case." Pellagra "spread most rapidly in districts where unsanitary methods of sewage disposal have been in use." The commission's researchers stuck with the infection hypothesis even though they, like others, could not transmit pellagra from patients to rhesus monkeys and could not incriminate *Simulium* flies or other insects beyond the general observation that flies swarmed around privies.

That same day—September 26, 1914—Goldberger wrote his wife from Jackson, Mississippi, that he had begun a test diet in two local orphanages."[28] He had changed the breakfast cereal from grits to oatmeal. He had increased the amounts of meat, milk, eggs, beans, and peas. He had kept everything else the same. With this small step Joseph Goldberger leaped toward his permanent place in the history of medicine.

On November 11 Goldberger squared off with the Thompson-McFadden Commission at the annual meeting of the Southern Medical Association in Richmond. Representing the commission was Dr. Philip A. Garrison.[29]

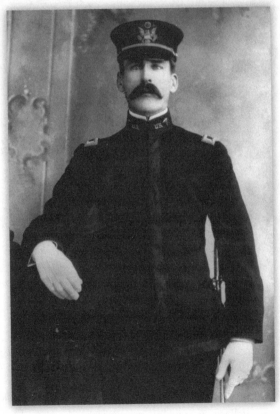

Dr. James Adams Hayne (1872–1953), shown here in uniform during the Spanish-American War, became state health officer for South Carolina. At the 1914 meeting of the Southern Medical Association he called Goldberger's version of the dietary hypothesis "an absurdity."
Courtesy: Waring Historical Library, Medical University of South Carolina, Charleston, S.C.

Garrison was gentlemanly, but Adams Hayne, South Carolina's state health officer, was not. Hayne called Goldberger's dietary-deficiency hypothesis "an absurdity."[30]

On November 19 Goldberger wrote his wife as he was about to leave Columbia: "My trip has been really disappointing in one thing, in that I missed seeing Dr. Babcock. He is out of town. He is one man I would like very much to meet and talk with. I shall try to come by this May again just to see him—if nothing more."[31] Goldberger acknowledged Babcock as the elder statesman of the American pellagra effort.

To solidify his case for the dietary hypothesis, Goldberger needed not only to prevent pellagra by dietary manipulation but also to cause it. In February 1915 he began a study of eleven white male prisoners at the farm of the Mississippi State Penitentiary, about eight miles east of Jackson and commonly known as the "Rankin Farm," where there was no history of pellagra among the inmates. Governor Earl Brewer had offered to pardon prisoners who volunteered for a feeding experiment. Goldberger watched the men for about six weeks on their usual diet. He then put them on an experimental diet weighted toward grits, cornbread, rice, gravy, fried mush, cabbage, collards, and cane syrup. To negate the possibility that they could get pellagra from biting insects, he kept them indoors and behind screens.[32]

By the summer of 1915 the Mississippi orphanage experiments were going well, as were similar studies on two wards at the Georgia State Sanitarium in Milledgeville. On July 24, 1915, Goldberger wrote his wife: "Our work is going along nicely. We are trying to decide how to extend it." He continued: "I know that our work is sound and I know that our results will carry convictions to sound minds. I am satisfied that the best opinion is already with us. Dr. Babcock of Columbia S.C. has practically expressed himself to that effect. Let the heathen rage!"[33]

Meanwhile Babcock planned for the third triennial conference of the National Association for the Study of Pellagra, destined to be an inconclusive showdown between Goldberger and the Thompson-McFadden Commission.

The 1915 Triennial Conference— "The Diet of the Well-to-Do"

Babcock again had primary responsibility for assuring a successful meeting, and the South Carolina State Hospital for the Insane would again be the venue. Fortunately for Babcock and for Nora Saunders, the asylum was no longer a hostile environment. Their ordeal of 1913-14 had renewed public attention on the horrific conditions, and Blease had been succeeded by a new governor, Richard Irvine Manning. Manning was a progressive, and progressives now controlled the legislature.[34]

In January 1915 Manning shared with the General Assembly his "intense interest ... in the care of the mentally ill in the South" and his desire to "place this hospital among the very best in the country." Henceforth the governor would appoint the regents, who would appoint the superintendent, who would appoint everyone else. The asylum would be "solely for the support, custody and treatment of insane persons." State Park would continue to be developed. Funds would also be made available to upgrade facilities at the downtown campus.[35]

Manning's changes went beyond regulations and facilities. He swept house in the Board of Regents, replacing all the previous members. In the spring of 1915 Dr. Frederick Williams became superintendent. He insisted the job be split in two. The superintendent would be strictly an administrator. There would be a separate medical director. Dr. James Thompson, the lead conspirator in 1913-14, saw the writing on the wall. The 61-year-old Thompson, claiming fatigue from his many years as assistant physician, asked for and received a job as clerk in charge of medical records.[36] The remaining parties to the conspiracy against Saunders and Babcock—staff physicians Griffin and Fulmer, Blackburn the pathologist, and Toole the dentist—were not reappointed when their terms expired on July 1, 1915. Williams recruited their replacements mainly from the North. He procured salaries for three interns and a new position, Woman Physician.[37] The year 1915, the new regents later reported to the governor, became "the most eventful year in the history of the Institution." The regents further observed that "practically all of the recommendations [now implemented] ... had been made by Dr. J. W. Babcock during his Superintendency."[38] It was as though Babcock had dictated a wish list. And Babcock and Saunders could return to the asylum without seeing any of the conspirators except, perhaps, Thompson, who was squirreled away in the medical records department.

Babcock solicited papers for the upcoming pellagra conference, writing letters on stationery designed for the purpose. He invited Fleming Sandwith to submit a paper as he'd done before, but Sandwith replied from London that he had "nothing new to say, but I am still of [the] opinion that the disease is due to deficiency of nutrition and that it is in some ways analogous to Beri-beri. It is a great comfort to see that some of the best workers in America are now partially or completely converted to that view." He added

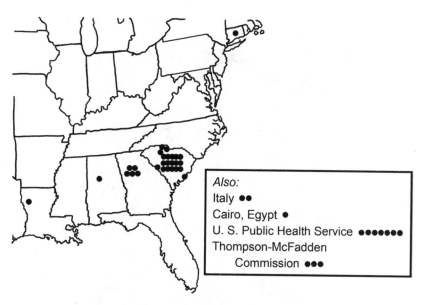

Also:
Italy ●●
Cairo, Egypt ●
U. S. Public Health Service ●●●●●●●
Thompson-McFadden
  Commission ●●●

Authors of papers presented at the third triennial conference of the National Association for the Study of Pellagra, October 21–22, 1915 at the South Carolina State Hospital for the Insane, reflected less geographic diversity than those at the 1909 and 1912 meetings (pages 106 and 177). (Each dot represents the hometown of the author or senior author of one paper.)

that "Sambon might [submit a paper]."[39] Sambon did not. As noted in the previous chapter, he apparently gave up on pellagra without telling anybody.

Babcock again heard from physicians with creative ideas. An Atlanta doctor planned to submit a paper on sensitization to corn and sugar-cane products as the etiology.[40] A Kansas physician claimed pellagra was a chronic acidosis caused by drinking water derived from clay soils.[41] A Missouri doctor claimed pellagra was caused by potassium poisoning due to meat preservatives.[42] However, the submissions were fewer than for the 1909 and 1912 conferences. The final program listed forty-one papers of which nearly half were from South Carolina, a higher percentage than at either of the two previous conferences. Babcock probably had to solicit papers from local doctors to fill the allotted time. Newspapers likewise showed less enthusiasm than before, the *State*'s announcement appearing on page six.[43] African American doctors were invited to "occupy the gallery at the meetings held at the State Hospital."[44] When the day arrived there were only about

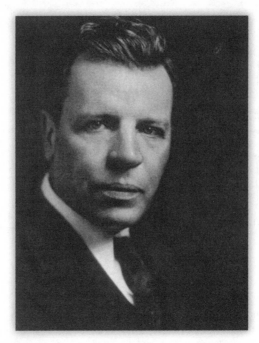

Dr. Edgar Sydenstricker (1881–1936), a political economist by training, helped Goldberger refute the Thompson-McFadden Commission's conclusions in Spartanburg County, South Carolina.
Courtesy: National Library of Medicine.

seventy-five attendees, far less than at previous meetings. Most American doctors, especially in the South, now knew the essential facts about pellagra. The Southern Medical Association and other groups now held sessions on pellagra at their annual meetings. A few organizations such as the predominantly black National Medical Association (but not the predominantly white American Medical Association) had started their own task forces.[45] Still, the speakers and attendees included a "who's who" of opinion leaders.

Governor Manning in his welcoming address honored, to applause, Babcock as "that man who sits among us and who is the father of the work in the treatment of pellagra."[46] Goldberger's paper was scheduled for the conference's second day. The first day's program contained two papers that presaged the eventual solution: "Vitamines and Pellagra" by Dr. Eugenio Bravetta of Italy and "The Rise in Cost of Food and the Alleged Increase in Prevalence of Pellagra" by Dr. Edgar Sydenstricker of the U.S. Public Health Service. Of interest to Goldberger was a summary of 200 cases of pellagra at the Epworth Orphanage in Columbia by Dr. Henry W. Rice. A child 9 years of age was much more likely to get pellagra than younger children, who got milk, or older children who, being expected to work, were more likely to get animal protein including lean meat. These data fit Goldberger's dietary hypothesis.[47]

The long and perhaps tedious first day concluded with an evening program at the Jefferson Hotel, consisting entirely of an update from the Thompson-McFadden Commission. MacNeal announced once more that the Spartanburg County data pointed away from a dietary etiology.[48] The fireworks began when MacNeal's paper became open for discussion.

Goldberger lit the first fuse: "Their [the Thompson-McFadden Commission's] very extensive dietary study ... failed to indicate the presence of either a pellagra-producing or a pellagra-preventing food in the mill village populations studied, and they express the opinion that no such things exist. Within the limits of time of this discussion it is of course impossible to go into details. All I can do, therefore, is to point out that by reason of the inadequacy of the method of analysis applied to their data, no conclusions whatever are permissible." And "as for the relation of pellagra to sewerage," Goldberger continued, "it need only be stated that this may [be] ... an instance of 'false correlation.'" Sydenstricker had implied the same thing: the privies were merely surrogate markers for low family income, which made preventative foodstuffs unaffordable.

Goldberger, like Carl Voegtlin the previous year, had stung MacNeal in a sensitive place. He like Voegtlin had accused MacNeal of faulty data analysis. Nor was Goldberger alone. Dr. Roy Blosser of Atlanta pointed out that while "Dr. MacNeal has presented a very clever lot of statistics," he had not taken into account "all the foods they [textile workers and their families] eat" and that "considering the immense amount of practical and experimental evidence we have to the effect that foods cause pellagra, it is absurd to attempt to formulate a new theory on such small evidence as has been brought forward by Dr. MacNeal."[49]

MacNeal sat silently taking notes. At last he rose to defend his methods. He cited a "little book by Davenport on Statistical Analysis" and offered "Dr. Goldberger the privilege of copying" his data. Compiling the data had been "an enormous amount of work," and it was necessary to "do something with the data besides theorize with it." MacNeal's tedious self-defense ended with an assertion that "the disease shows all the characteristics of ... transmissible disease and is, nevertheless, slightly contagious."[50] The animated discussion continued until one-thirty the next morning.

When the sleep-deprived delegates came down for breakfast they received a shock. On the front page of the *State*, wedged between stories about Mexican bandits along the Texas border and German advances in the Great War, appeared the headline, "CURING PELLAGRA BY DIET METHODS: Balanced Ration Needed to Stop Ravages; PROBLEM IN ECONOMY; Rise in Prices and Fall in Wages as Cause of Disease."[51] The story was based on a news release from *Public Health Reports* with the same dateline: October 22, 1915, a memorable day in the history of pellagra. Goldberger and his colleagues had just published the data from the two Mississippi orphanages and the two wards at the Milledgeville asylum.

Goldberger, with Drs. C. H. Waring and David G. Willets, reported that there had been 209 cases of pellagra at the two orphanages during the summer of 1914, but, since changing the diet, no new cases had occurred and only one patient had relapsed during a full year of follow-up. At the Milledgeville asylum none of 72 patients with pellagra relapsed during nine months on a balanced diet. Everything else had been kept the same at these closed institutions. Pellagra could be "prevented by an appropriate diet without any alteration in the environment, hygienic or sanitary."

Three points in this landmark report deserve emphasis. First, the authors claimed no originality except for designing and executing the studies. They cited a statement made forty-nine years earlier by the Frenchman Théophile Roussel that "Without dietetic measures *all remedies fail*."[52] Second, they faulted the Thompson-McFadden Commission for "the way in which they analyzed what is undoubtedly a very valuable mass of data." Finally, they had provided "those subject to pellagra with a diet such as that enjoyed by well-to-do people, who as a group are practically free from the disease." Society should "improve economic conditions; increase wages, reduce unemployment" and "make the other class of foods" (that is, other than carbohydrates) "cheap and readily accessible."[53] Therein lay the rub, or perhaps the *Simulium* fly or the stable fly in the ointment. Politicians, health officials, and taxpayers would prefer a solution that did not mandate broad social change and redistribution of wealth.

We can only imagine the buildup of excitement to Goldberger's paper, scheduled fourth that morning. When Goldberger finished, Siler conceded that "diet has a very great deal to do with pellagra," but restated the old argument that diet was merely "an important predisposing factor [to infection] bearing somewhat the relationship to pellagra that it does to tuberculosis." MacNeal again sat silently.

Babcock saw the gathering storm. He tried with his gentle humor to broker peace by alluding to John Godfrey Saxe's nineteenth-century version of an old fable:

Mr. Chairman, ladies and gentlemen: Possibly there will be nothing further to be said at this meeting upon the etiology of pellagra.

Some time ago Dr. Grimm of the United States Pellagra Hospital at Spartanburg, called my attention to a poem by Saxe. That poem, I think, should be learned by all students of the pellagra problem. I am very sorry I have not the poem with me, but you will all remember it better if you look it up yourselves. It is entitled, "The Eight Blind Men of Hindoostan." These eight blind men were each assigned as committees of one to report upon the elephant. The first blind man went out and examined the elephant's tail and came back with the information that the elephant was a rope. The second one, after examining its ears reported that there was no doubt about it, the elephant was a fan; the next man examined the elephant's leg and said that the elephant was undoubtedly a tree, and so on. Saxe said that each was partly in the right, yet all were in the wrong.

Gentlemen, I am satisfied if we learn the meaning of the poem of the Blind Men of Hindoostan, we shall all continue to study the great problem of pellagra with humility and with great respect for our fellow-workers.[54]

Adams Hayne then rose and immediately quashed Babcock's gentle plea for mutual respect among pellagra researchers.

Hayne had committed to the idea of an insect-borne infectious disease in 1912 if not earlier.[55] He was unimpressed by Goldberger's dietary experiments for "if you can give a man food in proper proportions, in such a way that he can assimilate it . . . you will strengthen his resistance and make him throw off the disease." Hayne insisted that "I am not trying to argue the cause of pellagra, but am simply stating that we can argue that a good, well balanced diet will help to cure pellagra, and possibly by making a person more resistant to disease . . . but don't let's put that down as the etiology. We are going round and round in a circle, and getting nowhere."[56] He made the valid point that if "you tell the health officer that the way to stop the thing is to make the whole people of the whole State change their mode of living, you will put a proposition up to him that is almost impossible." He would "much prefer dealing with the kind [of problem] he is accustomed to dealing with"—namely, communicable diseases.[57] Hayne withdrew his scheduled paper on "The Communicability of Pellagra." He and other southern health officers increasingly sided with MacNeal and the Thompson-McFadden Commission against Goldberger.

As the conference drew to a close Frederick Williams tried like Babcock to add a dash of humor: "I wish to make the suggestion: that before the meeting three years hence, that ... [pellagra researchers] thrash out and recommend the way to pronounce this disease. I have heard several different pronunciations and I would like to hear the proper way to pronounce it."[58] The "meeting three years hence" never took place. Williams had just made the last recorded comment at the National Association for the Study of Pellagra except for a motion to adjourn.

Goldberger left Columbia with grounds for optimism despite opposition from MacNeal, Hayne, and a few others. The *State* reported that many and perhaps most participants were "inclined to the theory of a possible error in diet."[59] Goldberger had identified two potential collaborators: Dr. Henry Rice of Columbia, whose studies at Epworth Orphanage held promise, and Dr. Carl A. Grote of Jasper, Alabama, a county health officer whose paper on "Diet as Cause and Cure" amounted to a demonstration project on how to rid a community of pellagra by diet alone.[60] From Columbia Goldberger went to Spartanburg and wrote his wife: "I have been very decidedly busy and I have much to tell you but will only write this [—] that 'Diet' wins by a large majority. We have the 'enemy' beat and they have half owned up in a public meeting. My fears that the 'conference' would bring about confusion and that it was therefore ill-timed proved to be wrong. Lavinder tells me that he was also afraid; in fact, he says that he was nervous about it until I read my paper. That he said 'did the business'; it spiked all the heavy artillery. In fact Dr. Hayne, the State Health Officer and one of the 'heavy artillery' for 'infection' withdrew his paper and bleated very gently when his turn to 'shoot' came around. To sum up: Dr. Lavinder congratulated me on 'putting it down.'"[61] The *State* congratulated Goldberger for his "practical demonstration of the ease with which pellagra can be prevented from occurring in institutions which have suffered severely, by the simple expedient of supplying a generous and nutritious diet to the inmates."[62]

Results from the Rankin Farm redoubled Goldberger's optimism. On October 29 he told his wife that prison volunteers were now getting pellagra.[63] Within two weeks he reported, with Dr. George Wheeler, that after six months on the test diet six of the eleven volunteers had features of pellagra including a rash that, interestingly, began on the scrotum. Two physicians experienced in pellagra confirmed the diagnosis. Two dermatologists excluded other causes of rash.[64] An editorialist praised Goldberger's gift of "a practical means of prevention and cure."[65]

Goldberger had now prevented and also caused pellagra by dietary manipulation. He had kept everything else the same at the two orphanages, the two asylum wards, and the Rankin Farm. All that remained was to identify the essential dietary substance(s), and, in the meantime, to convince

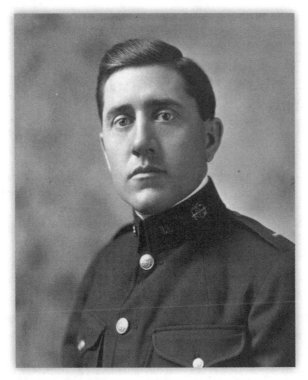

Dr. George Alexander Wheeler (1885–1981) worked with Goldberger on numerous projects, including the Rankin Farm experiment (in which prisoners developed pellagra on a restricted diet), the South Carolina upstate studies (demonstrating the correlation of pellagra with poverty), the canine "black tongue" demonstrations, and the prevention of pellagra at Epworth Orphanage in Columbia.
Courtesy: National Library of Medicine

people to drink more milk and to eat more meat, eggs, leafy vegetables, and other wholesome foods.[66]

Sambon's Sad Legacy

Goldberger's optimism was premature. He underestimated the backlash to his conclusion that poverty was the root cause. The result was tragic for thousands of Americans, most of them southerners. Although pellagra deaths fell precipitously after Goldberger's 1915 breakthrough, they increased during the mid-1920s, peaked during 1928, and became uncommon to rare only

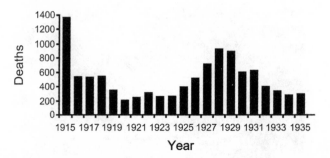

The annual number of deaths due to pellagra in South Carolina fell dramatically after Goldberger's 1915 report that poor diet was the main cause. However, deaths due to pellagra increased between 1925 and 1928, probably due to some combination of declining cotton prices and the boll weevil. These data come from the South Carolina State Board of Health, as tabulated by Milling, "Pellagra and the New Deal."

after food fortification with niacin became standard practice beginning in the late 1930s.[67] The backlash ultimately traces, in the present author's opinion, to the forcefulness of Louis Sambon's arguments that pellagra was an insect-borne infectious disease.

Reactions to Goldberger's "inconvenient truth" continue to fascinate social historians. Elizabeth Etheridge calls pellagra "an unappreciated reminder of Southern distinctiveness."[68] Mary Katherine Crabb describes "an epidemic of pride," an "irrational Southern response ... specifically related to the cultural identity and values of the South at this time."[69] Elizabeth Chacko tells how the discovery of the precise cause of pellagra and the implementation of control measures were delayed by "the conception of the South as the regional Other by Northern interests, a reluctance to acknowledge widespread deprivations in the region by Southern leaders, compounded by inadequate scrutiny of the racial and gender dimensions of the disease."[70] In 1921 health officials throughout the cotton belt opposed President Warren G. Harding's campaign for federal aid to relieve pellagra, denying that a crisis existed.[71] Congressman James F. Byrnes of South Carolina led the political assault on Goldberger, calling reports of southern poverty and hunger an "utter absurdity." Byrnes declined in advance an offer from the Red Cross to provide emergency aid.[72]

All of this makes good reading, and future historians might wish to compare and contrast the response to Goldberger's breakthrough in the early twentieth-century American South with denials in other times and places of the inconvenient truths of medical science, since, at least qualitatively,

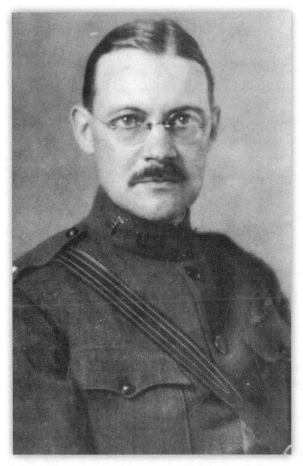

Captain Edward Bright Vedder (1878–1952) of the U.S. Army, an authority on
beriberi, worked briefly with the Thompson-McFadden Commission in 1916 and
wrote in favor of the dietary-deficiency hypothesis.
Courtesy: National Institutes of Health.

the response to Goldberger was not unique.[73] However, the focus here is
to conclude the story of James Woods Babcock and pellagra during his
lifetime, with three points of emphasis. First, those who opposed Goldberger's inconvenient truth drew their simulacrum of scientific legitimacy mainly
from the Thompson-McFadden Commission. As Michael Flannery points
out, the commission's reports "would be recited by Goldberger's opponents
like a well-worn catechism of faith."[74] Second, the opposition's tenacity
compelled Goldberger to spend much of 1916–22 strengthening the case
for diet and against infection. Finally, Goldberger's need to disprove the

Thompson-McFadden Commission almost certainly helped delay his demonstrating the curative and preventative power of brewer's yeast.

Ward MacNeal, his ego on the line, led the scientific counterattack on Goldberger. In early 1916 MacNeal challenged the diagnosis of pellagra in the Rankin Farm volunteers and even accused Goldberger of faking the results. In 1917 he brought out the Thompson-McFadden Commission's third and final report, a 454-page tome in which Goldberger isn't even mentioned.[75] The third report does, however, contain one article supporting dietary deficiency, written by U.S. Army Captain Edward Vedder. Vedder had studied beriberi and correctly saw the analogy with pellagra.[76] The last two articles in the third report consist of blame-the-victim studies on the role of heredity in pellagra by two eugenicists from Cold Spring Harbor, Long Island.[77] Allan Chase in *The Legacy of Malthus* calls the third Thompson-McFadden report "the medical fraud of the century," the centerpiece of the "Great Pellagra Cover-Up of 1916–33, which kept the medical benefit of Goldberger's work on pellagra from the entire nation for two decades."[78] Southern health officials, politicians, and others who preferred to deny that poverty caused pellagra had a champion in Ward J. MacNeal.

Goldberger had to respond. He devised studies of three general types. He exposed sixteen volunteers (including himself and his wife) to skin scales, blood, nasopharyngeal secretions, urine, and feces from pellagrins to buttress the case against infection. He coordinated labor-intensive field studies in mill villages in the South Carolina upstate to show that privies were merely surrogate markers of poverty.[79] He studied the effect of better diet in additional closed institutions. In January 1916 Goldberger wrote his wife that he was going to Columbia "to look at things there." He was especially interested in the Epworth Orphanage, where he and his new collaborator Henry Rice sought to eliminate pellagra with diet.[80]

One of Goldberger's best-known experiments, possibly his most famous, took place in April 1916 at the South Carolina State Hospital for the Insane.[81] From three pellagrins he took specimens of skin scales, urine, and liquid feces. He added wheat flour, rolled the mixture into pill-sized pellets—and swallowed the pellets, feces and all. The only side-effect was a self-limited case of diarrhea.[82]

On August 3, 1916, Goldberger wrote his wife: "I finished at Columbia yesterday. The orphanage [Epworth] is absolutely free of pellagra, the first time since the discovery of the disease there in 1908. I must confess that I had a little grippy "thrilly" feeling as I surveyed the place on leaving. The most skeptical must and will be impressed. Even Dr. Hayne told us that he is absolutely convinced that we can prevent pellagra!"[83] In December 1916

Goldberger asked his wife to include "Dr. and Mrs. J. W. Babcock, Columbia" on a list of ten persons to whom Christmas cards should be sent.[84]

The extent to which Goldberger and Babcock subsequently interacted is unclear, but Goldberger was often in South Carolina because of the field studies in the South Carolina upstate. These preoccupations almost surely delayed his exploitation of a new animal model: black tongue in dogs. It was not until 1925 that Goldberger and his colleagues reported that dried brewer's yeast, milk, and meat contained a pellagra-preventative factor or "factor P-P" (later named "vitamin G" in Goldberger's honor and now known as niacin).[85]

Two key observations were made in 1916, nearly a decade before Goldberger published on brewer's yeast. The first of these was a suggestion by a Concord, North Carolina, veterinarian that "black tongue" in dogs—characterized by severe inflammation of the mouth, gums, and teeth, weight loss, bloody diarrhea, and death—might be a canine analogue of human pellagra.[86] The following year two Yale University physiologists, Russell Chittenden and Frank Underhill, reported that they had caused a severe illness in dogs resembling human pellagra by feeding them a diet of boiled peas, cracker meal, and cottonseed oil or lard. Meat was curative.[87] Veterinarians soon suspected that black tongue and the Chittenden-Underhill syndrome were one and the same. At last there was an animal model for pellagra.

The second key 1916 observation was reported by Atherton Seidell, a biochemist working at the National Hygienic Laboratory in Washington, D.C., who formulated a vitamin preparation using brewer's yeast and suggested it might be tried in pellagra.[88] Later that year, Dr. Edward Jenner Wood of Wilmington, North Carolina, seconded the idea that Seidell's preparation should be tried in pellagrins.[89] Seidel's observation anticipated the wide use of brewer's yeast as a cost-effective therapeutic and preventative measure.

The story of pellagra during these years—that is, between 1915 and 1925—presents numerous complexities, involving as it does the question "what did they know and when did they know it?"[90] The Great War distracted many researchers, including Goldberger, who between September 1918 and April 1919 was assigned to work on influenza. But it was not until 1922 that Goldberger and his colleagues began to publish on black tongue in dogs. On the basis of autopsies on two Chesapeake Bay retrievers, with the assistance of a Spartanburg veterinarian, they confirmed to their satisfaction that black tongue and the Chittenden-Underhill syndrome were probably the same disease.[91] The contention here is that Goldberger might

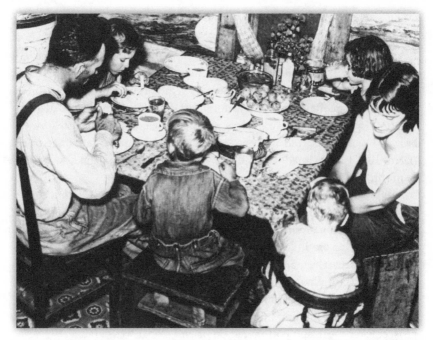

Textile workers and others in the South were reconciled to a diet based on the "three Ms"—meat (mainly fatback), meal (from degerminated corn), and molasses. The person most likely to get pellagra in this family would be the mother, since the father as breadwinner would get what little meat they could afford and the growing children would get the milk. Goldberger estimated that about 70 percent of pellagrins were adult women.
Courtesy: National Library of Medicine.

have tried brewer's yeast for canine black tongue and then human pellagra much sooner had he not felt obliged to show MacNeal and the Thompson-McFadden Commission wrong.[92] Goldberger's studies of the social and economic determinants of pellagra rank among the best studies of their kind—classics for students of public health[93]—but why were these studies even necessary? The pressing need was to find a cost-effective alternative to "the diet of the well-to-do."

A few southern physicians openly supported Goldberger.[94] However, general opinion among historians holds that Goldberger and his small team enjoyed little support from other doctors. In theory the National Association for the Study of Pellagra might have helped. The association could have continued to serve as a triennial clearinghouse for ideas and, more importantly, to foster fellowship and good will among researchers. However, the association had lost its momentum. Toward the end of the 1915 meeting Joseph Siler told members that "you have made a horrible mistake in electing me your presiding officer."[95] Siler also confessed: "I came down here in a very pessimistic frame of mind so far as pellagra is concerned. Seeing Dr. Babcock again and hearing the many excellent papers . . . put new life into me."[96] But to be an effective president Siler would have had to stand up to Ward MacNeal's bruised ego. It was probably to Siler's relief that he was made commander of the Laboratory Service of the American Expeditionary Forces in France. Babcock, for his part, had neither time nor resources to maintain the National Association for the Study of Pellagra. He preferred to avoid confrontation and to spend his energies where he might make a difference, as he had done throughout his life. He therefore focused on treating patients and teaching students. He started but did not complete the task of assembling the manuscripts from the 1915 meeting for publication, as had been done for the 1909 and 1912 national conferences.[97]

MacNeal never conceded. In 1922 he published on "The Infectious Etiology of Pellagra" and in a thinly veiled reference to Goldberger asserted

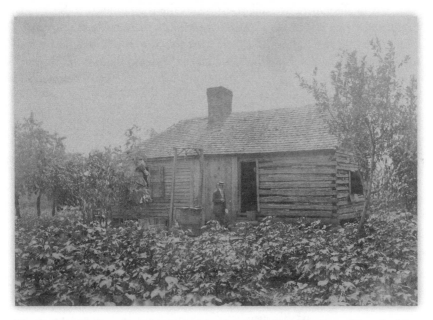

The rural poor often planted cotton right up to their front doors as shown in this photograph of a South Carolina sharecropper's house. Replacement of vegetable gardens with cotton contributed to pellagra in the South.
Courtesy: South Caroliniana Library, University of South Carolina, Columbia, S.C.

that "even public health officials make serious mistakes."[98] Public health measures—changing the eating habits of textile workers and their families and getting the rural poor to plant vegetables instead of cotton around their homes—lagged woefully behind. Even after Goldberger demonstrated the value of brewer's yeast, vigorous debate about the cause of pellagra continued until the late 1930s, when the preventative and curative value of niacin was finally demonstrated.[99]

Three observations should be made in defense of MacNeal and the others who opposed Goldberger.

First, today's powerful statistical methods were unavailable to that era's researchers. They did not enjoy, for example, software packages for multiple-variable linear regression analysis, which reduces the likelihood of false correlations ("confounders") such as the Spartanburg County privies. Now-familiar research protocols such as the case-control study and the prospective, randomized, placebo-controlled, double-blinded trial were rudimentary, if they existed at all.[100] And the argument that "the diet of the well-to-do" merely protected against infection still appeals to common sense; rapid weight loss impairs immunity even with adequate vitamin intake.

Second, Goldberger's studies, especially the Rankin Farm experiments, were not beyond legitimate scientific criticism. The eleven Mississippi prison volunteers did not uniformly develop the striking, nearly diagnostic rash on sun-exposed areas (notably, "Casál's necklace" and the rash on the back surfaces of the hands and feet). Keeping the volunteers indoors limited sun exposure, later shown necessary for full expression of pellagra and especially the rash.[101] Also, he had allowed the volunteers to drink coffee twice daily. As Nobel laureate Konrad Bloch points out, roasted coffee contains substantial amounts of nicotinic acid, which may have blunted the symptoms and signs of pellagra.[102] And MacNeal was correct in questioning whether the scrotal rashes represented pellagra, since we now know that scrotal rash is more typical of riboflavin (vitamin B_2) deficiency.

Finally, and most obviously, the vitamin-deficiency paradigm was new, while the germ theory—illustrative of efforts throughout history to find a unifying cause of all disease—was not. Early-twentieth-century researchers were understandably enthralled by the germ theory. Great reputations were to be won. As Daphne Roe observes: "Sambon's theory was not considered as illogical in his time as it is today."[103]

However, since Roe and Elizabeth Etheridge wrote their social histories of pellagra four decades ago, historians' perspectives on the germ theory have become more nuanced. The germ theory evolved and continues to evolve in the context of specific times, places, and diseases.[104] The histories of pellagra and beriberi have much in common (Appendix 2), but the impact of the germ theory was more pernicious in the case of pellagra—largely because of Sambon's novel idea about *Simulium* flies and an unidentified parasite. And since Roe and Etheridge wrote their histories much has come to light about Louis Sambon.

In 1904 Sambon presented on "The Elucidation of Sleeping Sickness" to the Epidemiological Society of London. A discussant politely challenged his claims for priority in "one or two matters." Sir Ronald Ross, who had received the Nobel Prize for proving that *Anopheles* mosquitoes transmit malaria, wrote in the margin of his copy: "This paper is full of carefully constructed falsifications in the true Italian manner. I have thrown away most of it as rubbish."[105] Sambon left sleeping sickness and turned to pellagra.

Sambon's elaborate hypothesis, combined with his stage presence and influence on Joseph Siler, triggered a series of events that led to the formation of the Thompson-McFadden Commission (see Chapter 5). Ward MacNeal's opposition to the dietary-deficiency hypothesis began with his commitment to Sambon's ideas, persisted despite the Thompson-McFadden Commission's failure to show transmission by *Simulium* flies, and accelerated after Voeghtlin, Goldberger, and others criticized his methods of data analysis and therefore his conclusions. Those opposed to the inconvenient truth that poverty was the root cause of pellagra could thank MacNeal, but their ultimate benefactor was Louis Westerna Sambon.

As it turns out, Sambon had two employers during those years. The London School of Tropical Medicine hired him as a lecturer. Henry Wellcome, the American-born London pharmaceutical magnate, hired him as a collecting agent during Wellcome's successful quest to build the world's largest museum of medical artifacts. Sambon enticed Wellcome to help finance his pellagra research. Sambon, according to fellow collector Charles Thompson, took advantage of Wellcome's good faith. Sambon began spending less time seeking artifacts for Wellcome and more time seeking personal glory through pellagra research. Thompson wrote: "From a long observation of Dr. Sambon's manner of work, I may point out that his chief drawback is a lack of staying power, and no method whatever, and there is the greatest difficulty in keeping him concentrated on any branch of work, even for a few days. It is in these points that failure is to be expected in carrying the investigation to a successful result."[106] The last correspondence pertaining to Sambon at the Wellcome Archives in London consists of letters written to him requesting immediate return of borrowed books and a camera.[107]

An historian of the London School of Tropical Medicine writes that Sambon's dashing around Europe and the United States claiming he had "proved" pellagra transmission by a *Simulium* fly seriously damaged his reputation. Undaunted, Sambon next tried to prove that cancer is caused by parasites after learning that a nematode parasite spread by cockroaches caused malignant tumors in rats. He used the same technique he had used for pellagra: constructing maps of where the disease occurred in Italy. The same historian adds that Sambon "had all the failings of a minor prophet."[108]

On August 30, 1931, Louis Sambon collapsed and died in a Paris café. A colleague wrote in the *British Medical Journal* that "the world of medicine has lost one of its brightest ornaments."[109] More perceptively the *Lancet* observed that although his ideas were seldom confirmed he "obtained ... considerable support for his views, of the correctness of which he always remained certain."[110] Some Britons saw through him but most Americans, unfortunately, did not.

"The Dreams of our Youth"

Babcock unlike Sambon prized service above showmanship to the end. His last years largely concerned his practice in Columbia, his voluntary teaching in Charleston, and his family, including the education of his daughters. His notebooks confirm that he remained a diligent student, seeking practical knowledge to help sick people. It does not seem too grandiose to say that he honored the ideals expressed in his presidential address to the Golden Branch at Phillips Exeter to be "of future usefulness" consistent with the "dreams of our youth" (see Chapter 1).

His notebooks demonstrate familiarity with new ideas in psychiatry and psychology by such Europeans as Sigmund Freud, Carl Jung, Alfred Adler, Pierre Janet, and Richard Krafft-Ebing and such Americans as Adolph Meyer and Morton Prince. His lecture notes for medical students and nurses document a carefully thought-out curriculum. He took the learners through categories of normal and abnormal mental processes: perception, consciousness, delusions, train-of-thought, volition, emotion, memory, and attention, defining basic concepts and even the idea of "the concept." He discussed dreams in terms that are now commonplace but were then part of the emerging psychoanalysis: "The dream is autosymbolic, i.e., it represents or solves symbolically some present mental conflict, not necessarily sexual, and past, very often infantile, experiences ... (Jung). According to Adler the conflict thus represented is usually between a real or supposed inferiority and a wish for greater power or superiority." He reviewed treatment modalities, including drugs, suggestion, isolation, psychoanalysis (including word association and dream analysis), occupation, and hypnosis, which he apparently did not favor. He warned against excessive use of diagnostic labels: "I am more and more concerned of the viciousness of making a diagnosis … the object of the examination. Too frequently, as soon as the name is given all interest ceases. If, on the contrary, the object is to try to find out the meaning of the patient's behavior, what he is trying to do, there is no more arbitrary limitation of interest." Focus not so much on the disease as on the *patient* with the disease—timeless advice for medical students and doctors.[111]

His growing interest in forensic psychiatry centered on the insanity defense. One of his daughters recorded that "dozens of small notebooks" contained interviews with "men and boys held for murder or other criminal charge."[112] He testified, for example, in the case of Hugh T. Bramlett, a contractor and member of a prominent Greenville, South Carolina, family, who in 1919 shot his mother-in-law and claimed that she had humiliated him to the extent that he was not responsible for his actions. Babcock examined Bramlett six times and declared him insane. The state introduced a score of witnesses to rebut charges of insanity. Bramlett was found guilty but the State Supreme Court later ruled a mistrial.[113]

Pellagra continued to be Babcock's special disease. His collection of reprints and notebooks is probably unsurpassed.[114] He recorded pellagra among troops during the Great War, "especially among those from countries in which the disease has long been recognized, such as Italy, Egypt, and adjoining Mediterranean territory." He consulted on cases at Camp Jackson (now Fort Jackson) near Columbia "in soldiers who had been passed by Southern examining boards." He observed that Italian physicians remained "divided on the subject of the etiology of pellagra," accepting neither Goldberger's nor Sambon's hypotheses. He was invariably nonjudgmental about others' opinions.

He nonetheless expressed his ideas on causation in an undated manuscript entitled "Treatment of Pellagra." Like nearly all of his contemporaries he stopped short of completely endorsing Goldberger's hypothesis, holding that "the cause of pellagra is complex and variable." However, he clearly grasped the essence of the vitamin-deficiency hypothesis and the role of monotonous diet: "Of these complex and variable causes in Italy and the United States we now suspect that alcohol may be one. In time the other causes may be affirmed; corn in Italy, Egypt, Rumania and the Southern States; oatmeal in the Northern States, Canada, England, and Scotland; sugar in Panama; beefsteak in St. Louis, beans in New Mexico, bacon in South Carolina, and oil in Atlanta; or whatever the monotonous dietary may be that fails to supply the ultimate vitamins or other elements necessary for

the maintenance of nutritive equilibrium." Based on what we know now—
that pellagra usually occurs in the setting of malnutrition with deficiencies of
multiple vitamins—he was prescient in his observation that the "variability
in the symptoms of pellagra in different localities and in different seasons
within the same localities may be associated with this variety of unbalanced
diets with their respective vitamins."[115]

He kept up with friends, including Tillman. The April 1917 issue of
Physical Culture contained an article by Tillman on "How I Restored my
Health and Vigor" in which he described a "congressional disease" brought
on by "eating [too much] and exercising too little."Tillman advised drinking
hot water, eating two meals a day with no snacking in between, deep breath-
ing, and walking two to three miles every day. "During my life," he wrote, "I
have been fortunate in having had the services of exceptionally good physicians; but I have come to believe that even these men, admirably educated
and trained professionally, did not know some of the things that I have been
learning in recent years."[116] Tillman died the next year, on July 3, 1918, after
a brain hemorrhage. Babcock wrote the inscription for his tombstone.

On August 11, 1921, his sixty-fifth birthday, Babcock visited his parents'
graves in Chester and requested he be buried there. In late December he
had a bad attack of influenza but recovered. In late February he developed
heart trouble, probably a myocardial infarction, which confined him largely
to bed. On March 3, 1922, he had a severe attack of chest pain and died.

His death was widely noted. The *State* called him "easily one of the best
known and most cultured physicians of South Carolina," who was "almost
to the hour of his death a diligent student in his chosen line or work and
was held in the highest regard by persons familiar with his scholarly attainments."[117] The *New York World* saluted him for identifying pellagra,[118] and
the *Boston Herald* observed that "such men as Dr. Babcock are an asset for
the welfare of the race."[119] The *Revista Pellagrologica Italiana* called him
"the first to recognize pellagra in the United States and to identify it with
Italian pellagra; but he had to struggle long and suffer many bitter checks
before the truth announced by him was imposed on the American medical
world and pellagra came to form part of official pathology."[120] The *American
Journal of Psychiatry* called him "*the* alienist of South Carolina," "the man who
identified pellagra in the United States," and a "close observer and accurate
diagnostician ... [who was] the sympathetic friend and adviser of every
physician with a difficult mental case through a large part of the Southland,
and after a consultation, was quite apt to send a reprint covering the case ...
. Generous to a fault, public spirited, kind, the friend of every one in trouble,
irrespective of race, color, creed or position in society, a man whom other men

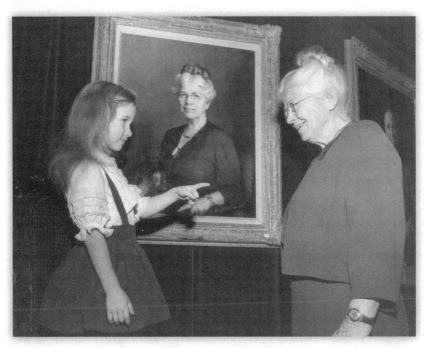

Dr. Connie Myers Guion (1882–1971), Babcock's sister-in-law, became the first female clinical professor of medicine in the United States and was described in the *New Yorker* as "the dean of women doctors in this country." A pavilion was dedicated in her honor at the New York Hospital.
Courtesy: Medical Center Archives of New York-Presbyterian/Weill Cornell.

loved."[121] The *Harvard Graduates' Magazine* reported: "Few Harvard men in the South have attained greater distinction or done more useful work."[122] His patient George Manly, who had done so many translations for him, wrote Kate Babcock that he "was one of those great hearted and forward looking men who sees the needs of those around them and delights in lending a helping hand and in working for the uplift of the community."[123]

Postscripts

Babcock's niece Connie Guion, whom he helped inspire to be a doctor, became one of her era's most distinguished and beloved physicians. She was the first woman in the United States to be named clinical professor of medicine. The *New Yorker* called her "the dean of women doctors in this country."[124] A social chronicle of New York City called her "a character

such as can only thrive in our city" who "treated entire families of Vander-
bilts, Whitneys, and Astors [who] were glad to be the victims of her old-
fashioned no-nonsense methods."[125] Her long and distinguished affiliation
with Cornell Medical College and the New York Hospital was recognized
in the naming of a new outpatient building. Also named for her was a new
science building at Sweet Briar College, where she had taught chemistry
before going to medical school.[126] She practiced medicine well into her
eighties, until her health failed.

Eleanora Saunders went from Columbia to Washington, D.C., where
she earned a Doctor of Philosophy degree from George Washington University while working at St. Elizabeth's Hospital. She then went to Towson,
Maryland, in greater Baltimore, where she spent the rest of her career at the

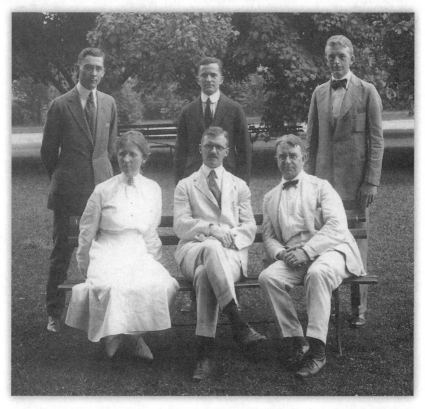

Dr. Eleanora Bennette Saunders (1883–1933), shown here in 1920 with other
medical staff members at the Sheppard and Enoch Pratt Hospital in Baltimore,
enjoyed a distinguished career after leaving South Carolina.
Courtesy: Sheppard Pratt Health System, Inc., Baltimore, Maryland.

Sheppard and Enoch Pratt Hospital. A history of that institution relates that she "lived for her work," was "self-effacing, a delightful companion with a happy sense of humor," and "of real assistance to the junior physicians, over whom she had general supervision."[127] She contributed to the psychiatric literature and wrote articles for laypersons such as "The Sick Person," "Psychiatry and Occupation," and "The Emotional Handicaps of Professional Women." Her last major scientific paper dealt with depression in old age.[128] She died of cancer at age 50 at the hospital where she worked.

Ernest Cooper, the earliest victim of James Thompson's conspiracy, left private practice in 1915 to become superintendent of a new sanatorium for tuberculosis on the State Park campus. He stayed there and is considered one of South Carolina's pioneers in the control of tuberculosis.[129]

James Thompson, long-time assistant physician at the state asylum, apparently spent the rest of his career in the medical records department. In his memoirs, written when he was nearly eighty, he said of Nora Saunders that she "was progressive in her work, always to the front of anything new . . . . It was remarkable the amount of work she accomplished. However, she did not get along with some members of the staff, and, unfortunately, she had backers in this matter and that increased the trouble. Dr. Babcock let her have full control over her work and never questioned the results, hence the friction with other members of the staff brought on an investigation, which resulted in Dr. Saunders and Dr. Babcock resigning."[130] Thompson conveniently overlooked his role as instigator of the conspiracy that triggered the infamous kangaroo court.

Claude Lavinder spent the rest of his career as chief medical officer at various Marine Hospitals of the U.S. Public Health Service. In 1916, while serving at the Marine Hospital on Ellis Island in New York, he was called to examine orphanages in three Southern states, one of which was in Columbia, South Carolina, for cases of pellagra.[131] Also that year he became involved in the great epidemic of poliomyelitis ("polio") that swept the northeastern United States. He worked with the famous epidemiologist Wade Hampton Frost and was senior author on the final report, now considered a classic.[132]

Joseph Siler enjoyed a productive career in the U.S. Army. During World War I he worked on typhoid vaccine, increased the number and the quality of the Army's laboratories, and taught medical officers how to deal with war-related medical and surgical problems. It was largely through his efforts that thousands of American physicians were exposed to the newer aspects of laboratory medicine. When they returned home they demanded laboratories for their hospitals. Siler received the Army's Distinguished Service Medal.[133] After the war he went back to the Philippines to resume his studies of dengue. He successfully transmitted dengue to U.S. Army volunteers by injecting the virus and thereby "closed the loop" in how this mosquito-borne disease is transmitted.[134] Siler's fellow U.S. Army researcher Edward Vedder, the pioneering beriberi researcher who was among the first to propose that pellagra was a vitamin-deficiency disease, likewise enjoyed a productive career as a U.S. Army medical researcher. When a new U.S. Army hospital (now a part of the Walter Reed Army Medical Center) was completed in 1932, one of the four pavilions was named for Siler and another for Vedder.

Ward MacNeal stayed at the New York Post-Graduate Medical School and Hospital as an infectious diseases researcher. He studied antibiotics and became an authority on bacterial viruses (bacteriophage).

Eight persons received Nobel Prizes for vitamin-related discoveries, and seven additional persons who worked on vitamin B_{12} received the prize for other contributions.[135] Christiaan Eijkman won the Nobel Prize for discovering an animal model of beriberi. Gowland Hopkins received the Nobel Prize for his work with "accessory food factors." Nobody received a Nobel Prize for discoveries related to pellagra or niacin, the deficient vitamin. Casimir Funk was bitter that Hopkins got more credit than he did. Hopkins suggested during his 1929 Nobel Prize acceptance speech that nobody really "discovered" the vitamins but that Funk had perhaps criticized him unfairly. Goldberger was nominated but passed over for the Nobel Prize several times, perhaps because the committee preferred to honor discoveries of new knowledge rather than applications of previously discovered knowledge.

Joseph Goldberger died on January 17, 1929, of an illness undiagnosed during life but found at autopsy to be carcinoma of the kidney. The front-page news story in the *State* called him an "Outstanding Contributor to Medical Science, Notably in Conquest of Pellagra."[136] He had come close to identifying the causative vitamin (see Appendix 3).

Babcock's friends formed a Babcock Psychological Club that met at Gittman's Book Shop on Main Street in Columbia, where his photographic portrait hung for years after his death. One of the members, Henry Bella-mann, later wrote the novel *King's Row* (1942), in which a thinly disguised Babcock appears in the character of Dr. Thaddeus Nolan.[137]

King's Row, which was made into a movie starring Ann Sheridan, Robert Cummings, and future President Ronald Reagan, depicts cruelty and mental instability in small-town America. (Reagan's character wakes up from an operation to find that a sadistic surgeon has amputated both of his legs. He exclaims, "Where's the rest of me!"—a line Reagan used for the title of his autobiography.) Dr. Nolan, patterned after Babcock, "had the face of a wise man, and a kind one," and was "a really great man in his position," a "fine,

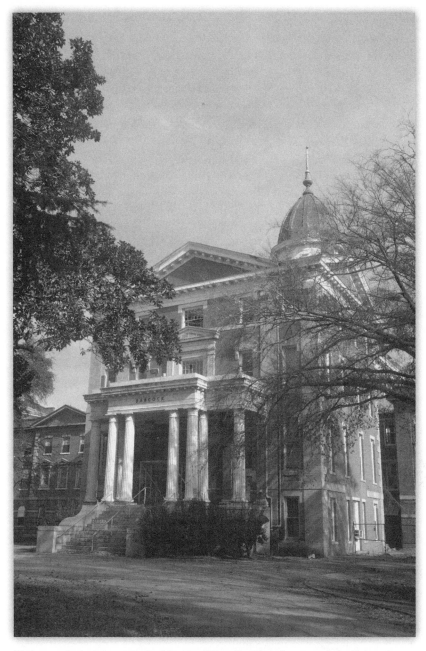

The central administration building or "New Building," renamed the Babcock Building, awaits restoration at the time of this writing. (Author photograph, with permission from the South Carolina Department of Mental Health.)

intelligent humanitarian."[138] Late in the novel the main character, Parris Mitchell, is a staff physician at the State Hospital for the Insane. When he is falsely accused of wrongdoing, Parris discusses his plight with Dr. Nolan:

> "It gives me a very strange feeling, Dr. Nolan, to think that anyone is 'after' me."
>
> "Yes, yes. That's natural. You'll get used to it the longer you remain in the service of the state."
>
> The undertone of irony and bitterness was strange and surprising coming from Dr. Nolan. Parris raised his eyebrows inquiringly.
>
> Dr. Nolan continued. "They 'honor' you with a state appointment. The work is harder than private work; the pay is far less. Then they sit back and watch for the first chance to get something on you."
>
> Parris started to speak, but Dr. Nolan interrupted. "Fact. They always speak of these 'soft state jobs' with 'good state money.' Well, I suppose it's a point of view. The doctors, even in a town with a state institution, are not very kind toward the staff doctors. Institutional work has advantages, of course, from a professional angle, but from any worldly consideration we have poor jobs, and we have to prove our rights to hold them after they're given to us. Now that's one side of the picture."

Bellamann, who came to Columbia in 1915 when Babcock was still smarting from the 1913–14 legislative investigation, probably heard the story of how Nora Saunders's determination to do Wassermann tests on her patients became Babcock's opponents' "first chance to get something" on him.

Kate Guion kept Waverley Sanitarium running smoothly until shortly before her death in 1943. She was succeeded by one of her daughters, Ferebe, and then by a grandson, Arthur Simons. Advertisements through the mid-1930s read in part: "Especial care given pellagrins."[139] In 1969 changing times forced Waverley's closure.[140] Simons donated the building to the Midlands Association for Retarded Children, begun two years earlier by Mary L. Duffie to provide daycare for children with special needs.[141] The organization, developed along the "cottage plan" (scattered buildings each housing small numbers of patients), was renamed the Babcock Center in honor of James and Kate Babcock and their daughter, Ferebe. One suspects Babcock would have been pleased to know that a cottage-plan facility for the disadvantaged bears his name.

The asylum property in downtown Columbia was eventually sold to a real estate developer. At the time of this writing the Babcock Building, formerly the "Main Building" or the "New Building," awaits renovation.

Perspective:
Asylum Doctor

IN 1930 TWO GRADUATE STUDENTS, one at the University of South Carolina and the other at the University of Chicago, chose the South Carolina State Hospital for their master's degree theses. The South Carolina student wrote of Babcock: "When it is considered how little he had to work with, his accomplishments at the hospital deserve much praise."[1] The Chicago student wrote: "Although Dr. Babcock was well-prepared for the position as chief officer of the institution, there was a marked lack of progress made during the twenty-two years of his administration. He displayed the qualities of the student, the historian, but failed at managing the institution."[2]

These opposite conclusions drawn from the same facts remind that we are all subject to observer bias, prisoners of the prevailing paradigms of our times and places to a greater extent than we'd like to think. Future generations, if they remember us at all, will see us differently than our contemporaries see us. Historians and biographers necessarily bring to their work preconceived ideas and—as the story of pellagra attests—so do scientists and clinicians. The present author read as a second-year medical student that "we must not explore the chest by percussing our ideas into it."[3] He later heard on the wards that "we see what we look for and we look for what we know."

Truisms aside, the present author confesses his inability to serve as an impartial judge or jury member in the case of James Woods Babcock, sharing too many career parallels and personality traits with his subject. He has sought to give readers enough facts to reach their own conclusions, especially in such hypersensitive areas as racial and gender disparities in health care. The following perspectives on Babcock in three areas—as an administrator, as a leader in the response to the pellagra epidemic, and as an exemplar of character traits worthy of emulation or avoidance, which is perhaps the ultimate purpose of biography, are proffered as merely that: one person's perspectives, with which readers may disagree, without argument.

Babcock as Administrator

Babcock's career as asylum superintendent serves up a cautionary tale for anyone aspiring to senior management without suitable training and temperament.[4] He accepted the job against better judgment after weighing his limitations against the opportunity to make a difference in his native state. The state's constitution, the asylum's Bylaws, the staff physicians' turf-protectiveness, and his own deference and desire to get along—traits evident from his school days—probably doomed him from the start despite his best efforts.

The extent to which we should apportion blame for deplorable conditions at the State Hospital for the Insane among Babcock, the regents, the governors, the legislators, and the state's philosophy of government—"from Wade Hampton onward, it had been accepted as an article of faith among South Carolina political leaders that the least expensive government was the best government"[5]—becomes a matter of judgment. In 1915 the *American Journal of Insanity* was unequivocal that Babcock had "struggled against the most difficult situation, made increasingly worse by lack of financial assistance and an apparent impossibility of awakening any real civic interest in the unfortunate insane of the state."[6] Babcock pleaded year after year for better funding and facilities but, marching in step to the chain of command, took lobbying the legislature as the regents' responsibility, not his. He became an agent for positive change mainly by accident. The 1909–10 and 1913–14 legislative hearings brought pyrrhic victories for Babcock, but progress at the asylum, as public attention drove legislation that propelled the troubled institution toward the mainstream of American psychiatry. His inability to make life much better for the African American patients, one of his main goals when he accepted the job, was no doubt a source of sadness. Their outcomes actually got worse during the years of his administration, first because of tuberculosis and then because of pellagra (see Appendix 1). However, he lived to see the new facility for blacks at State Park become a reality.

Babcock was too shy, passive, and sensitive for the nigh-impossible job description, which in today's terms made him both chief executive officer and chief medical officer of a large, complicated medical center. Abraham Lincoln's self-assessment of his presidency—"I claim not to have controlled events, but confess that events have controlled me," reflecting what a Lincoln biographer calls "the essential passivity of his nature"[7]—fits Babcock's tenure as superintendent. One close friend remembered Babcock's "highly sensitive and shrinking disposition: one had to know him well to appreciate him"[8]; another praised his "gentle and rare personality" but described a "truly painful sensitiveness that rendered him so easily misunderstood by those who knew him but slightly"[9]; and a third wrote that he "was full of sentiment and as sensitive as a child."[10] His personality was poorly suited to fight legislators for more money. And he might remind us that Oliver Wendell Holmes Sr. told graduating medical students, among other things: "Do not dabble in the muddy sewer of politics . . . . The great practitioners are generally those who concentrate all their powers on their business."[11]

Babcock as Leader in Response to the Pellagra Epidemic

His personality was, however, just right for his role as a catalyst in the American response to pellagra. His scholarly approach to medicine made him an eager bibliographer, textbook author, and devourer of the European literature. His warmth, geniality, graciousness, and self-effacement—traits that endeared him at Phillips Exeter Academy, Harvard College, the Tewksbury Almshouse, and McLean Asylum—made him a near-perfect host for local, regional, national, and indeed international meetings at a most improbable venue, the South Carolina State Hospital for the Insane. Attendees felt welcome and wanted to do as Babcock bid them, to "confer together in the interest of truth."[12] More than anyone else he was in close touch with the leading pellagra researchers on both sides of the Atlantic, hearing them out and playing no favorites. The singular exception was Ward MacNeal, who in 1915 torpedoed what the *Journal of the American Medical Association* had described in 1909 as a strikingly "scientific, humanitarian spirit," free of the prickly displays of pride and ego that often characterized medical meetings during that era.[13]

Babcock drew applause from contemporaries and receives credit down to the present day for founding and sustaining the National Association for the Study of Pellagra, but he downplayed his own importance. In a notebook he wrote: "I have not made a single discovery and my modest contribution is confined to a few elementary observations."[14] He was quick to praise others, including such South Carolinians as Joseph Jenkins Watson of Columbia, who independently confirmed pellagra by going to Italy; Frederick Williams of the State Board of Health, who promoted the Columbia meetings and mailed survey forms to all South Carolina doctors; and Harvey McConnell of Chester, who may have been the first to recognize pellagra in textile workers. Babcock through his modesty, idealism, hard work, and personal charm did much to galvanize a ragtag group of asylum doctors, private physicians, health officials, and federal employees into a force that established an American competence, fleshed out competing hypotheses, and set the stage for Joseph Goldberger. This response constitutes a largely unappreciated chapter in the coming of age of American medical science.[15]

Kenneth Carpenter writes in his history of beriberi that as "with other diseases, there have been simplified, semimythical accounts of one 'scientist-hero,'" and that we "can see now that it was fortunate that many researchers, from a number of countries, were all working on the problem of beriberi."[16] The histories of beriberi and pellagra present obvious parallels: (1) consensus for more than a century that the main problem was monotonous diet; (2) flirtation with the idea of a disease-causing toxin; (3) enthusiastic search for a "germ"; (4) feeding studies in humans pointing to a dietary explanation; (5) use of an animal model to strengthen the case for dietary deficiency; and (6) eventual isolation of the deficient vitamin by chemists (see Appendix 2). These histories also illustrate the incremental nature of most human progress. Many workers from many nations placed bricks in the wall (for an incomplete list in the case of pellagra, see Appendix 3), and a few laid cornerstones for the ages. Differences between the histories of beriberi and pellagra include the fierce opposition to Joseph Goldberger by politicians, health officials, and others opposed to the inconvenient truth that southern poverty was the root cause.

Babcock as Exemplar of Character Traits Worthy of Emulation

Babcock displayed in abundance several traits most people want in their public servants. He was scrupulously honest. Auditors for the 1909–10 Legislative Committee could not find the slightest hint of irregularity. James Thompson testified that Babcock would not accept so much as a bunch of lettuce or radishes that belonged to the state. The minutes of the Board of Regents reveal occasional attempts to snare him—for example, did he take pills from the asylum pharmacy over to the governor's mansion for Tillman?[17]—but accusers invariably left empty-handed. Babcock was not self-aggrandizing, declining proposals that his salary be increased by suggesting he was paid what he was worth. He was not self-promoting, never trumpeting his contributions to the pellagra effort. He was not vindictive, tolerating a not-so-loyal opposition from his staff physicians. And he was altruistic, spending his own money to research pellagra and even to buy supplies for the asylum.

As a humanitarian he tried to treat everyone alike. "Kind to all, partial to none," wrote admiring patients at the Tewksbury Almshouse."[18] "He never shows any favoritism," testified Thompson.[19] He found his closest friends among the intelligentsia—August Kohn, J. J. Watson, Julius Taylor, Francis Hopkins Weston, the regulars at Gittman's Book Shop, and, yes, Tillman—but he relished spending time with African Americans such as Page Ellington and the bugle-playing street vendor. As an early champion for women in medicine—employer of Sarah Allan, South Carolina's first licensed woman doctor; champion of Eleanora Saunders, for whom he fell on his sword—he probably has no equal in South Carolina medicine. He had little interest in "society." He seems to have internalized an ideal expressed by his favorite author, Rudyard Kipling (in *The Man Who Would be King*): "Brother to a prince and fellow to a beggar if he be found worthy."

Other traits worthy of emulation include generosity and courage. He gave away books almost as fast as he bought them, surely an uncommon trait among bibliophiles who border on bibliomania. He seldom said no to colleagues who wanted his consultative services. When pellagra struck, he devoted Sunday afternoons to seeing patients from all parts of the state at no charge. During his last years he made taxing trips to Charleston to teach a small group of students, with no expectation for reimbursement. Examples of physical courage include an occasion on which he climbed out onto a fourth-story roof to coax a suicidal patient into coming down.[20] And his moral courage went on public display during his ardent defense of Saunders.

During the 1910 legislative hearings a farmer-legislator from Chester County called Babcock "one of the great men of South Carolina," predicting "time will see a monument erected commemorating his goodness."[21] During those same hearings a Columbian wrote to the newspaper that while the "clergymen of this city are most excellent men ... I believe Dr. Babcock has done more good for humanity than all of them together."[22] Governor Duncan Clinch Heyward called him "the most useful citizen of South Carolina."[23] Years later August Kohn, himself one of the great South Carolinians of that era, told his daughter that "Dr. Babcock was one of South Carolina's truly great men, and if had been left to him [Kohn], the people of this state would have given him every honor they had to bestow."[24] Whether Babcock deserves remembrance as a great man is for readers to judge, but in many ways he was clearly a great example of what a good man should be.

Asylum Doctor

James Woods Babcock was among the last of a breed, the "old asylum doctor."
By the time of his death newly trained psychiatrists sought to distance themselves from the crowded asylums. In 1925 the president of the American
Psychiatric Association spoke of "the old superintendent's vision and courage
and humanitarian instincts" as the foundation on which "a scientific psychiatry" might be constructed.[25] More recently a psychiatrist writes of "the
term *alienist*" . . . as "usually applied to those brave enough to work in the
huge asylums that had begun to spread across the United States and Europe
in the 19th century."[26] It is hard for us to imagine the sights, sounds, and
smells of the old asylums—the pathetic countenances, the moaning, cries,
and hallucinations, the stench arising from some of the wards. Most of the
old asylum buildings in America lie fallow, if they survive at all. Asylum
inmates have been replaced by the successfully treated, the partially treated,
and, all too often, by the homeless.

Returning to the epigram with which this book began, in many ways
"the Old South disappeared along with pellagra."[27] It is hard to imagine
a time when a capital city in the United States had muddy streets with
horse-drawn wagons, governors who endorsed lynching, juries that acquitted politicians who gunned down newspaper editors in broad daylight, and
a mental hospital that commanded a corner of the cityscape. It is hard to
imagine a time when most hospitalized patients in the United States were
asylum inmates, when there were no major tranquilizers, no psychotropic
drugs, and no community mental health centers. It is hard to imagine a world
without ubiquitous vitamins—vitamin-enriched flour, bottles of vitamins
filling shelves and even entire stores, vitamin-enriched foods from near and
far. Gone are the old asylums, the monotonous "3-M" diets, the brewer's yeast
tablets on dining tables, the connotations of place names like "Bull Street,"
a local equivalent of "Bedlam." But we can be reasonably certain that the
poor, the undernourished, the medically underserved, and the mentally ill
will always be with us, or at least for the foreseeable future.

Mortality and Full Recoveries (as Percentages of Patients Treated) by Race, South Carolina State Hospital for the Insane, 1891–1914*

Year	Mortality (%)			Full Recoveries (%)		
	Whites	Blacks	Overall	Whites	Blacks	Overall
1891	13%	24%	18%	12%	9%	11%
1892	12	22	17	9	9	9
1893	15	29	17	9	9	9
1894	10	20	15	7	10	8
1895	11	21	16	10	10	10
1896	14	27	20	8	8	8
1897	9	20	13	8	8	8
1898	13	26	18	9	8	8
1899	13	21	16	9	9	9
1900	12	26	18	9	8	8
1901	12	20	15	6	7	6
1902	12	23	17	8	7	8
1903	14	22	17	8	7	8
1904	13	15	14	5	8	6
1905	11	21	16	5	3	4
1906	10	25	17	7	6	6
1907	11	22	16	5	3	4
1908	9	24	16	8	6	7
1909	9	21	14	7	4	5
1910	9	24	16	8	6	7
1911	11	24	17	9	5	7

(continues)

Year	Mortality (%)			Full Recoveries (%)		
	Whites	Blacks	Overall	Whites	Blacks	Overall
1912	14	31	22	6	4	5
1913	13	22	17	7	6	6
1914	20	31	25	4	4	4

Summaries for Babcock's Era as Superintendent (complete years, 1892–1913)

1892–1898	12%	22%	17%	9%	9%	9%
1899–1906	12	22	16	7	8	6
1907–1913	11	24	17	7	7	7
All Years	12%	23%	17%	7%	7%	7%

Summaries for Years Before and After Babcock's Era as Superintendent

1886–1889	12%	20%	16%	10%	9%	10%
1915–1922	12%	19%	17%	5%	4%	4%

*Spreadsheets with these data, and also the methods for this analysis, are in box 8, folder 34, Babcock papers, SCL. The data are from annual reports; these reports do not provide the numbers of full recoveries for 1915–1917.

Parallels in the Histories of Beriberi and Pellagra

	Beriberi	Pellagra
Cause	Deficiency of thiamine (vitamin B_1)	Deficiency of niacin (vitamin B_3)
Origin of the term	"Extreme weakness" (Sinhalese); others	"Rough skin" (Italian)
Principal manifestations	Peripheral neuritis and wasting (dry beriberi); heart failure (wet beriberi)	Dermatitis (symmetric, sunburn-like rash), diarrhea, dementia
Original place(s) of appearance	Asia	Spain, France, Italy, and Eastern Europe
Setting that led to eventual cure	Dutch West Indies	American Southeast
Presumed racial differences in susceptibility	Japanese were thought to be more susceptible than Russians during the Russo-Japanese War.	Blacks were generally thought to be more susceptible than whites in the American South.
Probable cause of epidemic form	Polished rice	Degerminated corn
Early explanation	Diet based mainly on rice	Diet based mainly on corn
Idea that toxins were the cause	Bacteria produce a beriberi-causing toxin (1886); others	Moldy corn contains a pellagra-causing toxin (early-nineteenth century)
Impact of the germ theory of the disease	An infectious agent exists in peripheral nerves and is transmitted from person to person by an agent, possibly an insect (1902)	The likely cause is a parasite, transmitted by an unidentified insect, quite possibly a fly of the genus *Simulium* (Louis Sambon, 1905).

(continues)

	Beriberi	Pellagra
Development of an animal model	Polyneuritis in chickens (fowl polyneuritis) (Conrad Eijkman, 1895)	Black tongue in dogs (Chittenden and Underhill, 1917)
Hero figure	Christiaan Eijkman, 1895	Joseph Goldberger
The hero figure's good fortune (or lucky break)	Eijkman's chickens were being fed leftover cooked rice without his knowledge.	Goldberger was assigned to pellagra shortly after Casimir Funk's "vitamine" hypothesis went public.
Major problems with the hero-myth	Eijkman did not appreciate the full significance of his experiments and returned to the germ theory, despite mounting evidence against it.	Goldberger did not "invent" the dietary-deficiency hypothesis (nor did he claim to have invented it). Numerous observations pointed away from an infectious cause.
Main contributions of the hero figure	Discovery of the animal model (fowl polyneuritis)	Design and execution of studies using dietary manipulation to establish the essential cause; relentless campaign to promote balanced diets; demonstration of the preventative and curative value of brewer's yeast
Identification of the deficient vitamin	Robert Runnels Williams (1933)	Conrad Elvehjem (1937)

APPENDIX 3

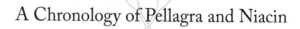

A Chronology of Pellagra and Niacin

Date	Event
~ 5000 B.C.E.	Wild corn appears in Latin America in appreciable quantities.
~ 2300 B.C.E.	A more modern form of corn has evolved, apparently by hybridization.
~ 1500 C.E.	Corn cultivation begins and spreads in the Old World as a result of Columbus's voyages.
1735	Don Gaspar Casál, of Oviedo, Spain, describes a disease among Asturian peasants which he calls *mal de la rosa* (from its characteristic erythema). He considers it a variety of leprosy. Affected persons are poor, subsist largely on maize (corn), and seldom eat fresh meat.
1755	Dr. François Thiéry, a French physician, publishes the first description of pellagra, having learned about the disease from Casál during his visit to the Asturias in 1750.
1771	Dr. Francesco Frapolli, of Milan, Italy, describes a disease among Italian peasants, which he calls pellagra (from the Italian words *pelle* for skin and *agra* for rough).
1789	Dr. Gaetano Strambio, director of a sixty-bed pellagra hospital in Legnano, Italy, publishes his first treatise on pellagra. He performs the first autopsies on pellagrins and describes pellagra without skin lesions ("pellagra *sine* pellagra").
1807	Dr. Francesco-Luigi Fanzago reads a memoir before the Academy of Padua, Italy, in which he states that maize is the sole cause of pellagra because it provides insufficient nourishment.
1810	Dr. Giovanni Battista Marzari suggests that a corn-heavy diet is inadequate because the cereal is deficient in gluten, by which he apparently meant that it was low in nitrogenous material. Two schools of thought soon arise: *Zeists*, who support the corn theory of Marzari, and *anti-Zeists*, who discredit it.

(continues)

269

Date	Event
1814	Dr. Pietro Guerreschi suggests that pellagra is caused by eating moldy corn. This causes a split among the Zeists. Some think that pellagra is due to corn's being an incomplete nutrient; others think that only spoiled corn causes pellagra.
1843	Dr. Carlo Calderini suggests pellagra is always hereditary and that imported or foreign corn is the cause in whatever country pellagra appears.
1844–1845	Dr. Ludovico Balardini suggests pellagra is due to spoiled corn. He reports that corn infected with the fungus *Sporisorium maidis* makes chickens sick.
1845	Dr. Théophile Roussel of France establishes that *mal de la rosa* (as described in Spain) and pellagra (as described in Italy) are one and the same disease.
1848	Roussel tells the French Minister of Agriculture that changing the peasants' diet might prevent pellagra.
Late 1840s	Dr. Cesare Lombroso of Italy begins to champion the corn theory, and devotes the next twenty-five years of his life to it. He later claims to have caused pellagra in humans and animals by injecting an alcoholic extract of damaged corn. He also proposes arsenic as therapy.
1864	Two cases of pellagra are reported at the annual meeting of American Asylum Physicians, held in Washington, D.C., and later published in the *American Journal of Insanity*.
1866	Dr. Pretenderis Thypaldos, Professor of Medicine at the University of Athens, reports an outbreak on the island of Corfu. He suggests that the residents of Corfu began to get pellagra only after they began importing corn from distant areas.
1866	Roussel writes on the basis of his experience and critical review of the literature that "Without dietetic measures *all remedies fail*." [italics are Roussel's]
1873	Austrian Chemist Hugo Weidel isolates nicotinic acid in sufficient quantities to determine its crystalline structure.
1882	Dr. Geoffrey Gaumer describes pellagra in the Yucatan and concludes that it is due to eating the cheapest imported corn on the market.
1894	German chemist Carl Engler synthesizes nicotinamide.
1898	Dr. Fleming M. Sandwith of London reports that since 1893 he has seen more than 500 cases of pellagra in Egypt, usually in laborers who lived on a monotonous diet and were exposed to the sun. He bars patients with pellagra from eating corn in any form and prescribes a balanced diet.

Date	Event
1901–06	The Beall degerminator is developed and marketed in the U.S., leading to widespread degermination of corn in the preparation of cornmeal. Since the germ contains most of the niacin, this almost certainly plays a major role in the subsequent epidemic of pellagra.
1902	Cases of pellagra are reported from Atlanta and Chicago.
1905	Louis Sambon, an Italian-born physician working in London, speculates that pellagra is caused by an infectious agent (probably a parasite) transmitted by an insect (probably a fly of the genus *Simulium*). Sir Patrick Manson lends support.
1906	Dr. Guido Tizzoni of Italy claims to have isolated a bacterium, *Streptobacillus pellagrae*, from blood and fecal matter of pellagrins.
1907	Dr. George H. Searcy of Alabama reports 88 cases of pellagra with 57 deaths at the Mount Vernon Hospital for the Colored Insane.
1907–1908	Dr. James Woods Babcock and his colleagues suspect pellagra at the State Hospital for the Insane in Columbia, S.C. Later, Babcock and another Columbia physician, Dr. Joseph Jenkins Watson, independently go to Italy and conclude that pellagra there is the same as in South Carolina. Babcock organizes a conference on pellagra (October 29)—the first such conference in an English-speaking country.
1908	Pellagra is reported at the Georgia State Sanitarium in Milledgeville (40 cases and 23 deaths).
1909	Babcock organizes the first national conference on pellagra in Columbia, S.C. (November 3-4). Participants establish a National Association for the Study of Pellagra and elect Babcock president. Dr. George Zeller of Illinois reports epidemic pellagra at the Peoria State Hospital.
1910	Babcock and Dr. Claude Lavinder bring out an English translation of Armand Marie's treatise on pellagra. This is the first substantial monograph in English on the disease.
1910	Sambon, funded by the British Pellagra Commission, goes to Italy to obtain further evidence for his speculation that pellagra is a specific infectious disease transmitted to humans by flies of the genus *Simulium*, and is therefore found especially along the banks of swift-flowing streams. In his party is Captain Joseph Siler of the U.S. Army.
1911	A Belton, South Carolina, mill worker named Ezxba Dedmond, who believes he is in partnership with God, manufactures "Ez-X-Ba River, the Stream of Life" as a cure for pellagra—one of numerous "wonder cures" for pellagra.

(continues)

Date	Event
1911	The Illinois Pellagra Commission concludes that pellagra is probably an infectious disease, for which "deficient animal protein in the diet" might be a predisposing factor.
1911–12	Casimir Funk, a Polish-born biochemist working in London, isolates a concentrate from rice polishings that cures polyneuritis in pigeons. Believing the critical substance to be an amine, he calls it a "vitamine" (*vita* for life, hence "an amine essential for life"). Funk suggests that pellagra like beriberi and scurvy is caused by dietary deficiency. He publishes his "vitamine hypothesis."
1912	Funk isolates nicotinic acid (niacin) but does not establish its relationship to pellagra.
1912	The second conference of the National Association for the Study of Pellagra takes place in Columbia, S.C. (October 3–4). Sandwith suggests through a submitted paper that the cause of pellagra might be deficiency of a specific dietary substance—in retrospect, a refinement of Marzari's 1810 hypothesis. Rupert Blue, Babcock, and others second this idea.
1913	Sandwith publishes a paper entitled, "Is pellagra a disease due to deficiency of nutrition?" He refers to other diseases now known to be caused by vitamin deficiencies: beriberi, scurvy, and rickets. He discusses tryptophan (a niacin precursor) at length.
1913	Members of the Thompson-McFadden Commission conclude in their first progress report that pellagra is probably an infectious disease. Sambon uses the occasion of the announcement of this report (a meeting in Spartanburg, S.C., on September 3) to promote his version of the infection hypothesis.
1914	The Thompson-McFadden Pellagra Commission reports that a survey of more than 5,000 persons in Spartanburg County, S.C., shows no relationship between pellagra and diet. The researchers again posit an infectious agent.
1914	Dr. Joseph Goldberger replaces Lavinder as the principal U.S. Public Health Service investigator of pellagra in the South. Goldberger quickly concludes that inadequate diet is the likely cause. He designs and begins controlled experiments to establish his case.
1914	Dr. W. F. Lorenz reports that patients with pellagra at the Georgia State Sanitarium improved within about four weeks of instituting a generous diet; hence, "a generous diet seems to have a decidedly favorable effect upon the course of pellagra."

Date	Event
1915	The third conference of the National Association for the Study of Pellagra takes place in Columbia, S.C. (October 21–22). On the second day participants learn that Goldberger and his colleagues have prevented pellagra in two orphanages and two asylum wards by dietary manipulation alone. Dr. Carl Grote reports controlling pellagra in Walker County, Alabama, by dietary modification. Drs. James Adams Hayne of South Carolina and Ward J. MacNeal of the Thompson-McFadden Pellagra Commission emerge as Goldberger's most vocal opponents.
1916	Goldberger reports that sixteen volunteers (including himself and his wife) ingested (or allowed themselves to be injected with) numerous substances from pellagrins and that none got the disease.
1916	Goldberger reports the production of pellagra in six of eleven prisoner-volunteers by dietary manipulation alone (the Rankin Farm experiment). However, the rash that developed in these volunteers is somewhat atypical for classic pellagra.
1916	A North Carolina veterinarian reports that canine black tongue may be an analogue of (and therefore a potential animal model for) human pellagra.
1916	Atherton Seidell, a biochemist working at the National Hygienic Laboratory in Washington, D.C., formulates a vitamin preparation using brewer's yeast. He suggests it might be tried in pellagra.
1917	Russell H. Chittenden and Frank P. Underhill at Yale University report that giving dogs a diet consisting of boiled (dried) peas, cracker meal, and cottonseed oil or lard produces a condition closely resembling human pellagra. They hypothesize a deficiency of "some essential dietary constituent or constituents." Veterinarians soon suspect that black tongue and the Chittenden-Underhill syndrome are one and the same condition.
1920	Goldberger reports additional data bearing on the experimental production of pellagra in Mississippi prison volunteers.
1922	Goldberger begins to study black tongue in dogs as a model of pellagra.
1925	Goldberger and a colleague report on "a heretofore unrecognized or unappreciated dietary factor which we designate as factor P-P," which "may possibly play the sole essential rôle in the prevention (and causation) of pellagra."

(continues)

Date	Event
1926	Goldberger and his colleagues show that a "pellagra-preventive factor" (which also prevents black tongue in dogs) is the heat-resistant portion of "water soluble vitamin B." "Factor P-P" was later named "vitamin G" in Goldberger's honor. (It is now known as niacin.)
1927	The American Red Cross begins to distribute yeast, at first in four states affected by a Mississippi River flood and later throughout pellagra-affected areas of the Southeast.
1928	Goldberger and George Wheeler report definitively that a heat-stable component of yeast prevents canine black tongue.
1928	The annual number of deaths due to pellagra in the United States reaches its highest point since 1915.
1929	Joseph Goldberger dies of carcinoma of the kidney at age 54.
1929–32	The annual number of deaths due to pellagra in the United States declines, probably because of the promotion of such antipellagra foods as milk, eggs, meat, and yeast, and also because of the economic impact of the New Deal.
1937	Conrad A. Elvehjem and colleagues at the University of Wisconsin report that canine black tongue is caused by deficiency of nicotinic acid, which is part of the vitamin B complex. They later isolate the "anti-black-tongue factor" as nicotinic acid and nicotinamide.
1937	Dr. Tom Douglas Spies and his colleagues at the University of Cincinnati College of Medicine cure human pellagra with nicotinamide.
1938	Bakers voluntarily begin to enrich bread with high-vitamin yeast, leading to a rapid decline in the incidence of pellagra in the U.S.
1941	The Food and Nutrition Board of the National Nutrition Board recommends enriching bread and flour with thiamine, niacin, and iron.
1942	"Niacin" becomes a synonym for "nicotinic acid" and "nicotinamide" after representatives of the baking industry complain that "nicotinic acid" (connoting as it does "nicotine") might discourage people from buying their products.
1943–48	Five Southern states including South Carolina enact laws requiring the enrichment of all degerminated cornmeal and grits sold within their borders.

Date	Event
1945	Researchers at the University of Wisconsin report that high consumption of corn depresses the level of nicotinic acid in the body, and that white corn (the kind favored in the South) is worse than yellow corn in this regard.
1945	American biochemist Willard Arthur Krehl discovers that the essential amino acid tryptophan is transformed into niacin by mammalian tissues.
1945	South Carolina becomes the first state to mandate vitamin enrichment of flour. It was determined that flour could be enriched with the vitamin B complex for about three cents per twelve-pound bag.
1952	Researchers at Tulane University determine that the minimum daily niacin requirement for women on a corn diet is about seven milligrams.
1955	American biochemist Max K. Horwitt, taking into account the niacin-tryptophan relationship, proposes the concept of "niacin equivalents."
1955	Canadian scientist Ruldolf Altschul and his colleagues report that high doses of nicotinic acid lower serum cholesterol levels in humans. (Nicotinamide, the other principal form of niacin, does not have this effect.)
1960	Pellagra has been essentially eradicated in the United States. It now occurs mainly in persons suffering from alcoholism and other disorders that lead to unbalanced diets.
1961	Biochemists at Oxford University demonstrate that nicotinamide is the principal form of niacin absorbed from the gastrointestinal tract.
1977	Eighteen adults with pellagra are reported at the Johns Hopkins Hospital. Only four had the complete triad of dermatitis, diarrhea, and dementia, emphasizing the need for clinicians to maintain a high index of suspicion.
1982–1993	Pellagra is reported as a complication of Crohn's disease and other conditions causing malabsorption, drugs used for tuberculosis, and chemotherapy for cancer.
1993	An outbreak of pellagra with at least 28,276 cases is reported among 85,942 Mozambican refugees in Malawi. The attack rate is 7.8 times higher in women than in men. It followed a five-month cessation of groundnut distribution (the major source of niacin for these people).

(continues)

Date	Event
1999	A pellagra outbreak begins in and around Kuito, the capital of Bie province in Central Angola, in the context of an armed conflict. The attack rate is at least 3.6 per 1000 people, with 66 percent of the victims being displaced persons (of whom 83 percent were women).
1999–2003	Pellagra is described as a complication of HIV disease, anorexia nervosa, and homelessness.
2007	Researchers at the University of Birmingham, United Kingdom, suggest that pellagra may hold "a clue as to why energy failure causes diseases."
Present day	Biochemists and other researchers continue to study niacin and related compounds for better understanding of health and illness.

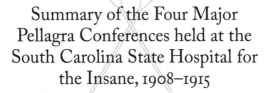

Summary of the Four Major Pellagra Conferences held at the South Carolina State Hospital for the Insane, 1908–1915

Year	1908	1909	1912	1915
Dates	October 29	November 3–4	October 3–4	October 21–22
Physician attendees	72	394	~ 150	~75
Papers presented (no.)	11	45	67	43
Authors (no.)[1]	11	48	75	44
Significance	First conference on pellagra in English-speaking nation	Formation of NASP[2]; stimulation of research	Public airing of the vitamin-deficiency hypothesis	Goldberger's breakthrough; opponents emerge
Dominant hypothesis	Corn has a central, but unclear role	Lombroso's spoiled-corn hypothesis	Sambon's infection hypothesis	Opinion begins to shift toward faulty diet
Sources of papers (residence of author, or senior author)				
South Carolina	7	17	12	20
N.C. or Georgia	4	4	11	5
Other Southeastern[3]		10	10	2
Other U.S.		4	12	1

(continues)

Year	1908	1909	1912	1915
U.S. P.H.S.[4]		2	3	7
Thompson-McFadden[5]			2	5
Other governmental[6]		1	2	
International		7	15	3

[1] Data are for unique authors; authors (or coauthors) of more than one paper are included only once in these tabulations.

[2] NASP: National Association for the Study of Pellagra

[3] Other Southeastern: Southeastern states (states that formerly belonged to the Confederacy) other than South Carolina, North Carolina, and Georgia; Other U.S.: states outside the Southeast, and also the District of Columbia, excluding physicians employed by the U.S. Government, who are listed separately.

[4] U.S. P.H.S.: U.S. Public Health Service (prior to 1912, the U.S. Public Health and Marine Hospital Service)

[5] Thompson-McFadden: Thompson-McFadden Pellagra Commission of the New York Post-Graduate Medical School and Hospital (includes physicians from government agencies on loan to the commission).

[6] Other governmental: U.S. government agencies other than the U.S. P.H.S. (for example, the U.S. Army and the U.S. Department of Agriculture), and excluding persons assigned by government agencies to work with the Thompson-McFadden Commission.

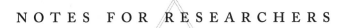

NOTES FOR RESEARCHERS

This project began, continued, and ended with students, most recently two graduate students exploring the history and architecture of the Babcock Building. History like science often raises more questions than it answers, and it occurred to the author that it might be useful to suggest projects for researchers at various levels. The six linear feet of James Woods Babcock papers in the South Caroliniana Library were catalogued during the course of this project and the author has placed therein various databases, illustrations, and a finding aid for governmental publications. Twelve potential projects are as follows.

The admission and discharge books of the South Carolina State Hospital for the Insane could be used to construct a database tracking individual patients. Researchers concerned about racial and gender disparities could analyze these data using present-day parameters such as length-of-stay and readmission rates, which might be of interest, especially if the archives of other asylums contain similar information.

Pellagra in the United States has not been well told from the perspective of patients and their families. A student (Louis Miller) drew the author's attention to the following reminiscence by a millworker: "The doctors patched me up. I was in a dread fix. Dr. Babcock treated me . . . I had pellagra inside and out. . . . the doctors can't cure all the time." The source was the Federal Writers' Project (Library of Congress); this and other repositories could be mined for reminiscences of how patients, families, and communities coped with pellagra.

To what extent, and at what rate, did American physicians change their opinions about the cause of pellagra after Joseph Goldberger's breakthrough? The author's database of 409 American authors of articles on pellagra published between 1907 and 1915, as referenced by the *Index Medicus*, could be extended. How many of these authors wrote on pellagra during the Goldberger era? Did they change their opinions? Did they campaign for better diets? Did they try to influence health officials and politicians?

What happened behind the scenes at the Thompson-McFadden Pellagra Commission, from which Ward MacNeal emerged as Goldberger's leading scientific opponent? Unfortunately, primary source materials have not been located. Separate collections of Ward J. MacNeal papers as indexed by the American Society for Microbiology and the University of Michigan are silent on this period of his life. In 1948 the New York Post-Graduate Medical School merged with New York University. An archivist at New York University searched diligently for materials pertaining to the Thompson-McFadden Commission but turned up nothing of interest. Such material if found would allow a researcher to refine and/or challenge the present author's narrative.

Goldberger and his small team assumed a task that would now be undertaken by "Big Science"—large-scale efforts by well-funded groups and coalitions of researchers. Alan Kraut's magisterial account of Goldberger's herculean efforts could be a starting point for projects along at least three lines. First, the scientific dimensions could be explored in greater detail (see, for example, note 90, page 349). Could pellagra have been solved sooner? To what extent did Goldberger exchange ideas with other researchers within the U.S. Public Health Service (such as Atherton Seidell and Carl Voegtlin), elsewhere in the United States, and abroad? Second, social determinants of resistance to Goldberger's conclusions could be contrasted with resistance to other new paradigms (familiar examples include Galileo, William Harvey, Darwin, and today's controversy about global warming; for examples during the early twentieth century, see note 73, page 347). Finally, those interested in the organization of science could compare and contrast the initial American response to pellagra to responses to other threats to public health. To what extent did the pellagra story between 1907 and 1925 constitute a watershed event in the professionalization of American medical science? And is it correct to assert that never again would American medical researchers be duped by the likes of Louis Sambon?

Of interest to the present author is the role played by practicing physicians in the advancement of knowledge. The arrival of Big Science during the mid-twentieth century markedly reduced the ability of practicing physicians to compete with full-time researchers in universities, government agencies, and industry. In 1908, when the first compendium of articles on pellagra in the English language appeared in the *Journal of the South Carolina Medical Association*, there were no full-time clinical faculty members at the state's only medical school. The present author previously showed that the subsequent proliferation of full-time faculty probably inhibited scholarship by practicing physicians in that journal. A researcher might undertake a qualitative and quantitative study of medical journals in this regard.

Those interested in the history of psychiatry will find useful material in the case records and annual reports of the South Carolina State Hospital for the Insane, and also in Babcock's lecture notes in the South Caroliniana Library. How did concepts and classifications of mental illnesses change over time? Did the Columbia asylum keep pace with others of that era? How do Babcock's lecture notes compare with similar collections of that era? How do they compare with present-day curricula for medical and nursing students? A student exploring these and similar questions would, at the very least, appreciate the relevance of medical history.

The inspiring story of Eleanora Saunders deserves telling and retelling. Unfortunately, no primary source material was found beyond that used in this book, either in the James Woods Babcock papers in the South Caroliniana Library or in the archives of the Sheppard Pratt Health System in Towson, Maryland. Still, the material on which Chapter 7 is based could be used to write an entertaining and informative screenplay, a short story, or perhaps a historical novel.

Dr. Allen Stokes of the South Caroliniana Library recently catalogued a major addition to the already extensive Christensen Family papers. That family's saga during the Civil War, Reconstruction, the conservative regime and Jim Crow, the Progressive Era, and beyond invites an instructive chronicle of progressive thought in South Carolina.

Finally, the recent sale of the Bull Street property suggests the need for a comprehensive, start-to-finish history of the South Carolina State Hospital for the Insane, building on previous accounts and notably that of Peter McCandless.

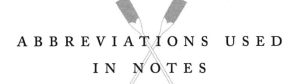

ABBREVIATIONS USED IN NOTES

Manuscript Sources and Libraries

CH	Case Histories, South Carolina State Hospital, South Carolina Department of Archives and History
CUL	Special Collections, University Libraries, Clemson University
MBR	Minutes of the Board of Regents, South Carolina State Hospital, South Carolina Department of Archives and History
SCDAH	South Carolina Department of Archives and History
SCL	South Caroliniana Library, University of South Carolina, Columbia
SHC	Southern Historical Collection, Wilson Library, University of North Carolina, Chapel Hill
WHL	Waring Historical Library, Medical University of South Carolina, Charleston

Unpublished Meeting Minutes

NASP Minutes (1915)	Minutes of the Third Triennial Meeting of the National Association for the Study of Pellagra

Reports of South Carolina Government and State Agencies, Meetings, Conferences, and Commissions

Acts and Resolutions	Acts and Joint Resolutions of the General Assembly of South Carolina
AR	Annual Reports of the South Carolina Lunatic Asylum/ South Carolina State Hospital of the Insane

(continues)

House Journal	Journal of the House of Representatives of the General Assembly of the State of South Carolina
Illinois Pellagra Commission	Report of the Pellagra Commission of the State of Illinois
Legislative Report (1910)	Report of the Legislative Committee to Investigate the State Hospital for the Insane
Legislative Report (1914)	Report and Proceedings of the Special Legislative Committee Appointed by Concurrent Resolution to Investigate the State Hospital for the Insane and State Park
Legislative Testimony (1909)	Testimony Taken Before the Legislative Committee to Investigate the State Hospital for the Insane at Columbia
NASP Transactions (1909)	Transactions of the National Conference on Pellagra Held Under Auspices of South Carolina State Board of Health at the State Hospital for the Insane
NASP Transactions (1912)	Transactions of the National Association for the Study of Pellagra. Second Triennial Meeting
Pellagra Conference (1908)	Conference on Pellagra Held under the Auspices of the State Board of Health of South Carolina at the State Hospital for the Insane
Reports and Resolutions	Reports and Resolutions of the General Assembly of the State of South Carolina
SBH/SHI	The State Board of Health and the South Carolina State Hospital for the Insane
Senate Journal	Journal of the Senate of the General Assembly of the State of South Carolina
Thompson–McFadden Report (1913)	Pellagra. First Progress Report of the Thompson–McFadden Pellagra Commission
Thompson–McFadden Report (1915)	Pellagra II. Second Progress Report of the Thompson–McFadden Pellagra
Thompson Report (1917)	Pellagra III. Third Report of the Robert M. Thompson Pellagra Commission

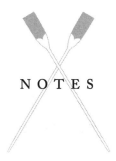

NOTES

NOTES TO PROLOGUE

1. Scurvy is caused by vitamin C deficiency, beriberi by thiamine deficiency, and rickets (and also osteomalacia) by vitamin D deficiency. Vitamin A deficiency causes night blindness and other symptoms.
2. Bollet, "Politics and Pellagra."
3. "Report of the State Board of Health" for 1910 (*Reports and Resolutions* [1910], 5: 1-102), for 1911 (Ibid. [1912], 2: 1307-76), and 1913 (Ibid. [1913], 1: 1049-1124).
4. See, for example, King, "The Conquest of Pellagra."
5. Kraut, *Goldberger's War*, 242–43.
6. Kuhn, *Scientific Revolutions*.
7. Johnson, *Good Ideas*, 34.
8. Review of *Where Good Ideas Come From.* These are not, of course, new concepts. See for example, Osler, *Growth of Truth*, and, for a contemporary popular account, Gladwell, *Outliers*.
9. Osler, *Principles and Practice*, 6th edition, 384.
10. Miller, "Case of Pellagra in Maine." Like other historians, Kraut confirms that the meetings of the National Association for the Study of Pellagra were "largely through the efforts of James Woods Babcock, whose articles had first called national attention to the disease" (Kraut, *Goldberger's War*, 117).
11. For more recent commentary on Babcock's importance to the pellagra effort, see McCandless, "James Woods Babcock," and Frankenburg, *Vitamin Discoveries*, 38.
12. "Notes and Comment. South Carolina and Her State Hospital."

NOTES TO CHAPTER I

1. For Babcock's understanding of his ancestry, see autobiographical sketch dated September 1882, Babcock papers, box 5, folder 9, SCL.

2. "Christmas Presents" (newspaper clipping, undated), Babcock papers, box 6, folder 2, SCL.
3. "Chester Doctors, 1861–65," *Chester* (S.C.) *Reporter*, May 8, 1905.
4. Zuczek, *State of Rebellion*, 91.
5. Autobiographical sketch dated September 1882, Babcock papers, box 5, folder 9, SCL.
6. Thomas P. Ivy, "The People's Forum: Dr. Babcock, Famous Alienist," *News and Observer* (Raleigh, N.C.), March 14, 1922.
7. "Obituary notice of James Woods Babcock, M.D., L.L.D."
8. Henry W. Cunningham to Babcock, February 6, 1905, Babcock papers, box 5, folder 8, SCL.
9. "Inaugural Address of James W. Babcock, delivered Sept. 15th 1877," Records of the Golden Branch Society, archives of Phillips Exeter Academy.
10. Information provided by Edouard L. Desrochers of Philips Exeter Academy, August 2, 1999.
11. Autobiographical sketch dated September 1882, Babcock papers, box 5, folder 9, SCL.
12. Eliot, "Defect in Football"; Eliot, "Evils of College Football"; "Eliot Against Basket Ball. Harvard President Says Rowing and Tennis Are the Only Clean Sports," *New York Times*, November 28, 1906.
13. Blanchard, *Harvard Athletics*, 44–46.
14. *Boston Globe*, May 8, 1881. The members of the crew were (photograph of crew in racing shell on page 10, left to right) Henry Thomas Oxnard of Boston (coxswain), Xanthus Henry Goodnough (stroke), George William Perkins, Frederic Warren, Charles Randall Dean, Babcock, Henry Hamilton Sherwood, Henry Reese Hoyt, and Morton Stimson Crehore (bow).
15. Untitled, undated address given by Babcock (September 1909), Babcock papers, box 4, folder 7, SCL.
16. *Boston Globe*, supplement, May 14, 1881.
17. Untitled address by Babcock given in September 1909, and "Lessons Taught to the Athlete" (newspaper clipping, undated), both in Babcock papers, box 4, folder 7, SCL.
18. *Boston Globe*, May 15, 1881.
19. *Boston Globe*, May 16, 1881. Prior to the invention of the sliding seat, oarsmen had leather pads sewn into their trousers for protection as they slid back and forth on a waxed board. Hoyt had no such protection.
20. H. W. Cunningham to Babcock, April 26, 1907, and F. L. Somerville to Babcock, April 27, 1907, both in Babcock papers, box 5, folder 8, SCL.
21. Babcock to Patrick Livingston Murphy, April 30, 1897, Patrick Livingston Murphy papers, collection 535, folder 6, SHC.
22. "Lessons Taught to the Athlete," Babcock papers, box 4, folder 7, SCL.
23. Undated notes made by Margaret Babcock Meriwether, Babcock papers, box 8, folder 1, SCL.

24. Harvard College, *Secretary's Report*; autobiographical sketch dated September 1882, Babcock papers, box 5, folder 9, SCL.
25. Allen Danforth to Babcock, July 1, 1882, Babcock papers, box 5, folder 8, SCL.
26. Studies suggest that by early adulthood most persons can recall several such situations that require the use of "wisdom" criteria, including knowing where to turn for help. See Baltes and Smith, "Toward a Psychology of Wisdom," and Gladwell, *Outliers*, 69–115.
27. Babcock to the Faculty of Harvard College [July 1882], Babcock papers, box 5, folder 8, SCL.
28. W. G. Farlow to Babcock, November 3, 1882, Babcock papers, box 5, folder 8, SCL.
29. Harrington and Mumford, *Harvard Medical School*, 3:1020, 1065, 1055. See also Ludmerer, *Learning to Heal*, 40, 48–57.
30. *One Hundredth Annual Catalog*.
31. Bryan, "Greatest Brahmin."
32. See Gibian, *Oliver Wendell Holmes*; and Podolsky and Bryan, eds., *Oliver Wendell Holmes*, especially the chapter by Weinstein ("Holmes's Depth Psychology"). The present author possesses Babcock's copy of Brown's *Life of Oliver Wendell Holmes*, which is marked in pencil in such a way as to indicate Babcock gave it a close reading.
33. Beecher and Altschule, *Medicine at Harvard*, 157–65. For extensive commentary on Putnam and Prince, see Hale, *Freud and the Americans*.
34. *One Hundredth Annual Catalog*; Harrington and Mumford, *Harvard Medical School*, 3:1077–78.
35. *Legislative Testimony* (1909), 362. Testifying more than two decades later, Babcock dated his employment at the Tewksbury Almshouse as January 1885. It is unclear whether this was a second stint at the asylum.
36. Ibid.
37. Babcock to William Frederick ("Brooks") Babcock, August 13, 1883, manuscript in the possession of Arthur St. J. Simons.
38. Taylor, *James Woods Babcock*, 5.
39. [Patients at the] State Almshouse Male Hospital, Tewksbury, to Babcock, August 29, 1883, Babcock papers, box 4, folder 10, SCL.
40. Babcock received his MD degree in June 1886.
41. Theodore C. Fisher to Babcock, September 14, 1885; C. Irving Fisher to Babcock, September 14, 1885; Eben Norton to Babcock, September 26, 1885; Babcock to Edward Cowles, December 2, 1885; Cowles to Babcock, January 4, 1886; all in Babcock papers, box 4, folder 10, SCL.
42. Shorter, *History of Psychiatry*, 33. For concise histories, see Duffin, "Wrestling with Demons"; Grob, *Mental Illness*, 3–29; and Grob, *Mad Among Us*, 1–53.
43. Tuttle, "McLean Hospital"; and Little, *McLean Hospital*, 13–14. The McLean Asylum for the Insane was renamed "McLean Hospital" in 1892. In 1895 it relocated to Waverley Oaks Hill, Belmont, Massachusetts.

44. Beam, *Gracefully Insane*, 1, 20–23, 51.
45. Sutton, *Crossroads*, 23–51.
46. Grob (*Mental Illness*, 68) writes that by Cowles's era McLean symbolized the new "scientific psychiatry." For a summary of Cowles's views on psychiatry and asylums, see Cowles, "Advanced Professional Work." See also "Dr. Edward Cowles."
47. Harlan B. Bean to Babcock, November 14, 1887, Babcock papers, box 4, folder 10, SCL.
48. Katherine Guion [Babcock], Medical Notebook, October 6, 1888–May 30, 1889, Babcock papers, SCL.
49. W. B. Fiske to Babcock, November 13, 1887, Babcock papers, box 4, folder 10, SCL.
50. Information in Babcock papers, box 5, folder 10, SCL.
51. Cowles to Babcock, March 16, 1890; Cowles to Babcock, March 21, 1890; both in Babcock papers, box 4, folder 10, SCL.
52. Sutton, *Crossroads*, 180–82.
53. Herbert B. Howard to Babcock, May 14, 1896, Babcock papers, box 5, folder 8, SCL.
54. Peter E. Griffin to Benjamin Ryan Tillman, May 5, May 8, May 19, and May 20, 1891, Governor Benjamin Ryan Tillman Papers, box 5, folders 5, 7, and 12, SCDAH; Tillman to Griffin, May 5, May 9, May 18, and May 20, 1891; all in Governor Benjamin Ryan Tillman papers, letter book (S526001), SCDAH.
55. W. F. ("Brooks") Babcock to Babcock, May 23 and May 24, 1891; Babcock to W. F. Babcock, May 25, 1891; W. F. Babcock to Babcock, June 4, 1891, all in Babcock papers, box 4, folder 20, SCL.
56. Thomas N. Berry to Babcock, June 3, 1891, Babcock papers, box 4, folder 20, SCL.
57. Berry to Tillman, June 6, 1891, Governor Benjamin Ryan Tillman papers, box 5, folder 22, SCDAH.
58. Tillman to P. E. Griffin, May 9, 1891, Governor Benjamin Ryan Tillman papers, letter book (S526001), SCDAH; Tillman to John S. Withers, June 8, 1891 (copy in Babcock papers, box 4, folder 20, SCL); Withers to Tillman, June 11, 1891, Governor Benjamin Ryan Tillman papers, box 5, folder 24, SCDAH.
59. Cowles to Tillman, June 20, 1891, Governor Benjamin Ryan Tillman papers, box 5, folder 28, SCDAH. A letter from Tillman dated three days earlier addressed to "Dear Sir" requests: "Will you be kind enough to counsel me in perfect confidence your candid opinion as to the fitness of Dr. Jas. W. Babcock for Supt. of our state Lunatic Asylum? What I particularly desire is your opinion of his business qualities & executive interest." The content of the letter strongly suggests that Cowles was the addressee (Tillman to "Dear Sir," June 17, 1891, Governor Benjamin Ryan Tillman papers, letter book [S526001], SCDAH).

60. John S. Withers told Tillman: "Dr. Babcock's relatives here were in full sympathy with the Farmers movement last year [that is, were Tillman supporters], while the relatives of some other applicants were very unfriendly to our cause" (Withers to Tillman, June 5, 1891, Governor Benjamin Ryan Tillman papers, box 5, folder 21, SCDAH).

61. Babcock to Berry, draft of letter, undated; Berry to Babcock, June 23, 1891; both in Babcock papers, box 4, folder 20, SCL.

62. A local newspaper attributed Sydney Eugene Babcock's death in 1892 to blood poisoning (sepsis) acquired from taking care of a man wounded while working on the Southern Railroad ("Chester Doctors, 1861–65," *Chester Reporter*, May 8, 1905).

63. Certificate of appointment, Babcock papers, box 4, folder 20, SCL.

64. J. Stevens Foster to Babcock, July 29, 1891, Babcock papers, box 4, folder 10, SCL.

NOTES FOR CHAPTER 2

1. Babcock's mentor Edward Cowles defined an "alienist" as "a general physician who is a student of neurology, and uses its anatomy and physiology; but he does a great deal more, for he must include all the bodily organs" (Cowles, "Advancement of Psychiatry"). The German physician Johann Christian Reil coined the term "psychiatrist," which, from its Greek roots, literally means "healer of the mind [or soul]." The French physician Philippe Pinel used the term *aliéntation mentale* to imply that the mental patient feels like a stranger (*alienus*) among the sane. Pinel suggested that the therapist could lead the patient back into society by journeying into the patient's world of "alienation." For discussion, see Weiner, "Madman."

2. For concise accounts of the history of psychiatry during this period, see Brown, "Neurology's Influence," and Grob, "Transformation of American Psychiatry." Grob's chapter draws from his four books on asylums in the United States. Grob generalizes: "Unlike asylum physicians whose outlook was shaped by a pietistic Protestantism, neurologists identified with the newly emerging scientific medicine" (Grob, *Mad among Us*, 132). See also references cited in note 43, Chapter 1.

3. Authors of short articles, pamphlets, masters' theses, and doctoral theses also address the history of the South Carolina asylum (see Bibliography).

4. See, for example, Babcock, "Public Charity in South Carolina"; Babcock, "Proud Record of South Carolina"; Babcock, "State Hospital for the Insane"; "Notes on the History of the State Hospital," which includes a manuscript by Babcock on Dr. James Davis (Babcock papers, box 9, folder 2, SCL); and "Notes on the History of Columbia" (Babcock papers, box 9, folder 3, SCL).

5. The extent of Mills's involvement was apparently unknown until the early twentieth century, when a set of the plans and elevations of the "Asylum at

Columbia, S.C." was found in the attic of the McLean Hospital, Waverley, Massachusetts, by Dr. George T. Tuttle. On one of the plans was written "Designed by Robert Mills, Eng. And Architect." Tuttle sent the plans to Babcock (Tuttle to Babcock, June 14, 1906, Babcock papers, box 11, folder 2, SCL). See also note by Margaret Babcock Meriwether, Babcock papers, box 9, folder 1, SCL; Bryan and Johnson, "Robert Mills' Sources"; Bryan, "Robert Mills: Public Architecture"; and Bryan, *Robert Mills*, 179–85. Babcock did not comment on the extent to which Mills relied on concepts developed by two English Quakers, William and Samuel Tuke, especially as they concerned the orientation and landscaping of asylum campuses.

6. Notebook entitled "Notes on Lunatic Asylum, etc.," Babcock papers, box 7, folder 2, SCL; "Governor's message, Stephen D. Miller," *Courier* (Charleston, S.C.), November 28, 1829.

7. Grob, *Mental Institutions*, 28.

8. Diary of Mrs. Henry W. Conner, quoted in Moore, *Columbia and Richland County*, 163.

9. "John Waring Parker, M.D.," unpublished manuscript, Babcock papers, box 7, folder 3, SCL.

10. The captured Union officers had been transferred from Charleston. They were kept initially at a makeshift prison near Columbia known as Camp Sorghum because of the molasses-heavy diet. Frequent escapes prompted the new prison on the asylum campus.

11. "John Waring Parker, M.D.," unpublished manuscript, Babcock papers, box 7, folder 3, SCL.

12. Notes on Thomas Cooper marked "1828" on the first page, Babcock papers, box 7, folder 3, SCL (see also notes on Cooper in Babcock papers, box 9, folder 4, SCL); Broussais, *Irritation and Insanity*. Cooper had no formal medical training but used "M.D." after his name based on an honorary degree.

13. Notes on D. H. Chamberlain marked "1875" on the first page, Babcock papers, box 7, folder 3, SCL.

14. For stunning photographs of many of these institutions, see Payne, *Asylum*.

15. Goffman, *Asylums*. The extent to which these occupational activities constituted therapy rather than exploitation is of course debatable.

16. See for example *AR* (1900), 14–15. Among the advantages of a cottage plan were better lighting, ventilation, noise control, and separation of violent patients.

17. Moore, *Columbia and Richland County*, 276–77.

18. For a summary of early South Carolina hospitals, see Waring, *Medicine in South Carolina, 1825–1900*, 180–89.

19. The Columbia Hospital began as a charity of the United King's Daughters. See Blackburn and Padgette, *Columbia Hospital*.

20. Rice, *Eighteenth Century*, 65. Rice's colorful description of Dr. Talley, although confirmed by Waring (*Medicine in South Carolina, 1825–1900*, 308–9), is perhaps unfair in that Talley was one of the state's most prominent physicians.

21. Bryan, "Profession or Business?"
22. Babcock to Tillman, July 8, 1891, Governor Benjamin Ryan Tillman papers, box 6, folder 2, SCDAH. Babcock asked for an extension of his arrival date from August 1 to August 15 so that he could visit other state asylums.
23. A. A. Moore, "State Board of Health, 1891. Report of the Committee on State Penal and Charitable Institutions." in *SBH/SHI*, 18–19.
24. MBR, September 18, 1891.
25. Eliot, "Character of a Gentleman."
26. *Rules and Regulations for the Government of The Lunatic Asylum.*
27. MBR, August 9, 1894.
28. Waring, *Medicine in South Carolina, 1825–1900*, 309–10; MBR, January 11, 1906. Bronze plaques in Taylor's memory in Trinity Cathedral and in Palmetto Health Richland hospital, both in Columbia, document his stature among his fellow citizens.
29. Thompson, *Shattered Minds*, 23. Babcock went to Europe during 1888 (see Chapter 1), but not for several years.
30. This division of labor and also of power between Babcock (superintendent) and Thompson (first assistant physician) reflected a national trend. In 1853 the Association of Medical Superintendents of American Institutions for the Insane (AMSAII) declared the superintendent should be the chief physician and also the chief executive officer; should "nominate to the board suitable persons to act as Assistant Physician, Steward, and Matron"; and should have "unrestricted power" over all aspects of patient care. In 1892 the AMSAII changed its name to the American Medico-Psychological Association (AMPA) and granted associate membership to assistant physicians, who would be granted full membership after three years of hospital experience. The AMPA became the American Psychiatric Association (APA) in 1921, at which time the *American Journal of Insanity* became the *American Journal of Psychiatry* (Grob, *Mad Among Us*, 73, 139, 162).
31. MBR, October 8, 1891.
32. MBR, August 11, 1892.
33. "First Annual Report, State Board of Health, 1880. Report on the Lunatic Asylum, Located in Columbia, S.C.," in *SBH/SHI*, 3–5.
34. A. A. Moore, "State Board of Health, 1888. Report of the Committee on State Penal and Charitable Institutions," in *SBH/SHI*, 12–15.
35. *AR* (1893–1894), 9–10.
36. Babcock to Katherine Guion, September 25, 1891; Katherine Guion to Babcock, copy of letter, undated; Babcock to Katherine Guion, October 2, 1891; all in Babcock papers, box 4, folder 12, SCL.
37. Babcock to Katherine Guion, October 8, 1891; Babcock to Katherine Guion, October 25, 1891; Babcock to Katherine Guion, undated (apparently an enclosure in Babcock to Katherine Guion, November 11, 1891); Babcock to Katherine Guion, December 27, 1891; all in Babcock papers, box 4, folder 12, SCL.

38. MBR, July 28, 1892.

39. "Babcock-Guion. An Interesting Marriage of a Popular Columbia Couple," Newspaper clipping (undated), Babcock papers, box 4, folder 12, SCL.

40. Campion and Stanton, *Look to This Day*, 70.

41. Standard biographies include Simkins, *Pitchfork Ben Tillman* and Kantrowitz, *Ben Tillman*.

42. For an insightful and entertaining account of Tillman's long shadow over subsequent generations of politicians, see Washington-Williams and Stadiem, *Dear Senator*, 59–64.

43. For the conventional narrative of Tillman's ascent to power see Bass and Poole, *Palmetto State*, 63–78. Cooper (in *Conservative Regime*) dispelled the idea that Tillman's supporters came from markedly different social and economic backgrounds than those of the Conservatives (also known as Bourbons or Redeemers). See also Edgar, *South Carolina in the Modern Age*, 24; and Edgar, *South Carolina: A History*, 430–52.

44. Hampton, who at the outbreak of the Civil War owned large numbers of slaves both in South Carolina and Mississippi, had a more tolerant view of blacks and their rights than did the Tillmanites. For an older study, see Jarrell, *Wade Hampton and the Negro*; for a recent account, see Andrew, *Wade Hampton*. Hampton unlike some of the politicians who followed was notable for his ability to manage ambiguity.

45. John Gary Evans, who succeeded Tillman as governor, reflected Tillman's views when he charged the members of the Constitutional Convention to insert a strong educational qualification for the right of suffrage, since "it is your duty ... to so fix your election laws that your wives, your children and your homes will be protected and Anglo-Saxon supremacy preserved" (*Journal of the Constitutional Convention*, 12).

46. Tillman, *Farewell*, 8.

47. Logan, *Betrayal*, 91.

48. Tillman, *Negro Problem*, 4.

49. *House Journal* (1891), 35.

50. Rubillo, *Hurricane Destruction*, 99–103.

51. See Davis, "Coosaw Rock Alchemy." Damages from a similar storm today would be measured in billions of dollars because of the major resorts and retirement communities on these islands, which include Hilton Head Island. For a concise review, see Marscher and Marscher, *Sea Island Storm*.

52. Tillman to Babcock, September 8, 1893, Babcock papers, box 5, folder 1, SCL.

53. Hennig, *August Kohn*, 80.

54. "The Sea Island Situation. Dr. Babcock Makes a Preliminary Report," *State* (Columbia, S.C.), September 6, 1893.

55. See Rose, *Rehearsal*. Northerners helped the former slaves become self-sufficient by farming the land abandoned by the plantation owners. Northern missionaries founded Penn School on St. Helena Island. The experiment

ended in 1865 when President Andrew Johnson returned the plantations to the previous white owners.

56. Babcock to Tillman, September 4, 1893, Governor Benjamin Ryan Tillman papers, box 23, folder 7, SCDAH.

57. "The Sea Island Situation. Dr. Babcock Makes a Preliminary Report," *State* (Columbia, S.C.), September 6, 1893.

58. Babcock to Tillman, September 5, 1893, Governor Benjamin Ryan Tillman papers, box 23, folder 8, SCDAH.

59. Fitzgerald, "Help These People Help Themselves." Other factors that appealed to Tillman's social conscience included offers to help from concerned citizens; monetary gifts including a $5,000 donation from the Citizens Permanent Relief Committee of Philadelphia; and the example of Dr. William C. Peters on St. Helena Island, who treated some 700 people free of charge and who "promised the colored people to stand by them in their distress and it is my purpose to do so, if I can provide for my family" (Peters to Babcock, September 7, 1893; Babcock to Tillman, September 9, 1893; both in Governor Benjamin Ryan Tillman papers, box 23, folder 14, SCDAH).

60. Tillman was a keen judge of men and had the capacity to value those who opposed him politically if he found them meritorious and trustworthy. August Kohn (1868–1930), who became one of Columbia's wealthiest and most influential citizens, was such an example. Kohn vigorously opposed lynching and was the acknowledged leader of an anti-Tillman faction known as "the Columbia ring." In an era of highly partisan journalism, Kohn was known for fair-mindedness; Tillman confided to a contemporary: "I knew Kohn was not of our party, but I could trust him implicitly" (Stokes, "The Kohn-Hennig Library").

61. Burton, "Introduction"; T. O. Powell to P. L. Murphy, April 17, 1897, Patrick Livingston Murphy papers, collection 535, folder 6, SHC.

62. James B. Meriwether, personal communication, October 12, 2004.

63. Howard, "James Woods Babcock."

64. MBR, January 9, 1908. This observation seems remarkable since, as noted in the text, tuberculosis caused about one in seven deaths. A possible explanation is that medical students of that era did not spend much time on the wards. Harvard's Oliver Wendell Holmes pleaded for more bedside teaching. William Osler generally receives credit for popularizing bedside teaching in the United States, beginning at Johns Hopkins in the early 1890s.

65. MBR, October 8, October 12, and October 30, 1893.

66. Babcock, "Prevention of Tuberculosis."

67. *AR* (1900), 2; *AR* (1907), 12. Identifying patients who were likely to be highly infectious was based almost entirely on physical examination, as chest x-rays and microscopic examination of expectorated sputum (the acid-fast-bacillus smear) were not in routine use.

68. MBR, January 9, 1908.

69. MBR, April 13, 1905. This remark was contained in a paper on "Evolution of Psychiatry" by Dr. William Francis Drewry of Petersburg, Virginia, presented at the fourth annual meeting of the Tri-State Medical Society of the Carolinas and Virginia.

70. Babcock, "Colored Insane."

71. John C. Calhoun buttressed his proslavery arguments by claiming the 1840 census demonstrated insanity to be more prevalent among free blacks than slaves, implying that "the African is incapable of self-care and sinks into lunacy under the burden of freedom" (quoted in Powers, "Worst of All Barbarism"). For the historiography of mental illness in African Americans in the post-emancipation U.S., see Summers, "Suitable Care."

72. For a study of the extent to which slaves' lives were regimented, see Smith, *Mastered by the Clock*. Historians have imploded most antebellum beliefs about slaves' resistance to various diseases and also to the pain of surgery. For example, the belief in an "African immunity" to malaria, held well into the twentieth century, has been largely discredited (McCandless, *Slavery, Disease, and Suffering*, 144–45). As discussed in chapter 5, Babcock seems to have been the first American physician to suggest that pellagra was at least as common in blacks as in whites, and that blacks had no special resistance to the disease.

73. For a recent account of how the "positive good" theory of slavery arising in South Carolina factored into the secession movement, see Kelly, *Longest Siege*.

74. Others included the Worcester (Massachusetts) State Hospital and the Eastern Lunatic Asylum in Williamsburg, Virginia. See Summers, "Suitable Care," 66n17; and Thielman, "Southern Madness."

75. See McCandless, *Slavery, Disease, and Suffering*, 231.

76. These included Ohio. The states with racially integrated asylums were mainly in New England, the mid-Atlantic, and the West. Grob writes that "the absence of segregation in the North grew largely out of the small number of black patients, and in a few hospitals segregation was imposed if the number warranted the practice" (Grob, *Mental Illness*, 220).

77. Babcock did not comment on whether segregation was right or wrong. He concluded by excerpting from a chapter on "The Present and Future of the Negro" by James Bryce, the British historian, jurist and politician, to the effect that discussing integration had become by the turn of the twentieth century beyond the pale of polite conversation among white American southerners (Bryce, "Present and Future").

78. Babcock, although not an office seeker, was by 1900 a councilor of the American Medico-Psychological Association (now the American Psychiatric Association) and secretary of the Southern Association of Asylum Superintendents (probably an informal subgroup of the national association).

79. See, for example, Powell, "Increase of Insanity," and McKie, "Brief History of Insanity."

80. For example, Babcock's fellow asylum superintendent Theophilus O. Powell wrote, "The rapid increase of insanity and consumption in this [the southern Negro] race, is due to a combination of causes and conditions. This race has developed a highly insane, consumptive, syphilitic and alcoholic constitution which predisposes them to diseases which they formerly were free from. In this disturbed and unstable condition they seem to be totally unable to resist the slightest exciting causes ("Increase of Insanity")."

81. See Horsman, *Josiah Nott*. Samuel Cartwright also wrote extensively on this subject, which was still respectable in academic circles in the early twentieth century. See Bean, "Racial Peculiarities."

82. For rich discussion, see Stephens, *Science, Race, and Religion*.

83. See Chase, *Legacy of Malthus*.

84. Jervey, "Passing of the Negro," in *Minutes of the Proceedings of the Fifty-Sixth Annual Meeting of the South Carolina Medical Association*. Jervey supported his conclusions with the results of a survey of 122 Southern physicians. These opinions reflected in part an acceptance of Herbert Spencer's concept of "survival of the fittest."

85. MBR, November 12, 1896.

86. Historian Rayford W. Logan applied "the nadir" to the years between 1877 and 1901, as indicated by his book title: *The Negro in American Life and Thought: The Nadir, 1877–1901*. Historians differ about the precise years, with some extending the period through 1940.

87. See Zuczek, *State of Rebellion*.

88. Calhoun, *Conceiving a New Republic*, 280.

89. Walter Hines Page to Horace E. Scudder, March 18, 1899, quoted in Tindall, *South Carolina Negroes*, 303.

90. Savitt, "Walking the Color Line."

91. W. F. Babcock to J. W. Babcock, May 24, 1891, Babcock papers, box 4, folder 20, SCL. "Brooks" addresses his older brother as "Buddie" in this correspondence.

92. Alice Babcock Simons, "Early Recollections."

93. Haller, "Race, Mortality, and Life Insurance." See also McCandless, *Moonlight*, 283.

94. *Legislative Testimony* (1909), 405.

95. MBR, July 13 and August 10, 1893.

96. *AR* (1899), 23. The bonds had been considered lost. The Dix Cottage housed approximately thirty white women.

97. *AR* (1902), 14.

98. Censer, *White Southern Womanhood*, 146–8, 280. For an in-depth analysis of the treatment of women at the South Carolina asylum, see McCandless, "A Female Malady?" (note 14 in this article references other histories of southern women in the nineteenth and early twentieth centuries).

99. MBR, August 9, 1894.

100. *Legislative Testimony* (1909), 12.
101. MBR, January 10, 1895.
102. MBR, July 13, 1899.
103. Worthington, "Psychiatrist and Humanitarian."
104. Allan, *Diary*.
105. Notes made by Margaret Babcock Meriwether, undated, Babcock papers, box 4, folder 19. An exchange between T. J. Mauldin and Dr. Julius Taylor during the 1914 legislative investigation (*Legislative Testimony* [1914], 434) suggests that Babcock and Ellington supervised new construction "without the aid of any outside architect, builder, or constructor." Other records indicate, however, a role for private contractors, notably a John Milady.
106. Biographical sketch of Page Ellington, undated, Babcock papers, box 4, folder 19, SCL.
107. Babcock to Tillman, September 28, 1910, Governor Benjamin Ryan Tillman papers, box 18, folder 264, CUL. Tillman during the 1850s began a close if paternalistic relationship with a slave named Joe Gibson, whom he continued to employ after emancipation and for whom he provided in his will (Kantrowitz, *Ben Tillman*, 85, 280).
108. Notes made by Margaret Babcock Meriwether, undated, Babcock papers, box 4, folder 19, SCL.
109. James B. Meriwether, personal communication, October 12, 2004.
110. Untitled handwritten notes, Babcock papers, box 4, folder 3, SCL.
111. *AR* (1890–1891), 11.
112. *AR* (1891–1892), 12.
113. Quoted in A. A. Moore, "State Board of Health, 1892. Report of the Committee on State Penal and Charitable Institutions," in *SBH/SHI*, 19–20.
114. Moore, "State Board of Health, 1898. Report of the Committee on State Penal and Charitable Institutions," in *SBH/SHI*, 29–30.
115. MBR, January 12, 1893, March 11, 1897, June 11, 1897, March 10, 1898, and elsewhere; *AR* (1898), 15; McCandless, *Moonlight*, 260–61. The regents and Babcock estimated the cost per bed to be about $75 and noted that the cost at some institutions was $1000 to $3000 per capita or even higher (*AR* [1898], 6, 15). For further discussion of the Parker Building, see Hellams, "South Carolina State Hospital," 113-14.
116. Quoted in Moore, "State Board of Health, 1900. Report of the Committee on State Penal and Charitable Institutions," in *SBH/SHI*, 34–35.
117. See, for example, Preskill, "Educating for Democracy."
118. Tetzlaff, *Cultivating a New South*, 118–21. For discussion of how and why most southern white reformers acknowledged "the need for white paternalism" as a basic requirement, see Link, *Southern Progressivism*, 58–91.
119. See, for example, Marks, "Epidemiologists Explain Pellagra."
120. Grob, *Mad Among Us*, 220–21.
121. See Babcock, "History of Columbia's Trees."

122. Thompson, *Shattered Minds*, 5.

123. Fires involved the laundry, carpenter shop, and dynamo room in 1897; the barn and its contents in 1899, with loss of nine mules; and the Taylor Building in 1903.

124. Thompson, *Shattered Minds*, 25–26.

125. *AR* (1905), 14. In 1896 the asylum obtained 110 acres known as the Wallace property; smaller properties known as the Jones tract (1902) and the Seegers tract (1903) were later acquired.

126. A. A. Moore, "State Board of Health, 1900" and "State Board of Health, 1902," in *SBH/SHI*, 34–37.

127. MBR, June 14 and October 11, 1906.

128. Quoted in A. A. Moore, "State Board of Health, 1903," in *SBH/SHI*, 38.

129. *AR* (1903), 9.

130. In 1906 W. J. Gooding, who had succeeded B. W. Taylor as president of the board of regents upon the latter's death, paraphrased the preceding remark by Babcock by calling the asylum "a conglomerate institution, which serves as the receptacle for undesirable members of all communities of our state" (*AR* [1906], 5).

131. *AR* (1891–1892), 6.

132. See McCandless, *Moonlight*, 266–69. Babcock persuaded the legislature to pass in 1894 an act empowering the superintendent to refuse admissions. The act also put the power of committal exclusively in the hands of probate judges. Although the act took away the power of the county commissioners to admit patients, the commissioners continued to exert considerable influence.

133. Thompson, *Shattered Minds*, 30–31.

134. MBR, June 11, 1908.

135. *Lunacy Laws of South Carolina*, 7, 15, 18.

136. James Woods Babcock, "Medical Certificates of Insanity" (unpublished manuscript), Babcock papers, box 4, folder 9, SCL.

137. This recurring problem prompted the United States Congress in 1986 to pass a law (EMTALA, also known as COBRA or the patient anti-dumping law) making it illegal to send medically unstable patients from a facility receiving federal funds to another facility.

138. "Babcock's Report," *State*, January 7, 1897.

139. "Dr. Babcock Gives Facts and Figures," *State*, January 15, 1900.

140. *AR* (1898), 7–8. See also *AR* (1899), 9–10.

141. *AR* (1900), 9. McCandless writes: "By the turn of the century, conditions at the South Carolina State Hospital approached the horrific. . . . In their quest to keep down expenditures . . . the hospital's administration sacrificed the patients' health, comfort, and even their lives" (*Moonlight*, 270–71).

142. For a succinct review of South Carolina's economic decline during the nineteenth century, including the impact of disease, see McCandless, *Slavery, Disease, and Suffering*, 274–79.

143. For this analysis, data were drawn from Klein, "Personal Income." Klein's data agree closely with those published by Richard A. Easterlin in 1957 (Easterlin, "State Income Estimates") and again in 1960 (Easterlin, "Interregional Differences"). The present author's analysis of these data is on file in box 8, folder 38, Babcock papers, SCL. For economic historians' discussions of methodology see Munyon, "Critical Review," and Mitchener and McLean, "U.S. Regional Growth."

144. Isaac Montrose Taylor to Patrick Livingston Murphy, January 27, 1900, Patrick Livingston Murphy papers, collection 535, folder 7, SHC. Taylor was an assistant physician to Murphy at the Morganton Asylum and the content of his letter suggests a desire to please his superior by making this and other comparisons. Taylor did not comment on Babcock's budget, although Taylor had written in 1891 that the approximate cost at North Carolina's three institutions was about $168 per capita, and that the cost was probably about $130 per capita for "the class of harmless and incurables" (Taylor, *Appeal for State Care*, 5–6.)

145. *AR* (1899).

146. In today's hospital terminology, the president of the Board of Regents functioned as chief executive officer (CEO), the superintendent as chief operating officer (COO), and the first assistant physician as a *quasi* chief medical officer (CMO). Babcock considered lobbying the legislature to be mainly the regents' responsibility, not his (see Chapter 4).

147. MBR, May 12, 1904.

148. Samuel Mather to Babcock, March 29, 1897; Herbert B. Howard to Babcock, April 7, 1897; C. Irving Fisher to Babcock, April 8, 1897; all in Babcock papers, box 4, folder 8, SCL.

149. Tillman to Babcock, April 16, 1897, Babcock papers, box 5, folder 1, SCL.

150. Samuel Mather to Babcock, April 20 and May 21, 1897; Babcock to Samuel Mather (copy or draft of letter), May 24, 1897; both in Babcock papers, box 4, folder 8, SCL.

151. T. O. Powell to Babcock, May 22, 1897; P. L. Murphy to Babcock, May 21, 1897; both in Babcock papers, box 4, folder 11, SCL.

152. Babcock to Murphy, May 21 and May 24, 1897, Patrick Livingston Murphy papers, collection 535, folder 6, SHC. In the second letter, Babcock indicated that his acceptance of the Cleveland job was contingent only upon settling on the salary.

153. Birth dates were: Margaret Woods Babcock, born January 25, 1895; Ferebe Eleanor Babcock, born February 2, 1897; and Alice Guion Babcock, born April 15, 1900. A first-born daughter, Katherine, died in early childhood in June 1895, which according to James B. Meriwether profoundly affected Kate Babcock. She became afraid to love her other children deeply, with the result that "most of the love they got came from their father" (James B. Meriwether, personal communication, October 12, 2004).

154. Simons, "Early Recollections."
155. D. C. Heyward to Babcock, February 16, 1903, Babcock papers, box 4, folder 26, SCL.
156. J. Perry Glenn, J. H. Taylor, W. R. Ray, and W. J. Gooding to Babcock, April 12, 1906, Babcock papers, box 4, folder 26, SCL. The nature of the incident is unclear.
157. MBR, April 3, 1899.
158. Babcock, "Communicated Insanity."
159. *AR* (1893–1894), 27. For further discussion of the classification of psychiatric conditions during the late nineteenth century, see Grob, *Mental Illness*, 35–38, and Horwitz and Grob, "Checkered History."
160. *AR* (1894–1895), 10–11. Although the text indicates that this was a study of 3,900 patients, the table provides data for only 2,692 patients. Calculations based on Babcock's data are as follows: for heredity as a cause of insanity, 26 percent of whites versus 13 percent of blacks (by chi-square test, $P < 0.0001$); for epilepsy, 12 percent for whites versus 15 percent for blacks ($P < 0.05$); for ill health, 12 percent versus nine percent ($P < 0.01$); for domestic affliction, 8 percent versus 9 percent (no significant difference); for intemperance, 11 percent versus 4 percent ($P < 0.0001$); and for religious excitement, 4 percent versus 7 percent ($P < 0.0001$).
161. *AR* (1900), 13.
162. Campion and Stanton, *Look to This Day*, 94.
163. Inscribed on inside back cover of a notebook marked "Memorabilia," Babcock papers, box 7, folder 1, SCL.
164. Thompson, *Shattered Minds*, 61–62, 65–66.
165. Ibid., 55, 62.
166. Ibid., 24.
167. Allan, "Diary," entries February 15 and 23, 1900. In the latter entry, Allan wrote, "Not a brilliant class, I'm afraid."
168. For discussion, see McCandless, *Moonlight*, 292–93. Between 1893 and 1913 there were 114 graduates of the nursing school (average 5.4 per year); of these, 45 graduated between 1893 and 1900 (average 5.6), 37 between 1901 and 1910 (average 4.2 per year), and 32 between 1911 and 1913 (average 10.7). The nadir occurred in 1901 (2 graduates) and the peak in 1913 (12 graduates). Thus, the number of graduates surged during Babcock's final three years as superintendent. These data are in file S190066, SCDAH.
169. In 1897 Alexander Murphy, son of the Morganton superintendent, wrote his mother: "What trouble is Dr. Babcock having that Miss Pitts and the other nurses went to Columbia?" (Alex Murphy to Mrs. P. L. Murphy, October 21, 1897, Patrick Livingston Murphy papers, collection 535, folder 6, SHC). Carrie Streeter concludes that Miss Susan E. Pitts and other nurses went to Columbia because Babcock needed "nurses who were well trained and supportive of current methods of practice." Susan Pitts headed the nurse training

school at the Morganton asylum, established in 1895 by P. L. Murphy. See
Streeter, "Theatrical Entertainments."

170. MBR, November 9, 1911. The nurses' association specifically pointed out
asylum students' deficiencies in obstetrical and surgical nursing. The bill passed
by the legislature at Babcock's instigation gave the asylum school's graduates
"all the rights and privileges of nurses graduating from any other training
school, hospital, or institution in this state" (1912 S.C. Act 417; in *Acts and
Resolutions* [1912], 738).

171. In 1892 and 1894, for example, two physicians resigned but in doing so
acknowledged their pleasant relationships with Babcock. See L. G. Corbett
to Babcock, October 15, 1892, and Marcus Heyman to Babcock, September
22, 1894, both in Babcock papers, box 4, folder 27, SCL. See also discussion
in note 20, page 312.

172. T. Grange Simons, "State Board of Health, 1902. South Carolina Hospital
for the Insane," in *SBH/SHI*, 36.

173. MBR, August 11, 1904.

174. C. C. Gambrell and H. T. Hall, "State Board of Health, 1907. Hospital for
the Insane," in *SBH/SHI*, 34–35.

175. Vaillant, *Adaptation to Life*.

176. One of Babcock's unpublished essays, probably prepared for presentation to
a local group, is entitled "The Physician as a Citizen" (Babcock papers, box 7,
folder 4, SCL), which is in essence a sketch of Dr. Henry Woodward, South
Carolina's first English settler.

177. The dates of these services were: City Board of Health, 1898–1903; Sewerage
Commission, 1901–1903; and Commission on Water and Waterworks,
1903–1907.

178. Undated newspaper clipping, Babcock papers, box 4, folder 30, SCL.

179. "Fortunate Columbia," undated newspaper clipping, Babcock papers, box 4,
folder 30, SCL.

180. "Loan and Exchange Formally Organized," *State*, July 7, 1903 and "New Bank
Report has been Approved," *State*, July 10, 1903. The new bank reportedly had
"the strongest capitalization in the state."

181. "Kosmos Club Founded 31 Years Ago, Maintains 'Town and Gown' Balance
in its Roster of 36 Active Members," *State*, March 21, 1936 (Sesquicentennial
Edition).

182. Benjamin Sloan to Babcock, December 26, 1904, Babcock papers, box 4, folder
7, SCL.

183. S. C. Mitchell to Babcock, September 18, 1909, Babcock papers, box 4, folder
7, SCL.

184. Quoted in "News from the Classes."

185. "Antique Treasures Hidden in Columbia. Dr. Babcock's Collection of Old
Furniture and Other Precious Relics of the Days that are no More—Seems to

have Cleaned out the Entire South for his Beauties," *State*, date undetermined (clipping in Babcock papers, box 4, folder 18, SCL).

186. The extent to which Babcock and his two friends took advantage of the owners of these pieces, who we can assume to have been mainly if not exclusively black farmers and sharecroppers, is unknown.

187. Taylor, *James Woods Babcock*, 5.

188. Babcock specifically encouraged Kohn to collect materials pertaining to the history of South Carolina. Kohn went on to amass the state's largest private collection of "Caroliniana," since donated to the South Caroliniana Library (Stokes, "The Kohn-Hennig Library"). For a compilation of some of Babcock's books at the time of his death, see Babcock papers, box 4, folder 4, SCL.

189. Taylor, *James Woods Babcock*, 7. Snowden (*Old Books*) records that Babcock's library concentrated in medical science, Americana, South Carolina history and literature, French works, notably Balzac, and English history and literature.

190. James B. Meriwether, personal communication, October 12, 2004.

191. "Dying Words of Gonzales Put in Evidence. 'I Sent no Messages,' Declared Wounded Man," *New York World*, October 1, 1903.

192. Anderson, "Eleanora Bennette Saunders."

NOTES FOR CHAPTER 3

1. The term *theory* is used throughout this book when it was so used by the persons in question. *Hypothesis* is used by the present author to denote a proposition, suggestion, or educated guess that has not been adequately tested by experiments or repeated observations.

2. Randolph, "Notes on Pellagra."

3. The discussion here follows the traditional view that pellagra is caused by dietary deficiency of niacin and tryptophan. For a provocative recent discussion, see Williams and Ramsden, "Pellagra." Some researchers suggest that human pellagra is a complex nutritional disorder caused by multiple deficiencies. For a thorough discussion of pellagra as "the first known electron transport disorder affecting the human nervous system," see Still, "Nicotinic Acid." See also Bruyn and Poser, "Pellagra." The description of pellagra as an electron transport disorder is more prevalent in the neurology literature than in the general medical literature. However, it seems reasonable because of the key role of NAD/NADH in the electron transport chain. One might alternatively consider pellagra an "electron transfer disorder" because of the wide role of NAD/NADH and NADP/NADPH in oxidation and reduction reactions. These perspectives are consistent with a definition given by Williams and Ramsden: "Pellagra is a curable dietary illness that unchecked leads to dementia, diarrhea, dermatitis and death due to lack of precursors of NAD(H)."

4. Nicotinic acid cannot be converted directly into nicotinamide, but both can be used to make NAD+ and NADP+. Nicotinic acid is also used to treat high cholesterol levels. Because nicotinic acid has flushing as a side effect, nicotinamide is the form commonly used as a food additive or vitamin supplement.
5. Elvehjem et al., "Relation to Nicotinic Acid"; Elvehjem et al., "Anti-black-tongue Factor."
6. Spies et al., "Treatment of Subclinical and Classical Pellagra."
7. Technically, "niacin" denotes nicotinic acid, while "niacinamide" denotes nicotinamide.
8. Reduction is the *gain* of electrons, as in the conversion of NAD+ to NADH. Oxidation is the *loss* of electrons, as in the conversion of NADH back to NAD+. NADH is thus an electron donor (reducing agent), while NAD+ is an electron acceptor (oxidizing agent).
9. Our critical dependence on a constant supply of ATP explains, for example, why we cannot do without oxygen for more than a few minutes and why cyanide poisoning kills so quickly. Oxygen deprivation shuts down aerobic respiration. Cyanide poisoning shuts down the electron transport chain. ATP is the "molecular currency of life" largely if not entirely because of its three high-energy phosphate bonds.
10. These paragraphs will strike some readers as inordinately complicated and others as inordinately simplistic, omitting as they do many key processes (for example, glycolysis, oxidative phosphorylation, and the pentose phosphate pathway) and molecules (for example, NADP/NADPH and FADH$_2$). The author consulted numerous sources and ultimately based this account mainly on his grandchildren's high school biology textbook (Postlethwait and Hopson, *Modern Biology*, 130–49).
11. Many authorities suggest that the "niacin equivalent" values of food—calculated from both the niacin and the tryptophan content—correlates better with pellagra-preventative value than niacin content alone. The statement that it takes 60 milligrams of tryptophan to make one milligram of niacin represents an average value; the extent of conversion depends on the body's relative needs. See Nakagawa et al., "Efficiency of Conversion," and Horwitt et al., "Niacin-tryptophan Relationships."
12. The combination of dermatitis, diarrhea, and dementia is sometimes called "Knowles's triad." Babcock and others noted numerous neuropsychiatric manifestations besides depression and dementia (Chapter 5).
13. Human pellagra is nearly always more complicated than experimental canine black tongue, since patients on impoverished diets typically have multiple nutritional deficiencies. Peripheral nerve damage (neuropathy) in pellagrins is due at least in part to thiamine (vitamin B$_1$) deficiency; sore tongue (glossitis) is due at least in part to riboflavin (vitamin B$_2$) deficiency.

14. Another, and complementary, explanation for the rarity of pellagra among Latin Americans was their habitual use of other vegetables such as beans, squash, chili peppers, and potatoes.

15. The words "epidemic" and "endemic" are often confused. "Epidemic" literally means "*upon* the people" and denotes the occurrence of a disease affecting many more people than would ordinarily be expected. "Endemic" literally means "*among* the people" and denotes the more-or-less stable and predictable occurrence of a disease within a locality. Thus, influenza A ("flu") is typically epidemic, whereas the common cold is typically endemic. The distinction between "epidemic" and "endemic" can be blurred. We could say, for example, that pellagra was "epidemic" in many U.S. asylums between roughly 1907 and 1910 (because it unexpectedly affected numerous patients) but thereafter became "endemic" (since it predictably affected a certain percentage of patients each year). "Pandemic" denotes an epidemic of world-wide proportions.

16. See, for example, Sydenstricker, "History of Pellagra," and Carpenter, "Effects of Different Methods."

17. For further discussion, see Chapters 5 and 6. In 1753 the surgeon James Lind reported that juice from lemons or limes eradicated scurvy, which had been endemic in the British navy. In 1884 the physician Takaki Kanehiro reported that adding meat and legumes to a diet weighted toward polished rice eradicated beriberi, which had been affecting the Japanese navy. For a concise review, see Jukes, "Prevention and Conquest."

18. The standard social histories in English are Etheridge, *Butterfly Caste*, and Roe, *Plague of Corn*. References cited in the present volume focus mainly on perspectives about pellagra since the treatises by Etheridge and Roe. The many good book chapters include Bollet, "The Pellagra Epidemics"; Etheridge, "Pellagra"; Frankenburg, "Dermatitis, Diarrhea, Dementia, and Death," in Frankenburg, *Vitamin Discoveries*, 33–55; and Lanska, "Historical Aspects." Among the better concise reviews in medical journals is Rajakumar, "Pellagra in the United States."

19. Casál's reputation as "the Asturian Hippocrates" led to his becoming personal physician to King Ferdinand VI, a severe manic-depressive. In Madrid, Casál met François Thiéry, physician to the French embassy, and told him about the strange malady among the Asturians. In 1755, seven years before Casál's observations were published posthumously, Thiéry published on pellagra and gave due credit to Casál.

20. Semba, "Thèophile Roussel."

21. Pellagra has recently been called the first known photosensitivity disease, although the precise relationship to sunlight remains unclear. See Wan et al., "Pellagra."

22. For a review, see Mariani-Costantini and Mariani-Costantini, "Pellagra in Italy." These authors point out how debates about the etiology of pellagra stimulated the emergence of a social conscience among Italian scientists.

23. The esteem with which Lombroso was held in the United States is evinced by his obituaries; see especially "Cesare Lombroso." Lombroso's fertile mind continues to attract scholarly attention. See Mazzarello, "Cesare Lombroso"; Monaco and Mula, "Lombroso and Epilepsy"; and Kushner, "Lombroso and the Pathology of Left-Handedness."

24. Sambon, "Geographical Distribution."

25. Sambon, "Elucidation of Sleeping Sickness." See also Livingstone, "Tropical Climate."

26. Manson became famous by showing that the tiny roundworms of filariasis (elephantiasis) are present in the bloodstream only during the night. "Following this discovery," writes Gordon C. Cook, Manson "became almost obsessed with the role of other filariae in the causation of human disease" (Cook, "Patrick Manson"). The parasite *Schistosoma mansoni* which Sambon thus named is known in much of the world as *Schistosoma mansoni sambon*.

27. "Importance of Rational Inductive Methods."

28. Rosenberg, *Cholera Years*; Rosenberg, "Explaining Epidemics."

29. The remembrance of history's largely forgotten *dramatis personae* of Acts One and Two constitutes a major purpose of this book.

30. Osler, *Principles and Practice*, 6th ed., 384. The first edition of this textbook (1892) became the standard and made its author the best-known physician in the English-speaking world. Lanska ("Stages in the Recognition") traces how case definitions of pellagra became more relaxed over time, resulting in an increase in diagnostic sensitivity (that is, *true-positive*: diagnosis of pellagra when the patient actually had pellagra) but a decrease in diagnostic specificity (that is, *false-positive*: diagnosis of the pellagra when the patient did not actually have pellagra).

31. Searcy, "Epidemic of Acute Pellagra." Searcy gave up his work in Alabama in the summer of 1908 and went west for his health. He hoped to return to Alabama to work on pellagra (George H. Searcy to Surgeon General Wyman, undated, box 148, NARA) but published little further on the disease.

32. Babcock, "State Hospital for the Insane."

33. MBR, January 1, 1908.

34. Ray et al., "Pellagra and Pellagrous Insanity." There is no evidence that anyone assisted Babcock in the writing of this paper.

35. "Pellagra in this Country." The author was probably Dr. J. W. Jervey, editor of the state medical journal.

36. An addendum expresses the logical concern that these patients might have had an unusual manifestation of hookworm: "After studying this case, Dr. Stiles' comment was 'If this is hookworm disease, its symptoms are entirely different from those I am familiar with, and without microscopic examination I should place her in the doubtful class as regards uncinariasis [hookworm].'" Charles Stiles was an authority on hookworm.

37. He had seen in consultation with J. J. Watson a 14-year-old married woman with classic symptoms and signs of pellagra. Dr. D. S. Pope had told him about two cases, one from his private practice and the other from the state penitentiary. Dr. L. K. Philpot had told him about three cases among children at the Epworth Orphanage in Columbia.

38. The word "syndrome" is modified Latin from the Greek *syn* ("with") plus *dramein* ("run")—hence, a cluster of symptoms (complaints related by the patient) and signs (abnormalities observed by the physician) that "run together."

39. "Pellagra in this Country." Just after this editorial came an announcement that South Carolina had created the position of State Health Officer. The first appointee was Dr. Charles Frederick Williams, who would assist Babcock in the fight against pellagra and would succeed Babcock as asylum superintendent ("State Health Officer").

40. "Hookworm Found in This State," *State* (Columbia, S.C.), January 15, 1908.

41. Babcock as Tillman's physician did not have means to monitor and treat hypertension and other risk factors for stroke. In 1910 Babcock advised Tillman to drink lots of buttermilk on the basis of a theory advanced by the great European scientist Eli Metchnikoff that lactic acid might prevent hardening of the arteries (Babcock to Tillman, July 7, 1910, Tillman papers, box 17, folder 256, CUL).

42. Tillman to Babcock, March 24, 1908, Babcock papers, box 5, folder 1, SCL. Absence of severe headache suggests the stroke was ischemic rather than hemorrhagic (Tillman to Babcock, April 5, 1908, Babcock papers, box 5, folder 1, SCL).

43. Tillman to Babcock, April 12, 1908, Babcock papers, SCL, box 5, folder 1. Tillman wrote a month after the stroke: "I do not feel sure of myself or my direction—that feeling of toppling over on the left side & of side stepping when I walk are still with me 'tho I can walk . . . by sheer will power." These and other letters indicate that Tillman was right-handed, as his handwriting was unimpaired despite a left hemiparesis. According to the newspaper, "Dr. Babcock himself had had a long illness" and was restored to health by the trip ("Finding a Cure for Pelagra [sic]," *State*, September 21, 1908). The present author has been unable to confirm that Babcock was ill; possibly his illness was simply what is now called "burnout."

44. Tillman to Babcock, April 23, 1908, Babcock papers, SCL, box 5, folder 1. In this letter Tillman, perhaps in denial, indicated that he was reluctant to travel abroad without Babcock because of unwillingness "to subject my wife to the risk of getting ill over there among strangers."

45. "Senator Tillman is Now 'Doing' Switzerland," *News and Courier* (Charleston, S.C.), August 2, 1908. Newspaper clippings from this trip are contained in Babcock papers, box 5, folder 1, and numerous letters from Dr. and Mrs.

Babcock to their daughters are contained in Babcock papers, box 8, folders 2 and 3, SCL.

46. Babcock, "The Diagnosis and Treatment of Pellagra." Babcock recorded some of these notes on small sheets of yellow paper. They now reside in a copy of Lombroso's monograph *L'Opera Pellagrologica*, having apparently been put there by Babcock (Babcock papers, box 8, folder 19, SCL).

47. Taylor, *James Woods Babcock*, 6.

48. Babcock's meeting with Fleming Sandwith in London is not mentioned in any previous accounts. Documentation consists of a letter from Babcock to one of the editors of the *American Journal of Insanity*, written just before Babcock sailed for home: "I have fully satisfied myself as to the identity of Pellagra as it exists in the Southern States and in Italy and Egypt. I studied many cases near Venice and Milan; and in London, Dr. Sandwith has been especially kind in reviewing the whole subject with me at the London School of Tropical Medicine" ("Notes and Comment" [anonymous], *AJI* 65, no. 2 (1908), 377–84). Babcock had known of Sandwith by reputation since medical school, having copied a regimen for acute dysentery by "Sandwith of Cairo" (Notebook entitled "Memorabilia," Babcock papers, box 7, folder 1, SCL).

49. "F. M. Sandwith"; "Fleming Mant Sandwith"; "The Late Colonel F.M. Sandwith."

50. Sandwith, *Egypt as a Winter Resort*.

51. Holland, "On the Pellagra." Holland read this paper before the Royal Medical and Chiurgical Society of London on June 24, 1817. Holland also drew an analogy between pellagra and scurvy. His autobiography includes observations about pellagra (Holland, *Recollections*, 140–41). Holland was preceded by Joseph Townsend, a British pastor who described encounters with pellagra during a two-year tour of Spain (Townsend, *Journey through Spain*, 10–11).

52. Sandwith, *Diseases of Egypt*.

53. As noted elsewhere, the red, smooth tongue in the later stages of pellagra is now generally attributed to riboflavin (vitamin B_2) deficiency.

54. Dr. Heyward Gibbes, Columbia's first internal medicine specialist, described Joseph Jenkins Watson (1872–1924) as "one of the keenest clinicians I have ever known" (Gibbes, "Fifty Years of Medicine"). A bronze plaque in Watson's memory at Palmetto Health Richland in Columbia, S.C., confirms his stature among contemporaries. Watson receives less attention in this book than he deserves because of the paucity of source material. Babcock had apparently suggested to Tillman that Watson go to Italy with their party, an idea Tillman welcomed (Tillman to Babcock, April 23, 1908, Babcock papers, box 5, folder 1, SCL). Perhaps Watson went separately because he had to limit time away from his private practice.

55. Watson was one of Babcock's closest friends (see Chapter 1). Babcock wrote: "Watson's studies of, and contribution to, the whole investigation are of great importance and value" (Babcock, "Diagnosis and Treatment"). Babcock and

Watson later made a joint presentation on pellagra at the New York Academy of Medicine ("Babcock and Watson Talk on Pellagra," undated newspaper clipping, Babcock papers, box 3, folder 19, SCL.) Babcock did not visit Lombroso in Italy, perhaps because such a visit did not fit into Tillman's itinerary. Likewise, he did not seek out Sigmund Freud in Vienna, perhaps in part because he frowned on Freud's theories with the exception of Freud's interpretation of dreams (James B. Meriwether, personal communication, October 12, 2004).

56. Hollis, *University of South Carolina*, 2:241. Kohn had been considered for the position but believed that as a Jew he was unelectable. He therefore promoted his close friend Babcock.

57. August Kohn to Babcock, June 10, 1908, Babcock papers, box 3, folder 18, SCL.

58. "Varsity President" (clipping from an unidentified newspaper), Babcock papers, box 4, folder 5, SCL.

59. The assembly hall was on the third floor of the Main Building (*Legislative Report* [1910], 95). There are also references to an "amusement hall"; lacking evidence to the contrary, the present author surmises that the assembly and amusement halls were one and the same.

60. *Conference on Pellagra . . .* October 29th, 1908.

61. Babcock had recently given a clinic in Charlotte, North Carolina ("Dr. Babcock on Pellagra. South Carolina Physician, Pioneer in Study of Mysterious and Insidious Disease, Gives Clinic at Presbyterian Hospital," *Charlotte News*, September 25, 1908).

62. One of these was a meeting of a committee of the South Carolina Medical Association to consider the establishment of an Anti-Tuberculosis League in the state ("Tuberculosis and Pellagra," *News and Courier*, October 31, 1908).

63. "Conference on Pellagra." See also "A Conference on Pellagra," *State*, October 29, 1908.

64. The Columbia newspaper reported that "among the many meetings of the fair week one of the most successful was the pellagra conference" ("The Pellagra Conference," *State*, November 1, 1908).

65. "The Pellagra Conference," *State*, November 1, 1908.

66. Moore, "Etiology of Pellagra."

67. Wood, "Pellagra—Some Problems." Wood was an early convert to the "infection hypothesis" but was later among the first southerners to accept Goldberger's thesis that dietary deficiency was the root cause of pellagra. See Jones, "Pellagra, Progress, and Public Polemics."

68. Watson, "Etiology of Pellagra"

69. Thompson, "Roumanian Theory."

70. Taylor, "Protozoan Theory."

71. Taylor, "Personal Experience."

72. McConnell, "Clinical Observations." Harvey E. McConnell (1866–1918) was one of the leading physicians of Chester, Babcock's home town. He was a founder of the Chester sanatorium and was noted for his charity work in

addition to his successful practice. He subsequently asserted he had recognized pellagra since 1903.

73. "Pellagra and Blind Staggers," *State*, November 1, 1908. The author, M. Ray Powers of Clemson College, was correct to the extent that blind staggers (technically known as equine leucoencephalomalacia) can be caused by mycotoxins (toxins produced by fungi). One mycotoxin-producing fungus, *Fusobacterium moniliforme*, is commonly found in corn and silage.

74. Babcock, "Diagnosis and Treatment." The recommendation by Babcock and many others to abstain from corn (in addition to adding more variety to their diets) may strike today's readers as illogical, but it was later shown that corn might have a "pellagragenic effect" independent of its "anti-nicotinic acid effect" (Goldsmith et al., "Studies of Niacin Requirement").

75. Lavinder to the Surgeon General [Walter Wyman], November 24, 1908, box 148, NARA.

76. "Thirtieth Annual Report of the State Board of Health of South Carolina for the Fiscal Year 1909," *Reports and Resolutions* (1910, vol. 2), 1351–1471.

77. *Conference on Pellagra* (1908), 56–59.

78. "Message from the Governor," Wednesday, January 13, 1909, *Senate Journal* (1909), 37.

79. What is now the National Institutes of Health (NIH) began in 1887 as a one-room laboratory at the U.S. Marine Hospital in Stapleton, Staten Island, New York. This later became the Hygienic Laboratory. In 1891 it was moved to Washington, D.C., and in 1902 it was reorganized under the newly named U.S. Public Health and Marine Hospital Service. It was not until 1930 that the Hygienic Laboratory, its scope greatly expanded, was renamed the National Institute (singular) of Health (NIH). Thus, what might seem today as ludicrous—Lavinder's setting up a laboratory in the Old Building of the South Carolina State Hospital for the Insane where facilities were clearly inadequate for the purpose—can be explained in part by the absence of a large, centralized laboratory under the auspices of the U.S. Public Health Service, as currently exists both at the NIH in Bethesda, Maryland, and at the Centers for Disease Control and Prevention (CDC) in Atlanta, Georgia.

80. Henry Rose Carter is best known for demonstrating the "extrinsic incubation period" of yellow fever, a key link in the chain of evidence that led to proof of mosquito transmission by the U.S. Army Commission headed by Walter Reed (See also page 160). Lavinder wrote Carter's widow that "I almost feel that I have lost a second father. For indeed he <u>was</u> my professional father, having initiated me—a green youngster—into the first principles of clinical Medicine and [having] favorably introduced to me the Public Health Service as a career for medical men" (C. H. Lavinder to Laura Armistead Carter, September 29, 1925, Philip S. Hench Walter Reed Yellow Fever Collection, Claude Moore Health Sciences Library, University of Virginia).

81. The U.S. Marine Hospital Service was created by Congress in 1870 from a loose network of locally controlled hospitals in seaports and in inland ports on major waterways. In 1889 Congress created the Commissioned Corps of the U.S. Marine-Hospital Service, the officers having ranks and pay grades corresponding to those of the Army and Navy. In 1902 the name was changed to U.S. Public Health and Marine Hospital Service; in 1912 the name was shortened to U.S. Public Health Service.

82. MBR, May 11, May 18, and May 19, 1909; "Personal" [observations]; Etheridge, *Butterfly Caste*, 16–17. A letter from Babcock to Tillman indicates that Babcock wrestled with but overcame concern that by collaborating with Lavinder he might be upstaged by the federal government. The letter suggests Babcock had asked W. Bayard Cutting, Jr., the State Department's acting consul to the Italian government in Milan, for copies of various monographs written by the Italian authorities on pellagra: "Thinking over the communication about the pellagra literature, it occurs to me that if we bring in Dr. Lavinder's name as we have done and also the name of his service, it is possible that the State Dept. might attribute this letter to him when I was the real instigator. . . . Sorry to trouble you but the matter seems important for the future of pellagra work in the South" (Babcock to Tillman, July 12, 1909, Tillman papers, box 14, folder 215, CUL).

83. Lavinder to Walter Wyman, May 28, 1909; Lavinder to Wyman, January 29, 1910, Lavinder to Wyman, June 28, 1910; all in NARA, box 148; Etheridge, *Butterfly Caste*, 16–17.

84. "Rare Disease Found Here," *New York Times*, July 21, 1909.

85. "In the Corn Belt," *Daily Record* (Columbia, S.C.), August 16, 1909. The hospital in Bartonville opened in 1902 as the Illinois Hospital for the Incurable Insane and was renamed Illinois General Hospital for the Insane (1907) and then Peoria State Hospital (1909). The latter name will be used here for simplicity.

86. Lavinder et al., "Prevalence of Pellagra."

87. "Personal" [observations].

88. MBR, December 30, 1908.

89. "Meet to Discuss Dread Pellagra," *State*, August 7, 1909.

90. C. H. Lavinder, "Prophylaxis of Pellagra."

91. MBR, November 3, 1909.

92. "Programme for the Pellagra Conference," *State*, November 3, 1909; "The First Conference to Study Pellagra," "To Study Pellagra," and "Noted Scientists Gather Here," *State*, November 4, 1909; and "The Conference on Pellagra," *State*, November 5, 1909.

93. The first Carolina-Clemson game took place in 1896, the newspaper reporting of the spectators: "The din from their yells and horns sounded as if the inmates of an insane asylum had broken loose" ("A Superb Game," *State*, November

13, 1896). The contests were suspended between 1903 and 1908 because of a riot at the 1902 game.
94. Etheridge, *Butterfly Caste*, 18.
95. *NASP Transactions* (1909). For a concise summary, see Lavinder, "National Congress on Pellagra."
96. Goldberger, "Etiology of Pellagra."
97. Sandwith, "Introductory Remarks." *NASP Transactions* (1909), 14–19.
98. Kerr, "Notes on the Hematology of Pellagra" [*sic*].
99. Watson, discussion of Taylor, "Etiology of Pellagra."
100. Jones, discussion of Taylor, "Etiology of Pellagra."
101. Sandwith, "Introductory Remarks."
102. Watson, "Economic Factors."
103. Roe (*Plague of Corn*, 83) comments: "It is easy to ridicule Watson's chauvinistic attitude, but his opinions were shared by many of those at the congress."
104. De Jarnet, "The Corn Curse."
105. Rohrer, "Pellagra."
106. Watson, "Symptomatology of Pellagra."
107. Taylor, "Etiology of Pellagra."
108. Lavinder, "Hematology of Pellagra."
109. Siler and Nichols, "Pellagra Situation in Illinois." Eighty-five percent of 88 patients with pellagra had amebic parasites in their tools, compared with 49 percent of 101 patients without pellagra (by chi-square test, $P < 0.0001$). Other investigators confirmed this observation but stated that the amebic parasites were of the nonpathogenic type. Several nonpathogenic amebae closely resemble *Entamoeba histolytica*, the cause of amebiasis (amebic dysentery). The suggestion here is that nonpathogenic amebae multiplied much more readily when the intestinal mucosa had been damaged by niacin deficiency.
110. In 1902 Zeller became superintendent of a new, thirty-three-building asylum built according to the cottage plan. He took down the bars from windows and doors, removed mechanical restraints, banned the use of narcotics to subdue patients, limited work shifts to eight hours, allowed women to work in the male wards, segregated patients with tuberculosis, and introduced music and dancing. He used the bars that had been removed from the windows and doors to make an enclosure for wild animals (notably deer, bears, and coyotes) in a nearby ravine. This provided an animal park for the amusement of patients and visitors. People came from long distances to observe the "Zeller treatment." For further information on Zeller, see Lisman and Parr, *Bittersweet Memories*, and Ward and Parr, *Asylum Light*.
111. Zeller, "Pellagra."
112. Babcock, discussion of Zeller, "Pellagra." Silas Weir Mitchell, the eminent Philadelphia physician and writer remembered for the "Weir Mitchell treatment" of neurasthenia and other mental conditions (which involved enforced

bed rest, frequent feedings, and other measures) disparaged asylum superintendents (See Brown, "Neurology's Influence," and note 2, Chapter 2.

113. As noted elsewhere, Joseph Goldberger would later cite this observation, and would also cite the observation made at the conference by Dr. C. G. Manning of Bridgetown, Barbadoes, that whatever its cause pellagra was not contagious.

114. To the present author's knowledge, this argument (the development of pellagra in long-term asylum inmates) against Sambon's hypothesis has not been previously made, nor was it mentioned by Goldberger. It is unclear what fraction of pellagra cases reported from asylums were acquired in the asylums, as opposed to having been acquired before admission. However, it is clear that many (if perhaps not most) of these cases resulted from the monotonous diets served in these institutions.

115. The ABO blood groups had been discovered by the Austrian scientist Karl Landsteiner in 1900, but transfusion science was in 1909 still in its infancy.

116. Kerr came away with the impression that Zeller had been elected president, but this is not reflected in the published minutes. Zeller had, however, apparently offered to host the next national meeting in Peoria (J. W. Kerr to Walter Wyman, November 10, 1909, box 148, NARA).

117. "The Conference on Pellagra."

118. F. M. Sandwith to Babcock, November 27, 1909; miscellaneous letters to Katherine Guion Babcock; all in Babcock papers, box 8, folder 4, SCL. Sandwith told Babcock he had asked a German chemical supply house to send Babcock "a gratis supply of Arsacetin, as I thought you would like to be the first person to try it in pellagra." Many and perhaps most physicians were prescribing arsenical compounds for pellagra. It had been suggested that Arsacetin would be less toxic than the then commonly used arsenic preparation, Atoxyl.

119. MBR, October 14, 1909.

NOTES FOR CHAPTER 4

1. Beardsley, *History of Neglect*, 6.

2. MBR, June 11, 1908 and July 1, 1908.

3. Hunter A. Gibbes to the General Assembly of South Carolina, Columbia, S.C., January 11, 1909, Babcock papers, box 4, folder 22, SCL; MBR, January 14, 1909; "The Asylum Investigation," *Carolina Spartan* (Spartanburg, S.C.), May 26, 1909. Grob observes that at the turn of the twentieth century "psychiatrists found themselves under attack from a variety of individuals and groups, including other physicians, social activists, lawyers, state regulatory agencies, and former patients" (Grob, *Mental Illness*, 46). All of these forces came to bear on Babcock.

4. MBR, February 11, 1897. According to these minutes, "The Superintendent acknowledges that he is somewhat of a stamp crank, having been engaged in collecting rare stamps since he was a small boy, but he denies wasting time on them, and inasmuch as he does not waste time on making social calls, attending social gatherings, going to the theater and other places of amusement and recreation he cannot see why the small pleasures he derives from this source be denied him and made the subject for a Legislative investigation."
5. Edgar, *South Carolina in the Modern Age*, 34; Link, *Southern Progressivism*.
6. See for example Moore, *Carnival of Blood*.
7. Tetzlaff, *Cultivating a New South*, 70–74.
8. See Faust, "Accounting."
9. Helsey, *Beaufort*, 130–31, 146.
10. Christensen, "State Dispensaries." Tillman had pushed a state-run liquor dispensary as a compromise with prohibitionists. Abbie Christensen was an ardent prohibitionist (Anne Christensen Pollitzer, personal communication, August 28, 2013) and may have influenced her son in this regard. The State Dispensary closed in 1907, although six counties continued to control their own liquor trade.
11. Niels Christensen Jr to Niels Christensen Sr, January 14, January 18, and January 19, 1909, Christensen Family Papers, SCL. The regents ultimately completed a list of twenty-four reasons for an investigation (MBR, July 8, 1909).
12. MBR, February 11, 1909.
13. "Investigation will be Serious," *State* (Columbia, S.C.), April 30, 1909.
14. *Legislative Testimony* (1909). The eight days of testimony were spread out over a month, continuing through late May. For a collection of newspaper clippings pertaining to these hearings, see Babcock papers, box 4, folder 6, SCL.
15. The newspaper reported that the investigation had been prompted "at the request of the superintendent and regents" ("Investigating State Hospital," *State*, April 27, 1909), but it seems more probable that Babcock and Gooding made their request in reaction to a decision that had already been made by the legislature.
16. "Asylum Investigation Begun," *News and Courier* (Charleston, S.C.), April 28, 1909.
17. Niels Christensen Jr. to Abbie Holmes Christensen, May 9, 1909, Christensen Family Papers, SCL.
18. *Legislative Testimony* (1909), 35–150.
19. Ibid., 150–96, 257–67.
20. In 1930 a graduate student after reviewing this material concluded that Babcock "failed to get on peaceably with his co-workers and, failing to remain in good terms with them, he left the responsibility to them. The inevitable result was the neglect of the institution" (Johnson, "South Carolina State

Hospital," 104–35). The present author has a different take based on his experience as a physician. Thompson probably conveyed in numerous subtle ways that he did not want Babcock to visit his wards or make rounds on his patients.

21. Blackburn and Padgette, *Columbia Hospital*, 12.
22. "Senator Weston Replies," *State*, February 17, 1910.
23. Thompson, *Shattered Minds*, 63–64. Babcock began his cross-examination of Thompson with an expression of empathy: "I don't suppose anybody can appreciate more than I can the stress under which you have been laboring for some weeks past, and I am sorry to have to prolong your ordeal by asking a few questions" (*Legislative Testimony* [1900], 181).
24. "Hospital Physician Testifies," *News and Courier*, May 7, 1909.
25. MBR, September 11, 1906.
26. Waring, *Medicine in South Carolina, 1900–1970*, 162. Waring notes that Taylor "was a pioneer in setting up a small clinic in the slum areas around the Pacific Mills." Taylor said on one occasion that "the matter of life was more important than the separation of the races" (MBR, December 30, 1908).
27. *Legislative Testimony* (1909), 302.
28. "Hospital Physician Testifies," *News and Courier*, May 7, 1909.
29. *Legislative Testimony* (1909), 245, 251–52.
30. Ibid., 334.
31. The reluctance of white men to work alongside blacks became one rationale for Babcock's advocacy of separate asylum campuses. Such reluctance was of course a carryover from slavery (see Chapter 2). As one historian puts it, "Slavery undermined the dignity of manual work by associating it with servility and thereby degraded white labor wherever bondage existed" (McPherson, *Battle Cry*, 55).
32. *Legislative Testimony* (1909), 369–70, 374, 380, 382, 397.
33. Ibid., 388.
34. Emphasis on reducing length-of-stay became prominent in hospitals in the United States during the late twentieth century after insurers, including the federal government, began to reimburse based on diagnosis rather than hospital charges. With hindsight one can fault Babcock for not being more aggressive about pressing for earlier discharge for patients who had improved. However, few physicians welcomed mental patients into their private practices and there was no system of publicly funded mental health clinics.
35. *Legislative Testimony* (1909), 391–92.
36. Ibid., 5–18, 398–99.
37. Ibid., 402–3.
38. Ibid., 402.
39. Ibid., 404, 423, 435.
40. "The Hospital and the Doctors."

41. *Legislative Report* (1910). Signing the Majority Report were Christensen and George H. Bates from the Senate and George W. Dick and Wade C. Harrison from the House of Representatives. Signing the Minority Report were P. L. Hardin from the Senate, and Olin Sawyer and J. P. Carey from the House of Representatives. Hardin was a farmer from Chester County; Sawyer was a physician from Beaufort County. Also included in this volume is a 34-page architectural report from the Columbia firm of Shand & Lafaye. The architects made numerous recommendations for modernization and estimated the cost of new (but not fireproof) facilities to be about $600 per patient.

42. Ibid., 60. In 1910 there were 207 cases of pellagra at the South Carolina State Hospital for the Insane, versus only seven cases at the Kankakee State Hospital (Singer, "Pellagra in Illinois"). For information on the Kankakee State Hospital, see Grob, *Mad Among Us*, 113.

43. *Legislative Report* (1910), 8–9.

44. Ibid., 11.

45. Ibid., 17. Ironically, the vertical filing cabinet was invented in 1898 less than a mile from Babcock's asylum by Columbia businessman Edwin G. Seibels.

46. Moreover, the clerical staff was inadequate. See McCandless, *Moonlight*, 287.

47. Medical records of that era were skimpy by today's standards. For a review with bibliography, see Kirkland and Bryan, "Osler's Service."

48. *Legislative Report* (1910), 21–23.

49. Poor overall quantity and quality of the staff were not unique to the South Carolina asylum. See Grob, *Mental Illness*, 20–22.

50. *Legislative Report* (1910), 5, 41–42.

51. Ibid., 43, 47. Restraints were controversial within the psychiatric community (see Grob, *Mental Illness*, 18). Henry Andrews Cotton, who became medical director of the Trenton State Hospital at the age of 30, implemented several progressive ideas such as abolishing mechanical restraints and holding daily staff meetings to discuss patient care. Cotton is now seen as a controversial figure because of his obsession with infections as the cause of mental illness (see Scull, *Madhouse*). It is generally acknowledged that frequent use of mechanical restraint correlates with understaffing.

52. The physicians at the South Carolina asylum used essentially the same drugs as their colleagues elsewhere, especially tonics and stimulants. For discussion, see McCandless, *Moonlight*, 276–77.

53. *Legislative Report* (1910), 15, 27–28.

54. Mental institutions played a major role in the 1917 formation of the National Society for the Promotion of Occupational Therapy. See Peloquin, "Occupational Therapy."

55. *Legislative Report* (1910), 53.

56. The asylum's assembly hall was large enough to accommodate at any one time more than 300 people, as evinced by its being the site of the 1909 pellagra

conference. However, there is no evidence that, during Babcock's period at least, it was used to provide sophisticated entertainment for patients. Benjamin Reiss in *Theaters of Madness* demonstrates that during the mid-nineteenth century some publicly funded asylums experimented successfully with theatrical programs, debating societies, literary journals, and religious services, all by the patients, and that these activities contributed to the nation's cultural life.

57. *Legislative Report* (1910), 18, 35, 53.

58. Ibid., 47–48. The committee used statistics from the "Special Report of the Census Office" of the United States for the year 1904, chosen because it was the most recent year for which data were available and the figures were thought to be representative. It is unclear whether the methods used to determine death rates were uniform across the various states. In 1877 Dr. John B. Chapin reported results from a survey of British and American asylums over the previous thirty-year period. Chapin estimated that for every 100 patients admitted to an asylum, 29 percent would die by the end of one year, 34 percent would recover (many of whom would later relapse and be readmitted), and the rest would stay about the same. See Grob, *Mental Illness*, 14–15. See also Appendix 1 and McCandless, *Moonlight*, 283.

59. Ibid., 49–55.

60. Ibid., 76–77, 85–86.

61. Ibid., 84–85.

62. For additional information and perspectives on the 1909–10 investigation, see McCandless, *Moonlight*, 297–306.

63. "Senator Weston Replies," *State*, February 17, 1910.

64. According to Thomas Irby Rogers, a Babcock supporter, the Judiciary Committee was called to meet on short notice at 11:00 P.M. on a Friday evening. Rogers promptly told the committee that he didn't think "that a better man could be found in all the United States" than Babcock ("Ask Asylum Officers to Resign," *Sunday News* [*News and Courier*], February 13, 1910). See also "Christensen on State Hospital," *State*, February 18, 1910.

65. "Babcock Vindicated by State Senate," *State*, February 18, 1910.

66. "Testimony of Senator Rogers," Babcock papers, box 4, folder 24, SCL. That Rogers was a personal friend of Babcock's is evinced by a letter to Mrs. Babcock informing her of his plan to visit the couple and asking, "Please remember me to the Doctor" (T. I. Rogers to Katherine G. Babcock, March 30, 1910, Babcock papers, box 4, folder 24, SCL).

67. The press largely agreed. One editor pointed out that the investigation had turned up nothing new since "all these matters have been reported to the legislature by the superintendent annually for the past ten years," that Babcock had "repeatedly gone before the Ways and Means Committee and ... always stated what was needed," that "it was the duty of the legislature to provide the means," that "South Carolina has never had a more efficient,

conscientious official than Dr. Babcock," and that "Instead of asking Dr. Babcock to resign the legislature better beg him to remain"(Editorial, *Herald and News* [Newberry, S.C.], February 15, 1910).

68. "Asylum Officials Vindicated," *News and Courier*, February 18, 1910.

69. "The Asylum Bond Issue before the House," *State*, February 19, 1910. Using the architect's estimate of $600 per patient, the cost of entirely new facilities for 1500 patients would have been $900,000.

70. 1910 S.C. Act 597 (*Acts and Resolutions* [1910], 1066). The five-member State Hospital Commission would include the asylum superintendent, the chairman of the State Board of Health, and three at-large members. This legislation emanated from the House of Representatives. Although it was implied during discussions that the new campus would be for blacks and that whites would remain in the downtown Columbia campus, this arrangement was not stipulated in the legislation (*House Journal* [1910], 914–15, 933–34).

71. "Senator Tillman is Seriously Ill," *State*, February 18, 1910; "Tillman's Condition is Serious," *State* February 19, 1910; "Senator Tillman is now Improving," *State*, February 20, 1910; "Senator Tillman is out of Danger," *State*, February 23, 1910. Letters from Tillman's wife and daughter pertaining to his recovery are in Babcock papers, box 5, folder 1, SCL.

72. Babcock, Murphy, Powell, and Searcy apparently constituted a quartet of friends who attended meetings together (Powell to Murphy, April 28, 1897; Babcock to Murphy, April 30, 1897; both in Patrick Livingston Murphy papers, collection 535, folder 6, SHC).

73. The *News and Courier* published an editorial, reprinted in the state medical journal ("The Hospital and the Doctors"), calling for more input from the South Carolina Medical Association in appointments to the asylum's Board of Directors and in evaluating conditions.

74. Babcock's daughter Margaret wrote that 45 years later Dr. Robert Gibbes invited her and her husband to dinner, and that after dinner Gibbes took her aside and "with a great deal of dignity and diffidence he said to me, 'Margaret, I want you to know before I die that I had a warm admiration for your father and would like to count him as my friend. I deplored my brother Hunter's instigation of the 1909 investigation of the Asylum, and tried to prevent him from doing what he did. I could not publicly accuse my brother of officiousness, and of course your father, who you know was [of] an intensely sensitive nature, felt that I as well as Hunter had treated him badly. There was the coolest formality between us after that and I have always regretted it deeply.' I was touched by this explanation and appreciated it, and think Daddy would have appreciated it, too" (Note by Margaret Babcock Meriwether, Babcock papers, box 4, folder 6, SCL).

75. Grob, commenting on the findings of the earliest surveys sponsored by the National Committee on Mental Hygiene, completed in 1915, states that

"there was general agreement that the quality of care and treatment in ... [the southern states] was considerably below that found elsewhere. South Carolina was perhaps typical. For years Dr. J. W. Babcock ... had been prodding the legislature to improve conditions. A legislative committee in 1910 not only conceded the accuracy of his complaints, but recommended the sale of the hospital and the erection of a new one" (Grob, *Mental Illness*, 159). Elsewhere, Grob adds: "The first surveys [1915] conducted under the Committee's auspices focused on the institutional insane in South Carolina, Texas, Tennessee, and Pennsylvania. That three of the four were Southern States was understandable; the poverty of that region created particularly troublesome problems insofar as expenditures for illness and dependency were concerned. In South Carolina, for example, Dr. J. W. Babcock ... had persistently called attention to deficiencies in his own institution, including an obsolete physical plant and inadequate operating funds" (Grob, *Mad Among Us*, 156).

76. In 1910—the same year as the legislative committee's report—a reviewer commented on the problems of overcrowding and understaffing in public asylums as follows: "In the development of institutional care of the insane, one of the chief problems has been to provide the individual the attention needed to bring about cure, and at the same time to furnish for the large and rapidly increasing numbers a shelter or asylum from neglect and brutality" (Russell, "The Medical Service").

77. Thompson, *Shattered Minds*, 63–64.

78. Tillman to Babcock, January 25, 1914, Babcock papers, box 5, folder 2, SCL.

79. MBR, July 8, 1909.

NOTES FOR CHAPTER 5

1. Osler, *Principles and Practice*, 7th ed., 384. Fleming Sandwith had written Babcock: "I told Osler some months ago of the pellagra situation with you, and he told me he would mention it in his new edition" (F. M. Sandwith to Babcock, August 26, 1909, Babcock papers, box 8, folder 8, SCL). See Searcy, "Epidemic of Acute Pellagra"; Wood and Bellamy, "Pellagra"; and Wood, "Appearance of Pellagra."

2. Marie's *Pellagra*, 3.

3. Lavinder to Walter Wyman, August 26, 1909, box 148, NARA.

4. Babcock and Lavinder wrote from scratch a chapter on the clinical manifestations. Sections by Eleanora Saunders and E. M. Whaley, both of the South Carolina State Hospital for the Insane, addressed the gynecologic and ocular aspects, respectively. Ten of the twenty new photographs were of South Carolina cases.

5. The contents of a folder entitled "Research Notes—English Bibliography" (Babcock papers, WHL) suggest Babcock did nearly all of the work on the bibliography.

6. Lavinder to Babcock, December 12, 1910, Babcock papers, box 8, folder 4, SCL. See also Etheridge, *Butterfly Caste*, 64.
7. James B. Meriwether, personal communication, January 28, 2004.
8. Babcock to Wyman, September 16, 1909, box 148, NARA.
9. Marie's *Pellagra*, 5.
10. George W. Manly to Katherine Guion Babcock, March 3, 1922, with note subsequently attached by Margaret Babcock Meriwether, Babcock papers, box 4, folder 13, SCL. Meriwether's note adds that "the huge ground floor room under Daddy's office (s-w corner) became Dr. Manly's 'office' & workroom. He mended books, made many little whittled devices (a 'Chinese Ring Puzzle' was one of his frequent gifts), [and] copied a great many papers in his fine pointed handwriting . . ." Because Manly is mentioned by name in the "Translators' Preface" and also in publicly-available archival material, and because the present author did not consult Manly's medical records, use of his name is judged not to violate the Health Insurance Portability and Accountability Act of 1996 (HIPPA). Manly made numerous translations for Babcock and in the present author's opinion deserves credit for his efforts against pellagra.
11. Apparently Babcock and Lavinder made little or no effort to secure a national publisher.
12. Marie's *Pellagra*, 121–22.
13. Ibid., 136–41. Sambon's argument reads:

> Pellagra is not due to maize, either good or bad, because (1) it is found in places where maize is neither cultivated nor eaten; (2) it is absent from many places where maize is the staple food of the population; (3) it has in many places either decreased or become more prevalent without any change in the food of the people; (4) its constant and peculiar distribution does not agree with the very irregular and ever-changing distribution of spoiled maize; and (5) in over a century and a half, since the maize theory was first suggested, no one has been able to prove it. The belief that the disease has everywhere followed the introduction of corn cultivation is unfounded. Pellagra was first recognized as a specific disease in the beginning of the eighteenth century, but this does not prove that it was not prevalent long before that time.
>
> Pellagra is a parasitic disease because: (1) for years the person affected may present some seasonal recurrences, which can only be explained by a parasitic agent with alternating periods of activity and latency; (2) it shows a constant and characteristic topographic distribution; (3) it shows a definite seasonal incidence; (4) its symptoms, course, duration, morbid anatomy, as well as its therapy, are similar to those of parasitic diseases; and (5) of two places, almost contiguous, one may be affected, the other not.
>
> Pellagra is an insect-borne disease because: (1) it is limited, like malaria, sleeping sickness, etc., to rural places and more especially to

the vicinity of certain bodies of water; (2) it has a definite seasonal incidence—spring and autumn; (3) it affects, to a large extent, a certain class
of people—the field laborers; (4) it is not contagious and neither food nor
water can account for its peculiar epidemiology; (5) within its epidemic
centers only adults who have visited the infection areas present the disease
and frequently only one or two members in a family are affected.

Pellagra is conveyed by *Simulium reptans* because: (1) *Simulium* is
found in the torrents and swift running streams of all pellagra districts;
(2) *Simulium* has the peculiar seasonal distribution of pellagra (spring
and autumn); (3) *Simulium* is found only in rural districts. It is unknown
in towns and villages. It does not enter houses; (4) *Simulium* explains
most admirably the peculiar limitation of the disease to field laborers; (5)
Simulium is the only blood-sucking insect which the British field commission has found in its visits to numerous pellagrous districts in Italy;
(6) *Simulium reptans*, like *Anopheles maculipennis* [the then-current name
for a malaria-transmitting mosquito], has a world-wide distribution and
explains the wide distribution of pellagra. It is found wherever pellagra
is found; (7) *Simulium* causes epizootics in animals in America and in
Europe; (8) Professor Mesnil has found a protozoal organism in *Simulium*.

14. In 1910 Dr. Howard D. King of New Orleans wrote: "Foremost among the
zeists—those who believe the use of damaged maize is responsible for the
disease—we find such eminent students as F. N. Sandwith, J. W. Babcock,
E. J. Wood, and C. H. Lavinder. . . . They present their side of the case with
ability and at times convincing earnestness; yet, on the other side, among the
antizeists, who believe that the malady may be and is caused by other factors
than the use of diseased corn, and notably by protozoa, we find Louis W.
Sambon and Sir Patrick Manson, who labor no less zealously to prove the
correctness of their theories" (King, "Etiologic Controversy").

15. Marie's *Pellagra*, 93–120. In retrospect, the symptoms in volunteers emphasize
the importance of randomized, placebo-controlled, double-blinded trials.

16. Lombroso additionally reported that a Professor von Dekenbach of St. Petersburg had determined that a "culture of oospora verticelloides, from corn,
produces phenomena in animals similar to those of pellagra."

17. C. Lombroso, "A Note to the Translators," September 1909, Babcock papers,
box 8, folder 17, SCL.

18. Marie's *Pellagra*, 124.

19. Ibid., 23–25. Sandwith later doubted the accuracy of Marie's assertion about
the appearance of pellagra in Corfu, since "it has been known since 1856
in that island" (Sandwith, "Pellagra in the Thirty-Five States"). Thypaldos
possibly overlooked confounding variables; for example, the Corfu residents
might have given up their vegetable gardens in addition to their cornfields to
make room for vineyards.

20. Marie's *Pellagra*, 188.
21. Ibid., 170. Etheridge utilizes the facial rash in her book title, *The Butterfly Caste*.
22. It is possible that the spots (macular lesions) on the palms and soles were due to secondary syphilis, since serologic testing for syphilis was not yet in routine use. In passing it should be noted that J. J. Watson described what may have been two new skin manifestations of pellagra (Marie's *Pellagra*, 169, 173).
23. Alsberg, "Agricultural Aspects."
24. "Pellagra.'London Lancet' Praises American Scientists' Work," *State*, February 5, 1911. Sandwith had written Babcock: "The Lancet of Jan 21 ought to have a short review of your book, which I am privately telling the medical libraries to buy" (Sandwith to Babcock, January 15, 1911, Babcock papers, box 1, folder 5, SCL). A collection of reviews is in Babcock papers, box 7, folder 1, SCL.
25. These data are on file in the Babcock papers, SCL, box 8, folders 42 and 43. The 118 American authors who wrote at least two articles accounted for 58 percent of the total number of articles.
26. Hyde, "Pellagra."
27. Wilkinson, "Pellagra."
28. Wolff, "Are the Jews Immune?"
29. During 1911 many people wrote Babcock inviting him to speak or to express opinions about the diagnosis and contagiousness of pellagra (Babcock papers, box 1, folders 6 and 7, SCL). Tillman arranged to have Babcock's paper on "The Prevalence of Pellagra," which had been published in the state medical journal, reissued by the Government Printing Office and sent Babcock 100 copies in franked envelopes (Tillman to Babcock, December 25, 1910, and January 20, 1911, Babcock papers, box 5, folder 1, SCL).
30. Wood, *Treatise on Pellagra*; Niles, *Pellagra*; Roberts, *Pellagra*.
31. Wood thanked Babcock and Lavinder "for many kindnesses" (p. viii). He also wrote a review article (Wood, "Appearance of Pellagra"). Niles cited Babcock seventeen times and included two photographs furnished by Babcock. Babcock corresponded with all three of these authors. The present author is indebted to Dr. Charles R. Roberts for showing him his grandfather's copy of Marie's *Pellagra*.
32. Lavinder to Babcock, October 25, 1911 and April 23, 1912, Babcock papers, box 8, folder 9, SCL.
33. Wood, "'Pellagra Sine Pellagra.'"
34. This statement refers to articles listed in the *Index Medicus* and is drawn from the author's data (see note 25, above). Between 1907 and 1915 Lavinder published 24 articles on pellagra, Siler 21, Bass 18, Cole 16, and Babcock 12 (a number matched by George C. Mizell of Atlanta, Georgia, who theorized that pellagra was caused by ingesting oils such as cottonseed oils). Charles Cassidy Bass of New Orleans was one of the few Americans who carried out

laboratory research on pellagra. Cole's publications on pellagra deal mainly with blood transfusions as a therapeutic modality.

35. Osler, "Books and Men."

36. Babcock grasped that one purpose of medical history is to explore hypotheses of causation, especially when an epidemic of a disease of unknown origin strikes a population. Medical historiography—that is, medical history as an academic discipline with its own purposes and methods—has advanced considerably since Babcock's era. For statements about the use of medical history to unravel the causes or essential natures of diseases, see Huisman and Warner, "Medical Histories," and Kushner, "Art of Medicine."

37. *AR* (1911), 13. The patients with "purpura or a scorbutic habit" might, in retrospect, have exhibited features of both pellagra and scurvy as part and parcel of generalized nutritional deficiency.

38. Babcock, "Prevalence and Psychology."

39. William Osler to Babcock, July 9, 1912, Babcock papers, box 6, folder 1, SCL.

40. Babcock, "Presidential Address," *NASP Transactions* (1912).

41. Babcock to Tillman, January 29, 1911, Tillman papers, box 19, folder 285, CUL; Notebook, "Andersonville Important," Babcock papers, box 1, folder 1. Dr. W. J. W. Kerr, who had been the chief surgeon at Andersonville, proposed in 1909 that pellagra rather than typhoid fever might have been the major killer during the summer of 1864 ("Pellagra Caused Deaths at Prison. Dr. Kerr, Surgeon at Andersonville, Reads Paper at Convention," *Atlanta Constitution*, November 11, 1909). Babcock concluded that the "actual occurrence of the disease has not been completely established from contemporary records" (Babcock, "Presidential Address," *NASP Transactions* [1912]). In 1916 Kerr disputed Goldberger's hypothesis but made a telling observation: "No surgeon or any one on the outside ever took the disease—yet we all had to eat exactly the same diet—every medical officer and all had the same to eat. We could not get anything else, so . . . if it had been corn-meal or bad provisions, the men on the outside would have had the same disease." (Kerr, "Cause of Pellagra"). More recently it has been suggested that poor nutrition rather than typhoid may have caused many and perhaps most of the deaths at Andersonville. For a short discussion of the possibility of pellagra at Andersonville, see Bollet, *Plagues & Poxes*, 159. However, the possibility of vitamin deficiencies is not discussed in a recent review of the historiography of Civil War prisons (Cloyd, *Haunted by Atrocity*).

42. See especially "Research, Notebooks, 2 of 3," Babcock papers, WHL; and material in Babcock papers, box 13, folder 5, SCL.

43. Babcock's translation is in Babcock papers, box 8, folder 6, SCL. The original copy of Babcock's translation is at the New York Academy of Medicine. Frapolli's treatise (*Mediolanensis Nosocomii majoris Medici Animadversiones in Morbum vulgò Pellagrum*) had not been previously available in English,

although occasional Englishmen, notably Henry Holland in 1817, were familiar with it.

44. For the role of photosensitivity in pellagra, see note 21, Chapter 3.
45. Notebook entitled "W.II.'09," Babcock papers, WHL.
46. Notebook entitled "LI," Babcock papers, WHL.
47. MBR, October 13, 1910. This observation raises at least two questions: Could Glenn's fatal illness have been something other than pellagra? Could Glenn have had another condition, such as alcoholism?
48. Caccini, "Pellagra." Caccini, who had taught in Rome before coming to New York City to work at the Harlem Tuberculosis Clinic, sent Babcock a reprint of this paper "thanking for many courtesies on your part."
49. The authority to require (mandate) reporting of conditions or diseases in the United States resides with state legislatures. Thus, anyone wanting accurate data had to conduct his or her own survey or write the respective state boards of health. For brief accounts of disease reporting in the United States, see "Mandatory Reporting of Infectious Diseases." See also "Historical Perspectives. Notifiable Disease Surveillance."
50. In 1911 Babcock wrote J. W. Kerr that he was compiling statistics and sending them to Lavinder, adding: "There is no doubt that the South Atlantic and Gulf States and Tennessee and Kentucky are in the midst of a very serious epidemic of pellagra" (Babcock to Kerr, August 25, 1911, box 148, NARA).
51. MBR, May 12, 1910.
52. Notebook, "Statistics on Pellagra," Babcock papers, WHL.
53. Lavinder, "Prevalence and Geographic Distribution."
54. MBR, May 12, 1910.
55. MBR August 11, 1910.
56. MBR, August 10, 1911. This appears to be Babcock's first use of the term "pellagraphobia," a term now commonly used by historians. The earliest use of this term uncovered by the present author came in a discussion at a medical meeting in Mobile, Alabama, in 1910 (Cole, in discussion of Mason, "Pellagra," *Transactions of the Medical Association of the State of Alabama*), in which the speaker said that he had not heard the term "pellagraphobia" before. A 1912 newspaper article entitled "Pellagraphobia New Disease" quoted Joseph Siler saying that "insanity attributed to pellagra was more often pellagraphobia" (*Chicago Record-Herald*, July 14, 1912). Later in 1912 at a national meeting in Washington, D.C., Babcock said: "We are bound to recognize that besides the disease pellagra, there is also a very serious disease, pellagraphobia" (Babcock, discussion of Hayne, "Pellagra," *Proceedings of the Twenty-Seventh Annual Meeting of the Conference of State and Provincial Boards of Health*). Laypersons were naturally concerned about the possibility that pellagra might be contagious. For example, a textile executive wanted Babcock's opinion whether it was "perfectly safe" to allow workers with suspected pellagra "to work alongside

the other hands" (W. E. Lindsay to Babcock, August 3, 1911, Babcock papers, box 1, folder 5, SCL).

57. MBR, August 10, 1911.
58. See Niles, *Pellagra*, 67–68. Although many authorities eventually concluded that pellagra was more prevalent in blacks, a commission of the predominantly black National Medical Association concluded that 90 percent of cases in the South were in whites (Green, "National Pellagra Commission").
59. The reduction in pellagra deaths in black females (as a percentage of all deaths due to pellagra) during 1912 and 1913, as compared to 1907-11, is significant whether analysis is performed by chi-square for trend using all of the annual data for 1907-13 ($P < 0.001$) or by chi-square using a two-by-two table (the sums for 1907-11 versus the sums for 1912 and 1913) ($P < 0.0001$).
60. MBR, May 11, 1911.
61. MBR, July 11, 1912.
62. Etheridge, *Butterfly Caste*, 2, 4.
63. S. C. Baker to Babcock, October 15, 1911, Babcock papers, box 8, folder 10, SCL.
64. B. G. Gregg to Babcock, October 24, 1911, Babcock papers, box 8, folder 10, SCL.
65. Case Book—Loose Notes, entry for June 1, 1911, Babcock papers, WHL. In the front of one of four notebooks filed under "Research Notes—Casebooks," Babcock made a checklist of twelve items: eruptions, pain, loss of weight, nausea, diarrhea, constipation, dizziness, cough, vomiting, profuse salivation, eye symptoms, and nervous systems.
66. Babcock, "Prevalence and Psychology."
67. Notebook entitled "Pellagra from Newspapers, etc," Babcock papers, WHL. The clipping was from the February 6, 1910, edition of the *Baltimore Sun*. Etheridge (*Butterfly Caste*, 30) paraphrases Babcock's excerpt.
68. For a more detailed account of pellagraphobia, see Etheridge, *Butterfly Caste*, 29–33.
69. Clippings from Luce's Press Clipping Bureau, Babcock papers, box 1, folder 3, and box 12, folders 1, 2, and 3, SCL.
70. *Vicksburg* (Miss.) *Herald*, June 9, 1912; *Memphis Commercial Appeal*, June 22, 1912; *Cincinnati Tribune*, December 11, 1911; *Greensboro* (N.C.) *Indus-News*, June 27, 1911.
71. "His Disease is Pellagra," *Baltimore Sun*, May 10, 1912.
72. *Rock Island* (Ill.) *News*, January 27, 1911; *New York Times*, June 8, 1912; *New Bern* (N.C.) *Sun*, November 12, 1909.
73. Notebook, "Pellagra from Newspapers, etc.," Babcock papers, WHL.
74. *Burlington* (Iowa) *Hawkeye*, April 9, 1911; *Phoenix* (Az.) *Gazette*, April 12, 1911.
75. "Pellagra from Newspapers, etc.," Babcock papers, WHL.

76. Salvarsan, also known as "compound 606," was the trade name for arsphena-mine, an organic arsenical compound. Historians consider it the first "modern" chemotherapeutic drug and also the first "blockbuster" drug. Naturally, there were attempts to try to Salvarsan for a wide range of conditions including pellagra.

77. "Pellagracide and Ez-X-Ba"; "Extract from a letter from Dr. Babcock under date of October 12 [1911]," box 148, NARA; Etheridge, *Butterfly Caste*, 38; Roe, *Plague of Corn*, 95–97. Dedmond whined to a newspaper that "Dr. Babcock refused to even allow me to treat one of the patients at my own expense. [He] Said I was not educated and that the patient might die" (Letter to the editor published under the heading "Mr. Dedmond Talks," *Clinton* (S.C.) *Gazette*, March 21, 1912). Dedmond also appealed to Tillman for support (E. W. Dedmond to Tillman, July 13, 1911, Babcock papers, box 5, folder 1, SCL). Another widely-marketed remedy of that era was "Baughn's Pellagra Remedy." Analysis revealed straw, dirt, iron sulfate, charcoal, and quinine sulfate.

78. Babcock, "Prevalence and Psychology."

79. Research notes—notebook, folder 2083, Babcock papers, WHL. Babcock's point here was that, in patients already diagnosed with pellagra, one should consider the possibility that insanity might be due to something else.

80. Lavinder to Walter Wyman, 2 September 1909, box 148, NARA.

81. For summaries, see Moran and Das, "William Beaumont," and Bryan et al., "Yellow Fever." See note 80, chapter 3 for information on Carter.

82. Sambon, "Geographical Distribution."

83. The importance of the Pellagra Investigation Committee, providing as it did funding for Sambon's 1910 trip to Italy which led in turn to Joseph Siler's tacit endorsement of Sambon's version of the germ theory and thus to Sambon's influence on the Thompson-McFadden Commission, has received little emphasis in previous accounts. Etheridge mentions it briefly (*Butterfly Caste*, 41). Roe gives an excellent short summary of Sambon's trip to Italy but does not mention the committee that made it possible (*Plague of Corn*, 84–87). The founding document of the committee reviews the then-recent history of pellagra, including the endorsement of Sambon's theory by three physicians (including Edward Jenner Wood and Julius Taylor) at the October 29, 1908, conference in Columbia, S.C. ("Pellagra Investigation Committee," Royal Society of Tropical Medicine and Hygiene Archives). Patrick Manson was knighted in 1903, William Osler in 1911; the present author has sometimes taken liberty with these dates for the sake of simplicity.

84. Sambon, "Progress Report."

85. "Pellagra Cases Clearly Studied," *State*, September 3, 1909.

86. Notebook, "C. H. Lavinder's Report to Surgeon General USPH & MH Service of Two Months' Study of Pellagra in Italy, 1910," in Research and Notes, Lavinder Report, 1910, received August 13, 1910. Babcock papers, WHL.

87. Gosio had devised a test for spoilage of corn (a modification is described in Black and Alsberg, *Deterioration of Maize*).
88. Lavinder, "Theory of the Parasitic Origin."
89. "Lavinder's Report" (note 86, above).
90. "Recent Investigations on Pellagra."
91. "Gnat Causes Pellagra," *New York Times*, May 14, 1910.
92. "Sand-fly Transmission of Pellagra." The editorialist elaborated: "The evidence on which Sambon supports his views is strong, but more will be required to satisfy the profession.... For example, it is necessary to know whether or not the species of sand-fly which Sambon considered the conveyer of the infection, or one closely enough allied to it to be similarly credited with carrying the disease, exists in this country; and if so, whether or not the occurrence of pellagra here corresponds with the distribution of this sand-fly."
93. Roberts, "Sambon's New Theory."
94. Sambon, "Progress Report."
95. Babcock to Tillman, February 26, 1911, Tillman papers, box 19, folder 287, CUL.
96. *Illinois Pellagra Commission*, 249.
97. Ibid., 3. For overviews of Ricketts's life, see Harden, "Koch's Postulates," and Gross and Schäfer, "100th Anniversary." It is unclear to the present author why prominent pellagra researchers at the Cook County Institutions at Dunning, Illinois, and at the Memorial Institute for Infectious Diseases, Chicago, did not participate in the Illinois Pellagra Commission. For examples of their work, see Clarke et al., "Studies on Pellagra," and Dick, "Inoculation of Monkeys."
98. See "In Memoriam. H. Douglas Singer."
99. Singer et al., "Attempts at Experimental Transmission," *Illinois Pellagra Commission*.
100. MacNeal and Allison, "Intestinal Bacteria," *Illinois Pellagra Commission*. This study, which occupies 42 percent of the report's 250 pages, reads like an exhaustive account of the normal fecal flora.
101. Rooks, "Protozoal Infection," *Illinois Pellagra Commission*.
102. Hirschfelder, "Cutaneous Tests," *Illinois Pellagra Commission*.
103. Forbes, "Black-Flies and Buffalo-Gnats," *Illinois Pellagra Commission*. Forbes confirmed the nuisance these insects pose to outdoorsmen, quoting from an 1850 account of Louis Agassiz's expedition to Lake Superior: "Neither the love of the picturesque ... or the interests of science, could tempt us into the woods, so terrible were the black-flies."
104. Siler and Nichols, "Investigations in Pellagra," *Illinois Pellagra Commission*; Wussow and Grindley, "Dietary Studies," *Illinois Pellagra Commission*; Singer, "Meat Used in the State Hospitals," *Illinois Pellagra Commission*.
105. "General Summary," *Illinois Pellagra Commission*.

106. Davenport, "The Hereditary Factor." Many of the key articles in the three reports (*Thompson-McFadden Report* [1913], *Thompson-McFadden Report* [1915], and *Thompson Report* [1917]) were also published elsewhere.
107. Novy and MacNeal, "Trypanosomes of Birds."
108. The suggestion that Siler's lectureship prompted formation of the commission is based in part on a newspaper article describing how Siler's lectures stimulated the interest of Thompson and McFadden ("Commission Ready to Study Pellagra," *New York Times*, May 26, 1912). The commission's first report relates that it was "through the instrumentality of Dr. George N. Miller" that the commission was funded. In 1912 MacNeal was promoted from lecturer to full professor. As noted in the text, the Thompson-McFadden Pellagra Commission ultimately became the "Robert M. Thompson Pellagra Commission," presumably because McFadden had stopped contributing.
109. Jonathan Wright to Rupert Blue, March 8, 1912, box 149, NARA. MacNeal wished to have Randolph M. Grimm loaned to him by the Public Health and Marine Hospital Service.
110. MBR, December 14, 1911; Randolph M. Grimm to the Surgeon General, February 2 and April 7, 1912, box 149, NARA. Grimm helped the Thompson-McFadden Commission by recommending, after consulting with Babcock and state health officer Adams Hayne, that the South Carolina Piedmont would be the best location.
111. See Koo and Thacker, "In Snow's Footsteps."
112. See Thompson and Subar, "Dietary Assessment."
113. Siler and Garrison, "An Intensive Study."
114. Allan H. Jennings and William van Orsdel King, two entomologists assigned to the commission by the U.S. Department of Agriculture, reported in detail on possible insect vectors and came to the conclusion that the stable fly was the best candidate (Jennings and King, "Intensive Study of Insects"; see also Jennings, "Two Years' Study of Insects").
115. Siler et al., "Summary of the First Progress Report."
116. Anderson and Goldberger, "Attempt to Infect the Rhesus Monkey."
117. Some historians have stated or implied that Goldberger went south in 1914 with no pre-formed ideas about the causation of pellagra, and that he soon saw what others had missed. As discussed more fully in chapter 8, Goldberger's co-authorship of this paper clearly indicates that he had been thinking about pellagra for at least three years. The citation in the *Index Medicus* reads: "Anderson (J.F.) An attempt to infect the Rhesus monkey with blood and spinal fluid from pellagrins. Pub. Health Rep. U.S. Mar. Hosp. Serv., Wash., 1911, xxvi, 1003" (Fletcher and Garrison, eds., *Index Medicus*, 886). Milton Terris, who prepared a bibliography of Goldberger's papers on pellagra, discusses the collaboration of Anderson and Goldberger on typhus and measles but omits the 1911 paper (Terris, *Goldberger*, 7–19). However, Goldberger's collaboration with Anderson on pellagra was known

to at least some of his contemporaries ("Attempts to Produce Experimental Pellagra"; Niles, *Pellagra*, 235–39; Deaderick and Thompson, *Endemic Diseases*, 308–11).

118. Lavinder, "Inoculation of the Rhesus Monkey."

119. Anderson to the Surgeon General, October 20, 1910, box 148, NARA.

120. See also note 80, Chapter 3. In 1900 it was shown that the infectious agent of yellow fever (later found to be a virus) was present in blood only during the earliest clinical stage of the disease, when symptoms and signs were nonspecific. Efforts to transmit yellow fever from patients with full-blown disease to uninfected persons were uniformly negative. Another example is syphilis; blood contains the causative spirochete only during the brief "secondary" stage of the disease.

121. John F. Anderson, J. D. Long, Reid Hunt, and C. H. Lavinder to the Surgeon General, November 23, 1910, box 148, NARA.

122. Ibid.

123. Lavinder to R. M. Grimm, April 17, 1911; Lavinder to the Surgeon General, August 12, 1911; both in box 148, NARA.

124. Lavinder to the Surgeon General, June 12, 1911, box 148, NARA. Babcock gave Grimm personal instruction on pellagra (R. M. Grimm to the Surgeon General, August 18, 1911, box 148, NARA).

125. Grimm to Wyman, September 23, 1911, box 148, NARA.

126. See Grimm, "Pellagra." For a summary of Grimm's work, see Etheridge, *Butterfly Caste*, 43–49.

127. Lavinder to the Surgeon General, November 6, 1911, box 148, NARA. These annual conferences had as their primary purpose the education of physicians through case presentations and discussions.

128. Babcock recognized the potential for interagency competition. He had, for example, advised authorities in Washington that "these organized bodies look with a jealous eye upon any action that may be interpreted as encroaching upon their authority" (Babcock to Wright Nash, August 12, 1911, box 148, NARA).

129. Garrison, "The Recent Pellagra Clinic."

130. When it was suggested to Lavinder that several southern medical societies might sponsor a symposium on pellagra for the purpose of generating new ideas, Lavinder objected on the grounds that it would take either him or Grimm away from their investigations (Lavinder to Kerr, June 10, 1911, box 148, NARA).

131. Lavinder to the Surgeon General, September 6, 1911; Wyman to Lavinder, September 14, 1911; both in box 148, NARA.

132. Lavinder to the Surgeon General, January 29, 1912, box 149, NARA.

133. Lavinder to J. W. Kerr, April 27, 1912, box 149, NARA. Lavinder added that Grimm was equally discouraged, thinking it "useless collecting one case after another when all show such sameness."

134. Lavinder to Babcock, May 8, 1912, Babcock papers, box 8, folder 9, SCL. Lavinder added that "the Siler commission [Thompson-McFadden Commission] . . . will have the best chance yet offered any one to do some real good work, and perhaps they may turn up something."

135. "Pellagra Work Now Under Way in U.S. Marine Hospital. Dr. Lavinder Does Not Accept Corn Theory for Disease," *Savannah Morning News*, August 24, 1911.

NOTES FOR CHAPTER 6

1. A standard, if perhaps dated, history of the vitamins is contained in McCollum, *History of Nutrition*. For a recent overview, see Frankenburg, *Vitamin Discoveries*. See also Carpenter, *Beriberi*; Carpenter, *History of Scurvy*; and Harvie, *Limeys*.

2. Among such "accessory food factors" are the essential amino acids and the vitamins. As noted in chapter 3, the essential amino acid tryptophan can be converted to the vitamin niacin, but the process is inefficient (since tryptophan is needed for the synthesis of proteins and other substances, such as serotonin). In 1906 F. Gowland Hopkins and a coworker, Edith G. Willcock, showed that young mice failed to thrive on a diet containing zein (a class of protein found in corn) as the only source of nitrogen. When tryptophan (an amino acid not present in zein) was added to their diet, the mice lived longer although they did not maintain growth. They concluded that tryptophan "is directly utilized as the normal precursor of some specific 'hormone' or other substance essential to the processes of the body" (Willcock and Hopkins, "Importance of Individual Amino-acids").

3. Carpenter, *Beriberi*. See also note 17, Chapter 3.

4. For discussion, see Kamminga, "Credit and Resistance." The idea that beriberi was "linked" to polished rice but not "caused" by the substitution of polished for unpolished rice finds a parallel in the pellagra debate. Many students of pellagra agreed that it was "linked" to a corn-predominant diet, but not necessarily "caused" by it. In both cases, the missing paradigm was of course the vitamin hypothesis.

5. Carpenter, *Beriberi*. Eijkman's genius was to explore *why* the chickens became sick.

6. Fischer's research career was winding down. Funk found himself working alongside Emil Abderhalden, Fischer's energetic if unfocused young assistant, who was testing synthetic diets in dogs. This experience introduced Funk to nutritional deficiency diseases.

7. Funk, "Etiology of the Deficiency Diseases." Carpenter (*Beriberi*, 99) implies that Martin gave Funk permission to publish research papers as the sole author with the stipulation that he needed Martin's prior approval of each manuscript. However, a solicited review article did not need such approval. Some authors

date Funk's formulation of the vitamin hypothesis to 1911 on the basis of a coauthored paper on beriberi (Cooper and Funk, "Causation of Beriberi"). See, for example, Piro et al., "Casimir Funk." For Funk's perspective, see Funk, "Nicotinic Acid and Vitamin B."

8. Babcock to Tillman, May 2, 1912, Tillman papers, box 20, folder 300, CUL. Tillman acted on this request (Tillman to Babcock, May 7, 1912, Babcock papers, box 5, folder 1, SCL). Babcock's correspondence in preparation for this meeting was extensive (Babcock papers, box 8, folders 9 and 10, SCL).

9. MBR, August 8, 1912.

10. MBR, September 11, 1912.

11. Each dot in the figure represents the hometown of one author (or, in the case of papers with more than one author, the hometown of the senior author; there were in all 70 different authors for the 62 papers). The two papers from the Thompson-McFadden Commission include Siler from the U.S. Army, Garrison from the U.S. Navy, MacNeal from the New York Post-Graduate Medical School, and Jennings and King (both from the U.S. Department of Agriculture). For the 1909 conference, 16 of 41 papers came from South Carolina, versus 12 of 62 papers at the 1912 conference (P < 0.01 by chi-square test). The program committee apparently consisted of Babcock and two Columbia colleagues, Joseph J. Watson and James Adams Hayne. Physicians throughout the nation were encouraged to submit papers (see "National Conference on Pellagra").

12. Cole, "Treatment of Pellagra," *NASP Transactions* (1912); Martin, "Soamin and Salvarsan," *NASP Transactions* (1912); Cranston, "Use of Salvarsan," *NASP Transactions* (1912); Brownston, "New Serum Treatment," *NASP Transactions* (1912).

13. Etheridge, *Butterfly Caste*, 51–52. Etheridge adds that the participants "carefully avoided the issue of what caused pellagra" when it came to writing resolutions.

14. Gosio and Antonini, "Etiology of Pellagra," *NASP Transactions* (1912); Reed, "Diplodia Zeae and Some Other Fungi," *NASP Transactions* (1912); Alsberg and Black, "Metabolism of Moulds," *NASP Transactions* (1912). The latter investigations pointed out the great diversity of molds, which might have been another reason to suspend judgment on the spoiled-corn hypothesis.

15. Mizell, "Etiologic Factors," *NASP Transactions* (1912); Adler, "Lesions Resembling Pellagra," *NASP Transactions* (1912).

16. Jennings and King, "Causation of Pellagra," *NASP Transactions* (1912). Jennings spearheaded the Thompson-McFadden entomologic studies. In 1914 he reported these observations in more detail (Jennings, "Summary of Two Years' Study"). King, who became famous as an entomologist, was a graduate student at the time of the 1912 report.

17. Roberts, "Analogies of Pellagra," *NASP Transactions* (1912).

18. Hunter, "Pellagra and the Sand-fly," *NASP Transactions* (1912).

19. Wood, "Geographical Distribution of Pellagra," *NASP Transactions* (1912).

20. Beall, "Pellagra in Texas," *NASP Transactions* (1912).

21. Babes, "Recent Hypotheses," *NASP Transactions* (1912). This statement by Babes runs counter to a statement (perhaps written by Sambon) in the 1910 document by the British Pellagra Committee (note 83, page 324): "Professor Babes, of Bucharest, Roumania, hitherto a pronounced champion of the maize theory, has also become a supporter of the protozoal theory of Sambon." Possibly, Babes changed his mind.

22. It is unclear how many of the eight international papers were read *in absentia*, since the published list of registrants includes only the members of the association. The published version of Babes's paper contains a discussion suggesting he was present.

23. Blue, "Problem of Pellagra," *NASP Transactions* (1912).

24. Sandwith to Babcock, August 4, 1912, Babcock papers, box 8, folder 10, SCL.

25. Sandwith, "Pellagra in the Thirty-Five States." In presenting this paper to the Society of Tropical Medicine and Hygiene on December 5, 1911, Sandwith said that while he had studied pellagra for nineteen years it was only the second time he had spoken on the disease in Great Britain. He observed that Sambon's "brilliant theory as to the possible cause of pellagra has of course aroused much interest in the United States," but did not express support for it.

26. In 1913 Funk thanked "Dr. Standwith" [sic], among others, for permission to reproduce photographs of patients with pellagra in the first edition of his treatise on the vitamines (Funk, *The Vitamines*, 9).

27. Sandwith, "Can Pellagra be a Disease Due to Deficiency of Nutrition?" *NASP Transactions* (1912).

28. Sandwith, "Is Pellagra a Disease due to Deficiency of Nutrition?"

29. Goldberger is said to have sometimes made marks in journal articles. The present author therefore inspected the copy of Sandwith's 1913 paper in the National Library of Medicine in Bethesda, Maryland, since this might have been the copy available to Goldberger in what was then the Library of the Surgeon General in Washington. The paper contains no marks.

30. Babcock, "Presidential Address," *NASP Transactions* (1912).

31. Babcock, "Medico-Legal Relations," *NASP Transactions* (1912).

32. MBR, October 10, 1912.

33. "The Pellagra Conference" [*Journal of the South Carolina Medical Association*].

34. Babcock, Discussion of Hayne, "Pellagra," *Proceedings of the Twenty-Seventh Annual Meeting of the Conference of State and Provincial Boards of Health of North America.*

35. Sandwith to Babcock, September 24, 1911, Babcock papers, box 1, folder 5, SCL.

36. Tucker, "Nervous and Mental Symptoms of Pellagra," *Transactions of the Forty-Third Annual Session of the Medical Society of Virginia.* A typescript of this editorial is in the Babcock papers, box 8, folder 4, SCL. Discussing another

paper at the same meeting, Tucker said that he had "no theory as to the cause, but study made him incline to the theory of infection, though [Rupert] Blue, Babcock, and Lavender [*sic*] lean to the belief that it is dietary, with apparent foundation" (Tucker, Discussion of Merrill, "Skin Symptoms," *Transactions of the Forty-Third Annual Session of the Medical Society of Virginia*). Tucker was one of the era's more prominent neurologists and psychiatrists (see "Beverley Randolph Tucker"). Babcock included Tucker among his five personal references in an application to the Navy in 1918.

37. Carl L. Alsberg to Babcock, October 23, 1912, Babcock papers, box 8, folder 10, SCL.

38. Alsberg as noted elsewhere was the point person for the U.S. Department of Agriculture's concern about the implications of pellagra for the corn industry. He had participated in the National Association for the Study of Pellagra almost from the beginning and closed this letter by thanking Babcock for "your kindness on this and many other occasions."

39. Lavinder, "Report of the Second Triennial Meeting."

40. Harris, "Experimental Production of Pellagra." For a summary of experimental attempts to produce pellagra in monkeys, see Day, "Nutritional Requirements of Primates."

41. Lavinder et al., "Attempts to Transmit Pellagra."

42. Telegram, Sambon to Babcock, August 20, 1913, Babcock papers, box 8, folder 7, SCL. Dr. Sambon reportedly "found it almost impossible to get any assistance in his work until Dr. J. W. Babcock and Dr. J. J. Watson of Columbia made it known that the disease was prevalent in America," whereupon "the medical journals of the country [Great Britain] and British physicians began to wake up ("Meet to Discuss Dread Pellagra," *State* (Columbia, S.C.), September 4, 1913).

43. "Prof. Louis Sambon Here. Comes from London to Address Southern Pellagra Conference," *New York Times*, September 1, 1913.

44. "Great Conference Convenes Today," *Spartanburg* (S.C.) *Herald*, September 3, 1913.

45. "Meet to Discuss Dread Pellagra," *State*, September 4, 1913.

46. Great Conference Convenes Today," *Spartanburg Herald*, September 3, 1913.

47. "The Informal Smoker was Pleasing Affair," *Spartanburg Herald*, September 4, 1913. The only new information Sambon presented at the Spartanburg meeting seems to have been his recognition of fifty-three cases in the British Isles, including Scotland. The *Columbia Record* (September 4, 1913) headlined: "Dr. Sambon Declares Pellagra Spreading Over All Parts of the World."

48. "Insect Carries Pellagra. English Scientist Says Spartanburg Conference Established This," *New York Times*, September 13, 1913. It seems likely that from Spartanburg Sambon went directly to Columbia (on or shortly after September 4), then went to Charleston, and then returned to New York by September 12 before heading for the British West Indies.

49. "Pellagra Conference" [*Southern Medical Journal*]. See also Green, "National Pellagra Commission."
50. "Pellagra Is Not Transmissible by Direct Contact," *Spartanburg Herald*, September 4, 1913.
51. "Pellagra Discussed by Eminent Doctors; its Cause a Mystery," *Greenville* (S.C.) *Daily News*, September 4, 1913.
52. MBR, September 11, 1913.
53. Wilson, discussion of Hayne, "History of Pellagra."
54. "Notes on Barbadoes," in folder marked "1914," box 149, NARA.
55. "No Buffalo Gnats but Finds Pellagra," *State*, November 15, 1913; "Buffalo Gnat is no Carrier of Pellagra," *Columbia Record*, November 16, 1913.
56. Siler to Babcock, April 18, 1914, Babcock papers, box 8, folder 4, SCL.
57. Claims were made for an infectious etiology of all four of the diseases postulated by Funk to be caused by vitamin deficiency (scurvy, beriberi, rickets, and pellagra). For discussion, see Ihde and Backer, "Conflict of Concepts."
58. Sydenstricker, "Impact of Vitamin Research."
59. Funk, "Studies on Beri-beri."
60. Funk, "Studies on Pellagra." As it later turned out, the vitamins in corn kernels are concentrated in the germ rather than in the skin (see chapter 3).
61. The concept that ideas behave as epidemics was recently popularized by Gladwell in *The Tipping Point*. He proposes three rules for ideas as epidemics ("the law of the few," the "stickiness factor," and "the power of context") and three types of individuals who affect the course of ideas ("mavens," "connectors," and "salesmen").
62. "The Late Colonel F. M. Sandwith."
63. "Fleming Mant Sandwith, M.D. Durh., F.R.C.P. Lond., C.M.G."
64. "F. M. Sandwith, C.M.G., M.D., F.R.C.P."
65. Livingstone, "Tropical Climate"; Wilkinson, "AJE Terzi and LW Sambon."
66. Manson-Bahr, *School of Tropical Medicine*, 132–36.
67. Taylor, "Sambon, the Man," *NASP Transactions* (1912).
68. Harrow, *Casimir Funk*, 46–47.
69. A decade earlier, Sambon and also Manson had heard and dismissed the idea that beriberi was a deficiency disease (Manson et al., "Discussion on Beri-Beri").
70. For discussion, see Griminger, "Casimir Funk."
71. MBR, August 10, 1911.
72. *Legislative Report* (1914), 383–84.
73. The author's tabulations are contained in box 8, folders 36 and 39, Babcock papers, SCL. According to the annual reports, the numbers of deaths due to pellagra between 1908 and 1915 were, sequentially, 33 (during 1908), 68, 106, 154, 228, 165, 356, and 327 (during 1915). The lower number of deaths during 1913 could, of course, have been an aberration. As noted elsewhere, the

substitution of rice for corn also led to recognition of beriberi at the asylum by Eleanora Saunders.

NOTES FOR CHAPTER 7

1. Tillman called Blease, among other things, "selfish, low, dirty, and revengeful." See "Why Blease Won," and Stone, "Bleaseism." This account relies especially on Burnside, "Governorship of Coleman Livingston Blease," and Brice, "Executive Clemency."
2. A table with data for admissions, discharges, deaths, recoveries, and "elopements" by year for the period 1891 through 1914 has been placed in box 8, folder 33, Babcock papers, SCL.
3. MBR, June 9, 1910.
4. MBR, July 14, 1910. Babcock told the regents: "It would seem that a time has arrived when some definite action must be taken. . . . It is emphatically no fault of yours or mine that such action was not taken during the session of the General Assembly a year and a half ago."
5. MBR, February 10 and February 21, 1910. Babcock had suggested the state buy 1,000 to 3,000 acres "in the healthy sandhills not far from Columbia," in which there should be "group cottages as our climate demands" (notes for an undated, untitled address, Babcock papers, box 4, folder 21, SCL). "State Park" appealed as a name especially because it "did not carry with it any suggestion of asylum, hospital, or colony" (*Reports of the State Hospital Commission* [second annual report, 1911], 10). The choice proved felicitous. The property became the campus for the state's tuberculosis hospital (now closed). It is now the site of the State Bureau of Laboratories and the South Carolina Department of Archives and History.
6. MBR, November 10, 1910.
7. The cottage plan traces to Gheel, Belgium, where during the Middle Ages townspeople opened their homes to pilgrims seeking intercession from Saint Dympha, the patron saint of mental illness. For discussion of how the cottage plan at Gheel influenced late-nineteenth-century thought in the United States, see Tuntiya, "Forgotten History."
8. *Reports of the State Hospital Commission* (first report, 1910–11), 6.
9. Board of Regents to the Commission of the State Hospital (Resolution), May 12, 1910, S190005, box 6, SCDAH.
10. MBR, September 13, 1912. The next year a regent recommended that the black men (rather than black women) be moved to State Park first (MBR, July 10, 1913).
11. *Reports of the State Hospital Commission* (second annual report, 1911). The trees at State Park were mainly scrub oaks and loblolly pines, but there were stands of the more valuable longleaf pine.

12. MBR, April 13, 1911, and July 11, 1912.
13. *AR* (1911), 15.
14. *AR* (1912), 10.
15. MBR, February 5, 1913.
16. In February 1914 the House of Representatives refused to pass a bill calling for sale of the downtown campus and removal of the entire asylum to the State Park campus. One representative "said he could not imagine who would buy the buildings" and proposed "confining the negro maniacs in the penitentiary and using the buildings at State Park for hospitals for tuberculosis and pellagra patients" ("Asylum Removal Fails by Fluke," *State* [Columbia, S.C.], February 7, 1914). This was not the first time such a suggestion had been made; in 1906 there had been rumors that the hospital's real estate would be sold and the asylum moved to the Congaree Swamp (MBR, February 8, 1906).
17. Strauss, *Medical Quotations*, 302.
18. Hurd, "Three-quarters of a Century." For a summary of American psychiatry during this period, see Grob, *Mental Illness*, 108–43.
19. A uniform system for classifying mental conditions was proposed in 1917 and adopted in 1918 (Grob, *Mental Illness*, 118–19). The idea that most psychiatric conditions can be framed as specific diagnoses remains somewhat controversial. See, for example, Dean, "Death of Specificity."
20. Psychoanalysis had little effect on American institutional psychiatry before 1920, especially outside of the Northeast (Grob, *Mental Illness*, 120). See Hale, *Freud and the Americans*.
21. In 1906 August Paul von Wassermann announced the serologic test that bears his name. In 1913 Hideyo Noguchi and J. W. Moore of the Rockefeller Institute for Medical Research in New York reported finding *Treponema pallidum*, the causative agent of syphilis, in the brains of victims of "general paresis of the insane." It was later concluded that Salvarsan was effective in the early stages of syphilis but disappointing in the late stages. Dr. Henry J. Nichols of the U.S. Army and a colleague published this observation in January 1913, the year Eleanora Saunders conducted her studies of syphilis at the South Carolina asylum (Nichols and Hough, "Demonstration of *Spirochaeta Pallida*"). At the time of this writing, no therapy, including high-dose penicillin, has been shown to convincingly alter the natural course of established neurosyphilis. In the wake of the notorious Tuskegee Study of Untreated Syphilis, it seems highly unlikely that a properly conducted randomized, double-blinded, placebo-controlled trial will ever be done (the Tuskegee Study, although seriously flawed, especially from the ethical perspective, nevertheless addressed a valid scientific question; see Benedek and Erlen, "Scientific Environment").
22. "Miss Saunder [*sic*] Wins First Honors," *State*, April 23, 1907.
23. *Legislative Report* (1914), 521.
24. Anderson, "Pioneer Women Physicians," (unpublished manuscript). See also Anderson, "Eleanora Bennette Saunders."

25. *Legislative Report* (1914), 425, 507–38.
26. In the winter of 1907–08 Saunders attended a six-week course in dermatology, neurology, and clinical microscopy in New York; in 1910, she completed a course in electrotherapy and hydrotherapy in Philadelphia; and in 1912 she took an extension course in nervous and mental diseases from Fordham University School of Medicine.
27. Anderson, "Pioneer Women Physicians" (unpublished manuscript); MBR, December 8, 1910.
28. "Nurses at Asylum Love Dr. Saunders," *State*, February 14, 1914.
29. Saunders, "Gynecological, Obstetrical and Surgical Aspects." She concluded that (1) women are more susceptible than men (about 75% of patients were women); (2) congestion and erythema of the vulva and vagina were nearly always present and were regarded by some as diagnostic; (3) symptoms could suggest cancer; (4) pregnancy and lactation could modify the course of the disease; and (5) many patients aborted after they developed pellagra. She was cited in the medical literature for the observation that pellagra can cause amenorrhea. Claude Lavinder reported that Saunders's paper "laid especial stress on the surgical side of the disease and the dangers of submitting patients to operation by reason of faulty diagnosis" (Lavinder, "National Conference on Pellagra").
30. See Miller, "Pellagra Deaths."
31. MBR, June 8, 1911.
32. See Brice, "Executive Clemency." One explanation for Blease's liberal clemency policy for whites is that, although he campaigned as a champion of poor whites, he favored small government and had no real social program to help them. He therefore sought to "give the poor devils a chance." Blease rationalized liberal clemency for blacks by saying they were needed for labor and, as an inferior race, had limited capacity for moral reasoning—hence, an understandable propensity to commit crimes. Brice concludes that Blease's administration was "certainly bizarre, but there is absolutely no proof to substantiate the charges of corruption." He suggests that Blease's motivations for clemency included a desire to help poor people and "a sincere concern for the unfortunate victims of an outmoded and inadequate system." As an example of Blease's racism, consider this attack on Niels Christensen Jr. (see Chapter 4): "I have heard the rumor that the father of the present senator from Beaufort County commanded at Holly Hill a negro company" ("Christensen Incident Subject of a Message," *State*, February 5, 1914). (The rumor was unfounded.)
33. Edgar, *South Carolina in the Modern Age*, 32–34.
34. Edgar, *South Carolina: A History*, 473.
35. Blease was expelled from the University of South Carolina for plagiarizing an essay. He then went to Georgetown University, where he received his law degree, and allegedly begrudged the University of South Carolina the rest of his life. Blease like many politicians used hyperbole when campaigning

for office and probably did not tell the whole truth when he denied further political ambition. However, there seems to be little or no evidence that he was by ordinary standards a liar.

36. *Legislative Report* (1914), 56–59; "Governor on Stand Gives his Version," *State*, February 8, 1914. Blease later hinted that Babcock had disclosed that someone had deceived him prior to his testimony, causing him to appear a "traitor to Ben Tillman's nephew" (Cole L. Blease, Message No. 21, *House Journal* [1914], 739–40, and *Senate Journal* [1914], 573–74).

37. "Address of Welcome by Governor Cole L. Blease at the Pellagra Clinic, Columbia, S.C., November 2nd, 1911," Babcock papers, box 3, folder 19, SCL.

38. *Legislative Report* (1914), 23–24. The minutes of the Board of Regents contain other examples of the working relationship between Babcock and Blease (MBR, August 8, 1912; November 11, 1913).

39. *Legislative Report* (1914), 155–57.

40. See Worthington, "Post-Flexner Survival." Worthington discovered that Wilson had written in a private account: "I had no difficulty whatever in getting along with the governor; and I think it was because I always took pains to recognize that he was the Governor of South Carolina."

41. *Legislative Report* (1914), 59–60, 69–70.

42. CH, February 9, 1911.

43. MBR, January 11, 1912. Between 1891 and 1914, 214 patients "eloped" (that is, escaped) from the asylum. These included 96 white men, 108 black men, 4 white women, and 6 black women. Thus, 95 percent of the escapees were men.

44. Donald, "James Higgins McIntosh." McIntosh was shot shortly after midnight on the day he was to confront the governor. The assailant was never identified. However, McIntosh's daughter, the late Nancy McIntosh Pearlstine, told the present author that her father was asked to identify a body in the morgue and suspected it was the assailant based on the corpse's smell—so close had McIntosh been to the assailant.

45. MBR, March 14, 1912.

46. Zuczek, *State of Rebellion*, 57.

47. MBR, September 14 and September 20, 1911.

48. *Legislative Report* (1914), 418.

49. Ibid., 22. In 1912 Major W. J. Gooding died and W. W. Ray was not reappointed when his term on the Board of Regents expired. Carothers, the new president of the Board of Regents, verified that friction between Babcock and Thompson began after the 1909 investigation and that friction later developed between Babcock and Griffin (*Legislative Report* [1914], 189).

50. As events played out, Saunders's detractors clearly used Cooper's return to the campus to teach her the Wassermann test as a smokescreen for what really bothered them: Saunders's superior performance and Babcock's confidence in her.

51. Blease later asserted: "One member of the Board of Regents informs me that the first friction between the Board of Regents and Dr. Saunders was that she handled these funds and refused to turn them over when requested to do so" (*Legislative Testimony* [1914], 63.) Had Blease investigated for himself, he would have found that Saunders received the funds on the regents' authority, and that she did not hesitate to give them back to the treasurer when asked to do so.

52. MBR, April 11, 1913.

53. *Legislative Report* (1914), 23. Allen, who later married and became Bessie Allen Sanders, testified (although not under oath) that she did not hear this remark and had burned her notes of the conversation (ibid., 148–51).

54. MBR, May 7, June 5, and July 10, 1913.

55. MBR, July 10, 1913. The minutes indicate that Bivens and Carothers met with Babcock, and Bivens then consulted Dominick, the assistant attorney general. It became clear during the 1914 legislative hearings that Bivens, who became an ardent opponent of Saunders, objected to her being the fund's custodian. Saunders established that she took care of about 600 women and, on cross-examining Bivens, asked pointedly: "If I am able to take care of six hundred women who are helpless, am I not able to take care of twenty-five hundred dollars?" (*Legislative Report* [1914], 405; see also "Bivens is Heard in Asylum Probe," *State*, February 19, 1914).

56. For a short biography, see Jenerette, *Ernest Cooper*. Medical school training during that era included basic laboratory tests such as complete blood counts and urinalyses, and many doctors did their own laboratory tests. It was not until 1919 that the Columbia Hospital (now Palmetto Health Richland) paid a pathologist (Blackburn and Padgette, *Columbia Hospital*, 94).

57. Ernest Cooper, "Report of Pathologist," AR (1911), 17. In looking for nocturnal parasites, Cooper was following a precedent set by Patrick Manson (see note 26, page 304).

58. *Pellagra Conference* (1912), 269–73. Cooper concluded, correctly, that amebae found in the stools of pellagrins were harmless commensal organisms.

59. *AR* (1912), 11.

60. *Legislative Report* (1914), 36, 52.

61. Ibid., 41, 75–76, 88, 142.

62. Ibid., 41.

63. Ibid., 104, 511–13. Saunders's hesitation to give the new drug to patients with structural brain lesions reflected her knowledge of the Jarisch-Herxheimer reaction—an acute febrile reaction to the initiation of drug therapy for late manifestations of syphilis.

64. *Legislative Report* (1914), 37.

65. Ibid., 325.

66. *Conspire*: "To combine secretly (*with*) for an unlawful or reprehensible purpose" (*Shorter Oxford Dictionary*, fifth edition, 2002; 1: 495). Taylor asserted that

Carothers and Settlemeyer had been "very disingenuous" in explaining why
Taylor had not been invited to the meeting. Carothers told Taylor that he
had "just not thought" to invite him. Settlemeyer told Taylor that none of the
members of the medical staff were invited, which was clearly incorrect (*Legislative Report* [1914], 417). The meeting probably took place on Wednesday,
September 10, since the Board of Regents was scheduled to meet the following
day and Carothers, Bivens, and Settlemeyer had to travel to Columbia from
elsewhere in the state.

67. *Legislative Testimony* (1914), 24–25.
68. Ibid., 316. When Babcock told Blease that if Dr. Saunders were to leave the
    asylum other women would probably follow, Blease said that "the decent
    women ought to leave now if what I heard was true. I am told . . . that women
    out there who are decent women, handle cases of syphilis and cases of gonor-
    rhea and other diseases which I would not want anybody kin to me that called
    themselves decent to handle" (ibid., 62). He testified that "I would rather
    scratch my finger nails off before I would let any of mine do it [let any of my
    white womenfolk diagnose and treat syphilis] or commit suicide and let them
    have the insurance policy, whichever would be best" (ibid., 316).
69. Blease to Babcock, November 10, 1913; Blease to Babcock, November 17,
    1913; carbon copies of the originals in the possession of Arthur St. J. Simons
    II. Copies of these letters have been placed in box 8, folder 45, Babcock papers,
    SCL. Blease paraphrased parts of the first of these letters during the legislative
    hearings in February 1914, telling Saunders directly, for example: "I believe
    you are a valuable woman, and a good woman. I believe you are a good woman
    at heart, but I think you made a fearful mistake when you flaunted in the
    face of these men that you would turn Dr. Blackburn down for Dr. Cooper"
    (*Legislative Report* [1914], 144).
70. *Legislative Report* (1914), 525–27. Babcock had previously notified Saunders's
    father by telegram. The minutes of the Board of Regents record that the special
    meeting was called on one day's notice "in regard to obstructions having been
    placed by some of the older officials" (MBR, December 11, 1913).
71. MBR, December 12, 1913; *Legislative Report* (1914), 33–34, 525–27.
72. Ibid.
73. J. L. Thompson to the Honorable Board of Regents, December 12, 1913
    (*Legislative Report* [1914], 105, 344 [the entire letter is reproduced in both
    places]). It is reasonable to assume this letter was written on the afternoon or
    evening of December 12, since it would have been unnecessary had Bivens's
    resolution calling for Saunders's removal passed.
74. MBR, January 6, 1914.
75. Coleman L. Blease to Babcock, January 16, 1914, Babcock papers, box 4,
    folder 17, SCL. Margaret Babcock Meriwether penciled onto this letter, "Dr.

Robert Wilson told me ... the governor had been drinking when he wrote the letter."

76. MBR, January 19, 1914. James A. Summersett did not vote on Bivens's resolution on the grounds that he was new to the Board of Regents and did not have all the facts.

77. Ibid.

78. Ibid; *Legislative Report* (1914), 35–36. An attorney for Eleanora Saunders was admitted to the room and declared the resolution against her unsatisfactory.

79. Blease observed in his final remarks to the 1914 legislature that although he had failed to get any major legislation passed during 1913 and 1914, he had retaliated by vetoing many measures passed by the Senate and House of Representatives. He concluded: "I do not wish all of you political success, but I wish you good health and Godspeed" (*House Journal* [1914], 1457).

80. *House Journal* (1914), 235–44 (Blease's message), 245 (resolution); *Senate Journal* (1914), 186–95 (Blease's message), 195 (resolution).

81. "Babcock Donates Fine Collection," *State*, February 9, 1914. The newspaper called Babcock "that friend of the institution of higher learning."

82. Tillman to Babcock, January 23 and January 25, 1914, Babcock papers, box 5, folder 2, SCL.

83. *Legislative Report* (1914), 335–38.

84. "[Dr. Griffin] Gives His Reasons for Making Charges," *State*, February 14, 1914. The newspaper carried in the same issue a letter to the editor signed by fifty-two nurses, concluding: "Dr. Saunders is in every sense of the word a gentlewoman. Her quick and tender sympathy for her patients is discernible to all who come in contact with her here. She is the same woman always, no matter what her own sorrows and grievances may be, dispensing cheerfulness and pleasant, kindly interest to every one with whom she comes in contact each day. We, the nurses of this institution, as a body, appeal to the men of this State, who are sitting in judgment of our worthy friend, not to remove her from our midst."

85. *Legislative Report* (1914), 135, 182, 256–66, 289–90. Griffin beefed that Saunders was "very disagreeable, discourteous, and rude."

86. *Legislative Report* (1914), 354, 420.

87. Ibid., 140, 486–507, 542.

88. See Grob, *Mental Illness*, 188–90, 292–96. By the 1920s much of the diagnostic and therapeutic efforts of psychiatrists at mental institutions focused on syphilis, since it was relatively common and potentially treatable. Between 1911 and 1919, about 20 percent of male first admissions to mental hospitals in New York State were for general paresis (syphilis), with the rates for females about one-third those of males.

89. *Legislative Report* (1914), 116–18, 216–17, 445–78. See also "Blackburn Examined as to Interference," *State*, February 19, 1914.

90. See Jenerette, *Ernest Cooper.*
91. *Legislative Report* (1914), 102.
92. Ibid., 105. At this point, Carothers introduced the letter dated December 12, 1913, that he had received from Thompson, claiming that Saunders had usurped his authority.
93. *Legislative Report* (1914), 109–10.
94. "The War Against the Woman," *State*, February 19, 1914. To clarify, O. L. Saunders is listed in the legislative directory as a merchant, not a farmer.
95. *Legislative Report* (1914), 422, 507–38.
96. As noted earlier, Blease came into office determined to dismiss Babcock. He asked his family physician, Dr. W. G. Houseal, whether he would accept the position if offered. Houseal said no. Tillman made much of this incident to no avail (*Legislative Testimony* [1914], 17, 58; see also *Senate Journal* [1914], 186–95). On at least two occasions, Blease declined Babcock's offer to resign. Blease considered nobody to be indispensible. He later wrote (*House Journal* [1914], 742; *Senate Journal* [1914], 576) that he "didn't know that Dr. Babcock . . . was the only man in the world who could run the Asylum," but that "I could have had him out before this [February 1914] if I had so desired. I have his resignation in my hand today and all I would have to do is accept it." Blease testified that he'd done all he could to keep the peace (See "Governor on Stand Gives his Version," *State*, February 8, 1914). However, on the first day of the hearings (February 3, 1914), Blease acknowledged his part in the resolution passed by the regents on January 19, condemning Babcock and Saunders for their actions but not calling for their removal.
97. *Legislative Report* (1914), 367–78.
98. Ibid., 380–82.
99. Ibid., 147.
100. Ibid., 5–10.
101. "Dr. Saunders Exonerated by Legislative Probers," *State*, February 26, 1914.
102. "Dr. Babcock May Resign as Head of State Asylum," *News and Courier* (Charleston, S.C.), March 1, 1914.
103. MBR, March 12, 1914; "Dr. Babcock Likely to Remain on Job," *News and Courier*, March 13, 1914; "Dr. Babcock Likely to Remain," *Keowee Courier* (Pickens, S.C.), March 18, 1914.
104. Blease to Babcock, March 12, 1914; Babcock to Blease, March 12, 1914; Blease to Babcock, March 13, 1914; all in Babcock papers, box 4, folder 17, SCL.
105. "Give Loving Cup to Dr. Saunders," *State*, March 6, 1914.
106. E. B. Saunders to the Board of Regents [of the State Hospital for the Insane], March 13, 1914, Babcock papers, box 4, folder 17, SCL; MBR, March 13, 1914.
107. MBR, March 26, 1914; MBR May 14, 1914.

108. J. T. Searcy to Babcock March 18, 1914; W. B. Glenn to Babcock, March 14, 1914; W. S. Shelor to Babcock, March 15, 1914; Franklin B. Wear to Babcock, March 18, 1914; W. D. Partlow to Babcock, March 18, 1914; all in Babcock papers, box 4, folder 17, SCL.
109. J. F. Siler to Babcock, April 18, 1914, Babcock papers, box 8, folder 4, SCL.

NOTES FOR CHAPTER 8

1. "Notable Columbians: Dr. J. W. Babcock," *State* (Columbia, S.C.), February 10, 1936. The extent to which Babcock wanted his old job back is unclear. When Richard I. Manning became governor in 1915, Tillman lobbied for Babcock's reinstatement as superintendent (Tillman to Babcock, February 26, 1915, Babcock papers, box 5, folder 2, SCL; see also Grob, *Mental Illness*, 159–60).
2. Quoted in "Dr. J. W. Babcock."
3. In 1910 only 3.2 percent of psychiatrists attending the annual meeting of the American Psychiatric Association were in private practice; by 1921 7.3 percent of the registrants were in private practice; and by 1933 31 percent of American psychiatrists were in private practice (Shorter, *History of Psychiatry*, 161, 180–81).
4. "Babcock to Join Medical Faculty," *Evening Post* (Charleston, S.C.), June 3, 1915; W. Grady Callison to Babcock, June 15, 1918, Babcock papers, box 4, folder 15, SCL.
5. James B. Meriwether, personal communication, October 12, 2004.
6. [August Kohn,] "Dr. J. W. Babcock Dies in Columbia," *News and Courier* (Charleston, S.C.), March 4, 1922.
7. Waring, *Medicine in South Carolina, 1900–1970*, 181–82.
8. Rupert Blue to Joseph Goldberger, February 7, 1914, Goldberger papers, box 1641, folder 16, SHC.
9. Blue to Goldberger, February 17, 1914, Goldberger papers, box 1641, folder 16, SHC.
10. The standard biographies are Parsons, *Trail to Light*, and Kraut, *Goldberger's War*. The many short biographical sketches include Elmore and Feinstein, "Joseph Goldberger," and Schultz, "Joseph Goldberger." For Goldberger's more important papers, see Terris, *Goldberger*.
11. Elmore and Feinstein, "Joseph Goldberger."
12. Frankenburg, *Vitamin Discoveries*, 40.
13. Kraut states: "At a time when most physicians regarded the germ theory as the causal explanation or paradigm, for all forms of disease, Goldberger hypothesized that pellagra was triggered by a flawed diet" (*Goldberger's War*, 7). For a brief summary of the germ theory in this context, see pp. 83–84.
14. 1910 S.C. Act 304 (*Acts and Resolutions* [1910], 613–22). For brief discussion, see Etheridge, *Butterfly Caste*, 44. State Commissioner of Agriculture E. J.

Watson stated at the 1915 pellagra conference in Columbia that 108 of 240 "odd shipments of corn meal" to South Carolina in 1914 were spoiled, but that his department had "been unable to find a single dangerous sample of corn meal made from corn grown and cured in our own state" (*NASP Minutes* [1915], 32–41).

15. "Pellagra in California."

16. Parsons, *Trail to Light*, 280.

17. After the story broke that Goldberger had prevented pellagra by dietary manipulation alone, *The State* (October 25, 1915) echoed Goldberger's tributes to previous physicians who championed diet as the cause. The newspaper pointed out that "in the history of medicine some of the greatest discoveries have not in reality been discoveries." Cited examples included Edward Jenner's work on vaccination against smallpox and Walter Reed's work on mosquito transmission of yellow fever; in both instances, the investigators designed experiments to prove what others had suspected.

18. Siler, Garrison, and MacNeal, "Pellagra. A Summary of the First Progress Report."

19. "Pellagra Spread by Bad Sewerage," *State*, January 3, 1914. This report, presented before the American Association for the Advancement of Science, featured the observation that pellagra seldom occurred in "districts completely equipped with [a] water carriage system of sewage disposal." The authors failed to take into account household incomes.

20. "State Must Help Combat Pellagra," *State*, January 27, 1914. The commission was listed as "The Robert M. Thompson Commission" on the program of the 1915 triennial conference of the National Association of Pellagra and also in the third progress report in 1917.

21. "Pellagra Bill Passes Senate," *State*, February 19, 1914; "Pellagra Measure Killed in House," *State*, March 4, 1914. Robert Wilson Jr, chairman of the State Board of Health, had repeatedly called for a state pellagra commission.

22. "Doctors are Worried," *State*, January 18, 1915. The newspaper reported that Babcock had "received a letter from Dr. Siler in which he expresses grave doubts [because of insufficient funding] of the continued researches of the Thompson-McFadden pellagra commission" and that Babcock strongly endorsed the commission's work. It is likely that Babcock communicated with Tillman in this regard. A pellagra hospital had been proposed earlier (for background, see Tillman to Babcock, July 17, 1913, Babcock papers, box 5, folder 1, SCL).

23. Goldberger, "Etiology of Pellagra." Goldberger's classic paper begins: "The writer desires to invite attention to certain observations recorded in the literature of pellagra the significance of which appears entirely to have escaped attention." However others, including Adams Hayne, (see note 55, below) had commented on the observation that staff members of institutions where

pellagra was highly prevalent did not get the disease. They pointed out that the patients could have been bitten by an insect prior to being admitted to the institution; hence the staff would not necessarily have been exposed.

24. Goldberger wrote that "at the South Carolina State Hospital for the Insane, where Babcock (1910 Ann. Rept.) states that cases of pellagra develop in patients who have been there for years, no case so far as the writer was able to ascertain has occurred in the nurses or attendants." The present author cannot find this statement in the 1910 *Annual Report* or in other reports by Babcock to the Board of Regents. It is unlikely that Goldberger obtained this information directly from Babcock, since they had not yet met. Blue had asked Goldberger to inspect asylums in the South (Blue to Goldberger, April 22, 1914, Goldberger papers, box 1641, folder 16, SHC). Possibly, Goldberger was in Columbia during April or May of 1914, missed seeing Babcock, but spoke with others.

25. Voegtlin, "Treatment of Pellagra." Voegtlin later became the first director of the National Cancer Institute ("Carl Voegtlin, 1879–1960").

26. Goldberger, "Cause and Prevention of Pellagra."

27. Siler, Garrison, and MacNeal, "Further Studies of the Thompson-McFadden Commission. Summary of the Second Progress Report." Among the visitors to the commission's field laboratory in Spartanburg listed in this report were Babcock, Sambon, and consultants from the U.S. Public Health Service, the U.S. Department of Agriculture, the French Department of Agriculture, and Cambridge University.

28. Goldberger to Mary Farrar Goldberger, September 26, 1914, Goldberger papers, box 1641, folder 16, SHC.

29. The four papers presented at the half-morning symposium on pellagra were not published, nor was the lively discussion that followed. The papers included "Treatment of Pellagra by Proper Diet, With a Report of Eleven Cases," by Dr. Y. A. Little of Milledgeville, Georgia ("Southern Medical Association, Minutes of the Eighth Annual Meeting").

30. "Pellagra's Cause Remains Mystery," *State*, November 17, 1914. One of Goldberger's colleagues later told Mary Goldberger, "No one takes him [James Adams Hayne] seriously in these meetings" (Kraut, *Goldberger's War*, 249). For biographical sketches of Hayne, see Beardsley, *History of Neglect*, 142–48; and Bryan, "Not Like his Father." Beardsley (p. 146) points out that in 1930 Surgeon General H. S. Cumming said that South Carolina would be a poor place for a pellagra demonstration project because of the attitudes shown by Hayne and a few others. However, in 1932, Hayne credited Goldberger for demonstrating that pellagra was caused by dietary deficiency (Hayne, "History of Pellagra").

31. Goldberger to Mary Farrar Goldberger, November 29, 1914, Goldberger papers, box 1641, folder 16, SHC.

32. Goldberger and Wheeler, "Pellagra in the Human Subject."
33. Goldberger to Mary Farrar Goldberger, Goldberger papers, box 1641, folder 16, SHC.
34. See Edgar, *South Carolina: A History*, 475–76. Edgar suggests that Manning secured more cooperation from the legislature than any governor in the history of South Carolina.
35. *House Journal* (1915), 286–305 (Manning's address, January 29, 1915); 1915 S.C. Acts 107 (*Acts and Resolutions* [1915], 147–49.
36. Thompson served very briefly as superintendent after Babcock's resignation but was replaced shortly thereafter by Dr. T. J. Strait, who was then replaced by Williams.
37. *AR* (1915), 28; C. F. Williams to the Board of Regents, State Hospital for the Insane, Columbia, S.C., Superintendent's Reports to the Board of Regents, SCDAH.
38. *AR* (1915), 3–4.
39. Sandwith to Babcock, September 4, 1915, Babcock papers, box 8, folder 5, SCL.
40. G. M. Niles to Babcock, September 22, 1915, Babcock papers, box 8, folder 5, SCL. The paper on "The Etiology of Pellagra with Especial Consideration of the Phenomena of Sensitization to Maize and Sugar-Cane Products" was to be submitted by Dr. Roy Blosser of Atlanta.
41. E. M. Perdue to Babcock, October 16, 1915, Babcock papers, box 8, folder 5, SCL.
42. H. M. Evans to Babcock, October 17, 1915, Babcock papers, box 8, folder 5, SCL.
43. "Study Pellagra for Two Days," *State*, October 21, 1915. Since the transactions of this conference were never published, the actual number of presentations cannot be ascertained. Of the twenty papers from South Carolina listed in the program, fifteen were from Columbia and one each from Charleston, Clover, Edgefield, Union, and York. Judging from the paucity of papers, it is likely that Babcock had to solicit in-state papers to fill the program.
44. This announcement pointedly implied that black physicians were not welcome at the evening session scheduled for the Jefferson Hotel. For discussions of the impact of segregation on physicians of that era, see Beardsley, "Making Separate, Equal"; and Savitt, "Entering a White Profession." In 1890 there were in South Carolina 30 black physicians and 1,099 white physicians; by 1920 there were 85 black physicians and 1,257 white physicians.
45. Green, "National Pellagra Commission." For background on the National Medical Association, see Baker et al., "Segregated Medical Profession."
46. *NASP Minutes* (1915), 4.
47. Rice had presented the gist of his observations at the 1912 national conference (Rice, "Pellagra in Children"). On July 2, 1915, Rice told members of

the Columbia Medical Society that he had seen pellagra as early as 1901, and that the average age of 214 patients (117 males and 97 females) was nine years. The causative factors were "apparently poor nutrition and microorganisms." He reported that "proper feeding, or giving the well balanced diet, is giving the greatest satisfaction in the way of treatment." Rice later published his presentation to the 1915 conference (Rice, "Etiology of Pellagra"). Rice was a "deeply studious" and "most unusually well-informed" physician whose activities suggest a strong social conscience (Minutes of the Columbia Medical Society, March 9, 1914, July 12, 1915, July 11, 1933 [memorial], and elsewhere in these minutes, SCL).

48. "Experts Discuss Pellagra Study," *State*, October 22, 1915; *NASP Minutes* (1915), 144.

49. Joseph Goldberger and Roy Blosser, both in "Discussion of Dr. MacNeal's Address," *NASP Minutes* (1915), 68–72. Siler's response to Goldberger was, as usual, polite and gentlemanly. Dr. James D. Bozeman of Fort Worth, Texas, provided what may have been comic relief by proposing that pellagra had been introduced to the United States in 1905 by a shipload of Italian workers brought in to harvest oak trees from Alabama swamps (ibid., 81–83).

50. Ward J. MacNeal, in "Discussion of Dr. MacNeal's Address," *NASP Minutes* (1915), 88–94.

51. "Curing Pellagra by Diet Methods . . . ," *State*, October 22, 1915.

52. The reference is Roussel, *Traité de la Pellagra.* The original contains the italics.

53. Goldberger, Waring, and Willets, "Prevention of Pellagra." For historical controls in orphanages, they used data provided by Henry Rice of Columbia indicating that recurrence rates were between 58 percent and 76 percent.

54. Babcock, discussion of Joseph Goldberger, C. H. Waring, and David G. Willets, "A Test Diet in the Prevention of Pellagra," *NASP Minutes* (1915), 111.

55. In 1912 Hayne presented a brief paper with this same title ("The Communicability of Pellagra") at the annual meeting of state and provincial boards of health, held in Washington, D.C., in which he proclaimed:

> The State Board of Health has been the recipient of numerous letters, the burden of these letters being, 'Is this disease communicable?' . . . . The argument of the Italians that no cases have ever developed among hospital attendants and nurses . . . is specious, for we know that yellow fever is communicable; yet a case of yellow fever could be safely treated in a hospital where the stegomyia [the yellow-fever-transmitting mosquito] did not exist and the nurses and attendants would never develop the disease. The same facts are true of malaria, of Rocky Mountain spotted fever. . . . and many other known communicable diseases. . . . From the facts that have been presented to me, I must confess that I am compelled to believe this

disease is communicable, and that it is conveyed by some unknown biting insect from the sick to the well. It is our task to find out what the conveyer is. . . .

Hayne called for a federal commission to investigate the communicability of pellagra and added: "My guess is that this disease is spread either by some variety of simulium or by the stemoxis fly" (Hayne, "Communicability of Pellagra," *Proceedings of the Twenty-Seventh Annual Meeting of the State and Provincial Boards of Health*).

56. J. A. Hayne, discussion of Joseph Goldberger, C. H. Waring, and David G. Willets, "A Test Diet in the Prevention of Pellagra," *NASP Minutes* (1915), 113.

57. Ibid., 143–4. Goldberger probably did not help his cause by suggesting that many physicians weren't interested in a practical remedy:

> An interesting psychological phenomenon: I found that the profession are extraordinarily interested in the discussion of pellagra. I can get a rise out of the doctors any time the cause is mentioned of pellagra, and they will talk by the hour, but if one diplomatically suggests the very simple or practical device of treating the patient, they will change the subject.
>
> There is an adage to the effect that "the proof of the pudding is in the eating thereof?"and the only thing that I care to say in closing is, suppose we stop talking so much. We don't have to inject salvarsan, etc. (*NASP Minutes* [1915], 121).

58. Ibid., 158.

59. "Pellagra Cause Remains Unknown," *State*, October 23, 1915. The newspaper reported:

> When asked for an opinion of the comparative merits of the three conferences [the triennial meetings of 1909, 1912, and 1915, all held in Columbia] a leading physician said: "The first meeting devoted its attention to 'corn' as a cause of pellagra; the second to a possible 'protozoa' [parasitic] origin; and this meeting was inclined to the theory of a possible error in 'diet.' Scientifically, the meeting this week indicated a distinct advance over previous meetings."
>
> No positive conclusions as to the cause of pellagra were announced, although many were advocated by contributors of the various papers.

The reporter was apparently unwilling to take sides in the debate between Goldberger and the Thompson-McFadden Commission. The Committee on Resolutions, of which Goldberger was chairman and Siler a member, was officially silent on the cause of pellagra.

60. See Flannery, "Pellagra in Alabama." Goldberger spoke of the "great practical importance of the contribution made by Dr. Grote," adding: "His experience

in Walker County clearly indicates that we have in diet a practical means for combating pellagra in a community" (*NASP Minutes* [1915], 152).

61. Goldberger to Mary Farrar Goldberger, October 23, 1915, Goldberger papers, box 1641, folder 18, SHC.

62. "Pellagra Study gives Impetus," *State*, October 25, 1915.

63. Goldberger to Mary Farrar Goldberger, October 29, 1915, Goldberger papers, box 1641, folder 18, SHC.

64. Goldberger and Wheeler, "Experimental Pellagra." The rash appeared on the backs of the hands in only two of the six cases, and on the neck in only one case. Ward MacNeal persistently challenged the diagnosis of pellagra in these subjects largely because the rash had been less than classic. For discussion of the later ethics controversy about the Rankin Farm experiment, see Harkness, "Prisoners and Pellagra."

65. "Studies of Pellagra."

66. Further grounds for optimism included a report from the Southern Medical Association's Committee on Prevention and Treatment of Pellagra stating that Goldberger's ideas and results were "most plausible, and that his is probably the only theory that has come anywhere near being proved" ("Pellagra Symposium").

67. For a statistical account, see Park et al., "Effectiveness of Food Fortification." For a social perspective, see Humphreys, "Four Once Common Diseases."

68. Etheridge, "Pellagra."

69. Crabb, "Epidemic of Pride."

70. Chacko, "Geography of Pellagra."

71. "South Resents Federal Alarm over Pellagra," *New York Times*, July 27, 1921.

72. Kraut, *Goldberger's War*, 192.

73. Early-twentieth-century examples include the irrational public responses to medical discoveries by Drs. Joseph James Kinyoun (the presence of plague in San Francisco) and Carlos Chagas (the parasitic cause, linked to poverty, of what is now called Chagas disease or American trypanosomiasis). Kinyoun was accused of maliciously faking the epidemic of plague; a lawsuit was brought against him; and it was even suggested in the California legislature that Kinyoun be hanged. Fellow Brazilians' attacks on Chagas may have cost him the Nobel Prize. For reviews, see Morens et al., "Plague in San Francisco"; and Lewinsohn, "Prophet in his Own Country."

74. Flannery, "Pellagra in Alabama."

75. Siler, Garrison, and MacNeal, "Introduction to the Third Report." The third report, unlike the first and second reports, lists "W. J. MacNeal, Ph.D., M.D." as the sole editor. Siler and Garrison had returned to active duty in their respective services. The absence of any mention or reference to Goldberger—other than an allusion to the effect that "the ancient theory of dietary deficiency" had been "again exploited by Sandwith and others in the recent literature"—bears silent witness to MacNeal's heavy editorial hand and opposition to Goldberger.

76. Vedder, "Dietary Deficiency." In 1913 Vedder suggested in passing that "pellagra, rickets, and other diseases" might be dietary deficiencies (Vedder, *Beriberi*, 313). In 1914 Vedder elaborated that "if pellagra is a deficiency disease, its relation to corn is precisely the relation of beri-beri to rice. That is, corn *per* se is not harmful, but that when certain kinds of corn are too exclusively consumed, a deficiency of some unknown substance or vitamine necessary to metabolism is created" (Vedder, "Further Remarks"). Vedder thus joined the short list of Americans, including Blue, Babcock, Tucker, and Alsberg, who mentioned the vitamin-deficiency hypothesis in print before Goldberger went south. MacNeal seems to have ignored him. For a biographical sketch see Williams, "Edward Bright Vedder."

77. Muncey, "Heredity of Pellagra"; Davenport, "Hereditary Factor in Pellagra." Muncey and Davenport listed their affiliations as the Eugenic Records Office at Cold Spring Harbor and the New York Post-Graduate Medical School and Hospital.

78. Allan Chase, A Few False Correlations = A Few Million Real Deaths: Scientific Racism Prevails over Scientific Truth," in Chase, *Legacy of Malthus*, 201–25.

79. George Wheeler coordinated most of the field studies. Edgar Sydenstricker coordinated the study designs and statistical analysis. Results include Goldberger et al., "Factors of a Sanitary Character"; Goldberger, Wheeler, and Sydenstricker, "Relation of Family Income"; and other publications reproduced or listed in Terris, *Goldberger on Pellagra*. For the final report, see Goldberger et al., *Study of Endemic Pellagra*. Of the original seven mill villages in this study, four were in Spartanburg County, two were in Oconee County, and one was in Chester County; "All had previously been studied more or less intensively by the Thompson-McFadden Commission." The study was extended to twenty-four villages in 1917, downsized to six in 1918, and reduced to a single community in 1919.

80. Goldberger to Mary Farrar Goldberger, January 27, 1916, February 9, 1916, and April 21, 1916, Goldberger papers, box 1641, folder 19, SHC.

81. For a review of Goldberger's work in the context of the history of self-experimentation, see Altman, "Dietary Deprivations."

82. Goldberger took skin scales and urine specimens from two pellagrins and liquid feces from a third. He mixed the skin scales with 4 milliliters (about a teaspoon) of urine and 4 milliliters of the liquid feces. To neutralize his stomach acid and thereby increase the likelihood of infection (if indeed a "germ" that caused pellagra was present), he swallowed sodium carbonate about thirty minutes before the ingestion and again about sixty to ninety minutes after the ingestion.

83. Goldberger to Mary Farrar Goldberger, August 3, 1916, Goldberger papers, box 1641, folder 19, SHC.

84. Goldberger to Mary Farrar Goldberger, December 17, 1916, Goldberger papers, box 1641, folder 19, SHC.

85. Goldberger and Tanner, "Pellagra-Preventive Action."

86. Spencer, "Black Tongue." Spencer based his deduction on the case of a dentist in Monroe, North Carolina, who cured himself of pellagra with diet, and on an analogy with beriberi. All of his cases "gotten hold of in the early stages of the disease" responded to a diet of milk, eggs, and raw meat.

87. Chittenden and Underhill, "Production in Dogs." For an example of the reservations about the Chittenden-Underhill syndrome as a model for pellagra, see Voegtlin, "Recent Work."

88. Seidell, "Stable Form of Vitamine."

89. Wood, "The Etiology of Pellagra."

90. For a review of some of the complexities of pellagra research during this era from a chemist's point of view, see McCollum, "Investigations on Pellagra," in McCollum, *History of Nutrition*, 302-18. More studies in monkeys also took place during this period. Two researchers in London produced symptoms suggesting pellagra in monkeys by feeding them a low-protein diet; giving the monkeys tryptophan was only partially effective as therapy (Chick and Hume, "Production in Monkeys").

91. Wheeler, Goldberger, and Blackstock, "Probable Identity."

92. For fuller discussion, see Kraut, *Goldberger's War*, 143–231.

93. Rosen, *Public Health*, 413.

94. Jones ("Pellagra, Progress, and Public Polemics") suggests that a current of acceptance of the dietary hypothesis emerged among southern physicians after 1915. See "Notes for Researchers" in the present volume, 280.

95. *NASP Minutes* (1915), 124. R. M. Grimm of the U.S. Public Health Service was elected first vice president and Dr. H. W. Rice of Columbia was elected second vice president. Babcock would remain as secretary and Hayne would be treasurer.

96. *NASP Minutes* (1915), 158.

97. The more important papers presented at the 1915 NASP meeting had already been published, and the more important discussions had appeared in the *Journal of the American Medical Association* ("Society Proceedings"). Babcock collected some of the manuscripts and made notes where they had been published (Babcock papers, box 7, folders 20 through 32, SCL). Correspondence documenting the expectation that he would assemble the manuscripts, but never completed the task, consists of: The R. L. Bryan Company to D. S. Masterson, December 18, 1916; The R. L. Bryan Company to the Office of the Surgeon General, Public Health Service, September 10, 1917; and D. S. Masterson to the R. L. Bryan Company, September 25, 1917, all in box 150, NARA.

98. MacNeal, "Infectious Etiology of Pellagra."

99. In 1931, for example, an editorialist wrote in the *Journal of the American Medical Association*: "It has again become 'open season' in the hunt for explanations [of pellagra]" ("Increasing Prevalence of Pellagra").

100. Some authorities date the present-day concept of the case-control study to Janet Layne-Claypon's 1926 study of breast cancer, and the concept of the randomized, prospective, placebo-controlled, double-blinded trial to the British Medical Research Council's 1946 trial of streptomycin for tuberculosis. There were of course earlier trials, famously including James Lind's study of citrus fruits for scurvy. For reviews, see Concato, Shah, and Horwitz, "Randomized, Controlled Trials"; Paneth, Susser, and Susser, "Case-Control Study"; and Doll, "Controlled Clinical Trial."

101. Smith and Ruffin, "Effect of Sunlight"; Wan, Moat, and Antsley, "Pellagra."

102. Bloch, "Two Centuries."

103. Roe, *Plague of Corn*, 86.

104. Full discussion of the historiography of the germ theory is well beyond the scope of the present volume. For a concise summary, see Tomes and Warner, "Introduction to Special Issue." For discussion of the germ theory as it affected the deficiency theory of disease, see Carter, "Germ Theory."

105. Handwritten note signed "R Ross" on "The Elucidation of Sleeping Sickness" by Dr. Louis Sambon. This copy, which is in the archives of the London School of Hygiene and Tropical Medicine, appears to be an offprint or reprint of Sambon's paper. The author is indebted to Matthew Chipping for drawing his attention to Ross's inscription. Ross was, however, a member of the British Pellagra Commission that helped finance Sambon's 1910 trip to Italy.

106. Notes by Charles Thompson, July 1911, quoted in Larson, *Infinity of Things*, 120. Although "Sambon's talents as a scholar and his connections in Europe made him too valuable to dismiss," Larson writes, his "colourful turns of phrase—'You must really forgive me. My life has been a veritable inferno.'—began to sound increasingly hollow."

107. Wilkinson, "AJE Terzi and LW Sambon."

108. Manson-Bahr, *School of Tropical Medicine in London*, 132–36.

109. "Louis Sambon, M.D."

110. "Louis Sambon, M.D. Naples."

111. Lecture notes, Babcock papers, box 10, folders 1 through 5, SCL.

112. One of Babcock's daughters [not stated], undated memorandum, Babcock papers, box 4, folder 14, SCL.

113. Babcock's colleague Isaac M. Taylor of Morgantown, North Carolina, was also an expert witness for the defense (Taylor to Babcock, September 12, 1919, Babcock papers, box 4, folder 14, SCL). The case is still cited for the court's decision that a wife is incompetent to testify against her husband (114 S.C. 389; 103 S.E. 755 [1920]).

114. Most of Babcock's reprints are in the Waring Historical Library at the Medical University of South Carolina, Charleston, and have now been catalogued. Papers by Goldberger are usually stamped "with the author's compliments."

115. J. W. Babcock, "Treatment of Pellagra," undated manuscript, Babcock papers, SCL. This manuscript was almost surely Babcock's text for an address at a medical meeting, as a Kentucky physician quotes several sentences from it almost verbatim (Harris, "Pellagra"). William Osler in the 1918 edition of his textbook (co-authored with Thomas McCrae) seems to give equal weight to Sambon's version of the infection hypothesis and Goldberger's version of the dietary-deficiency hypothesis (Osler and McCrae, *Principles and Practice*, 8th ed., 411–15). Likewise, a 1921 editorialist for the *Journal of the American Medical Association* declines to take sides between MacNeal and Goldberger ("What is the Cause of Pellagra?").

116. Tillman, "How I Restored my Health."

117. "Dr. J. W. Babcock Dies at Residence," *State*, March 4, 1922.

118. "J. W. Babcock Dies; Identified Pellagra," *New York World*, March 4, 1922.

119. "He Identified Pellagra," *Boston Herald*, March 11, 1922.

120. "Italians mourn Dr. J. W. Babcock," *State*, May 23, 1922.

121. Howard, "James Woods Babcock."

122. "News from the Classes."

123. George W. Manly to Katherine Babcock, March 3, 1922, Babcock papers, box 4, folder 13, SCL.

124. "Reconciled."

125. Hayes and Loos, *Twice Over Lightly*, 49–50.

126. Connie Guion taught at Sweet Briar in order to fund her younger siblings' educations, thus setting aside for a few years her ambition to be a doctor.

127. Forbush, *Sheppard and Enoch Pratt Hospital*, 155.

128. Saunders, "Depressions in Late Life."

129. Cooper, *South Carolina Sanatorium*; Cooper, *South Carolina and Palmetto Sanatoria*. The South Carolina Sanatorium for white men opened in 1915; five years later a separate sanatorium, named the Palmetto Sanatorium, opened for black men.

130. Thompson, *Shattered Minds*, 62.

131. Lavinder examined 1,015 orphans in Columbia, S.C., Milledgeville, Georgia, and Jackson, Mississippi, and found only two cases of pellagra, both of whom apparently had pellagra when they were admitted to the orphanages (Lavinder to the Surgeon General, June 3, 1916, box 149, NARA).

132. Lavinder, Freeman, and Frost, *Epidemiologic Studies*.

133. Citation for Joseph F. Siler for the Army Distinguished Service Medal, War Department, General Orders No. 59 (1922).

134. There are at the time of this writing four known dengue viruses. Dr. Scott B. Halstead examined four of Siler's volunteers more than four decades later to determine their immunity patterns (Halstead, "Experimental Dengues").

135. The eight persons who received the Nobel Prize for discoveries pertaining to vitamins were Henrik Carl Peter Dam (vitamin K, 1943), Edward Adelbert Doisy (vitamin K, 1943), Christiaan Eijkman (vitamin B_1, 1929), Walter Norman Haworth (vitamin C, 1937), Sir Frederick Gowland Hopkins (growth-stimulating vitamins, 1929), Paul Karrer (vitamins A, B, and E, 1937), Richard Kuhn (vitamins B_2 and B_6, 1938), and Albert von Szent-Györgyi (vitamin C, 1937).

136. "Dr. Joseph Goldberger Dies in Washington," *State*, January 18, 1929.

137. Henry Bellamann (1882–1945), born Heinrich Hauer Bellamann, is best known for *King's Row* but was also an accomplished musician. He came to Columbia in 1915 to teach at Chicora College for Women (later consolidated with Queens College, Charlotte, North Carolina). He was a key figure in a group of Columbians interested in psychology. Although Bellamann apparently never earned an undergraduate degree he later served as acting director of the Julliard Musical Foundation and became a professor of music at Vassar College.

138. Bellamann, *King's Row*, 533, 559, 591.

139. "Waverley Sanitarium, Inc."

140. "Requiem for a Gracious Gentlewoman."

141. "Babcock Center Opened," *State*, September 24, 1969.

NOTES FOR EPILOGUE

1. King, "South Carolina State Hospital," 5.

2. Johnson, "South Carolina State Hospital," 104.

3. Major and Delp, *Physical Diagnosis*, 225. The quotation is attributed to the German physician Friedrich von Müller.

4. For a critical review of Babcock's efficacy (or lack thereof) as superintendent, see McCandless, *Moonlight*, 244–313.

5. Bass and Poole, *Palmetto State*, 115.

6. "South Carolina and Her State Hospital."

7. Donald, *Lincoln*, 14–15.

8. "Pays Fine Tribute to Dr. J. W. Babcock" (Francis H. Weston, letter to the editor), *State* (Columbia, S.C.), March 4, 1922.

9. Taylor, *James Woods Babcock*, 4.

10. "Dr. J. W. Babcock Dies in Columbia" (signed "August Kohn"), *News and Courier* (Charleston, S.C.), March 4, 1922. See also chapter 4, note 74, page 316.

11. Holmes, "The Young Practitioner."

12. See p. 110.

13. See p. 111.

14. James W. Babcock, M.D., "Treatment of Pellagra." Unpublished, undated manuscript, Babcock papers, box 6, folder 1, SCL.

15. Nearly all accounts of the conquest of pellagra mention its first description in Spain, tell of its spread in the American South, and then relate the story of Joseph Goldberger, with little or no mention of how Americans before Goldberger fleshed out competing hypotheses. See, for example, Bordley and Harvey, *Two Centuries*, 247–50. Substantial growth in full-time clinical faculty in American medical schools and in the research capabilities of federal agencies—notably, the U.S. Public Health Service and the National Institutes of Health—began between roughly 1910 and 1920 and accelerated after World War II. The response to a major epidemic by such a diverse group of amateurs (that is, persons who were not fully trained as researchers) possibly has no parallel in the history of American medicine.

16. Carpenter, *Beriberi*, xii, 201.

17. MBR, February 11, 1897.

18. See p. 16.

19. See p. 123.

20. James B. Meriwether, personal communication, October 12, 2004.

21. Peter Lawrence Hardin, quoted in "Asylum Fight Continued," *State*, February 17, 1910.

22. Letter to the editor, *Columbia Record*, February 7, 1910.

23. "Gov. Heyward Comments on Dr. Babcock," *Columbia Record*, February 14, 1910.

24. Hennig, *August Kohn*.

25. White, "Presidential Address."

26. Dean, "Death of Specificity."

27. Warman, *Corn & Capitalism*, 173.

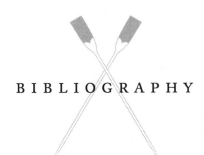

BIBLIOGRAPHY

Primary Sources

ARCHIVES AND COLLECTIONS

Claude Moore Health Sciences Library, University of Virginia, Charlottesville
Philip S. Hench Walter Reed Yellow Fever Collection

Harvard University Archives
Class records and reports

Medical Center Archives, New York-Presbyterian / Weill Cornell Medical College, New York, New York
Connie Myers Guion papers

National Archives and Records Administration, College Park, Maryland
Pellagra files of the U.S. Public Health Service, record group 90, file 1648

Philips Exeter Academy, Exeter, New Hampshire
Class records and reports
Records of the Golden Branch Society

Royal Society of Tropical Medicine and Hygiene Archives, London
Pellagra Investigation Committee (GB 0809)

South Carolina Department of Archives and History, Columbia
Admission and discharge books (S190026)
Admission books (S190025)
Admissions register (S190028)
Annual Reports (S190002)

Case Histories (S199021)

Commitment files (S190024)

Discharge books (S190034)

Governor Benjamin Ryan Tillman papers (S526001 and S526006)

Governor Richard I. Manning's Special Message on the State Hospital for the Insane to the General Assembly and a 1915 Report to the Governor (S190080)

List of admissions (S190027)

Minutes of the Mental Health Commission, 1828–2006 (includes Minutes of the Board of Regents, South Carolina State Hospital) (S190001)

Record of deaths (S190038)

School of Nursing, list of graduates, 1893–1943 (S190066)

South Carolina State Hospital for the Insane, Miscellaneous Papers, 1866–1917 (S190010)

Superintendent's Reports to the Regents (S190005)

South Caroliniana Library, University of South Carolina, Columbia

Christensen Family papers

James Woods Babcock papers

Minutes of the Columbia (S.C.) Medical Society

Southern Historical Collection, Wilson Library, University of North Carolina, Chapel Hill

Joseph Goldberger papers

Patrick Livingston Murphy papers

Special Collections, University Libraries, Clemson University, Clemson, South Carolina

Benjamin Ryan Tillman papers

Waring Historical Library, Medical University of South Carolina, Charleston

James Woods Babcock papers

UNPUBLISHED MANUSCRIPTS,
THESES, AND DISSERTATIONS

Allan, Sarah Campbell. "Diary from SC State Hospital, 1900." Waring Historical Library.

Anderson, Uta Puppel. "Pioneer Women Physicians in South Carolina: Sarah Campbell Allan and Eleanora Bennette Saunders." Undated manuscript [ca. 1995] in the possession of the present author.

Brice, James Taylor. "The Use of Executive Clemency under Coleman Livingston Blease, Governor of South Carolina, 1911–1915." Master's thesis, University of North Carolina, 1965.

Burnside, Robert Dantan. "The Governorship of Coleman Livingston Blease of South Carolina, 1911–1915." Ph.D. diss., Indiana University, 1963.

Fitzgerald, Jennifer. "'Help These People Help Themselves': Governor Benjamin R. Tillman's Response to the 1893 Sea Island Hurricane and Languishing Phosphate Industry in Beaufort County, South Carolina." Master's thesis, University of South Carolina, 2004.

Hellams, Wilton. "A History of South Carolina State Hospital." Ph.D. diss., University of South Carolina, 1985.

Johnson, Leila Glover. "A History of the South Carolina State Hospital." Master's thesis, University of Chicago, 1930.

King, Malvena Geraldine Sowell. "The South Carolina State Hospital and its Treatment of Mental Disease." Master's thesis, University of South Carolina, 1930.

Simons, Alice Babcock. "Early Recollections of My Father at the State Hospital. Dr. James Woods Babcock, 1891–1914." Undated manuscript in the possession of Arthur St. J. Simons II.

Thielman, Samuel Barnett. "Madness and Medicine: The Medical Approach to Madness in Antebellum America, with Particular Reference to the Eastern Lunatic Asylum of Virginia and the South Carolina Lunatic Asylum." Ph.D. diss., Duke University, 1986.

Tuntiya N. "The Forgotten History: The Deinstitutionalization Movement in the Mental Health Care System in the United States." Master's thesis, University of South Florida, 2003.

PUBLISHED REPORTS OF SOUTH CAROLINA GOVERNMENT AND STATE AGENCIES

Acts and Joint Resolutions of the General Assembly of the State of South Carolina

Annual Reports of the South Carolina Lunatic Asylum (until 1894–95, thereafter *Annual Reports of the South Carolina State Hospital of the Insane*)

Journal of the Constitutional Convention of the State of South Carolina. Columbia, S.C.: Charles A. Calvo, 1895.

Journal of the House of Representatives of the General Assembly of the State of South Carolina

Journal of the Senate of the General Assembly of the State of South Carolina

The Lunacy Laws of South Carolina: Directions for the Admission of Patients and the By-Laws Adopted by the Board of Regents of the Lunatic Asylum of South Carolina, October 8, 1891. Columbia, S.C.: Presbyterian Publishing, 1891.

Report and Proceedings of the Special Legislative Committee Appointed by Concurrent Resolution to Investigate the State Hospital for the Insane and State Park, January 1914. Columbia, S.C.: Gonzales and Bryan, 1914.

Report of the Legislative Committee to Investigate the State Hospital for the Insane. Columbia, S.C.: Gonzales and Bryan, State Printers, 1910. Also in *Reports and Resolutions of the General Assembly of the State of South Carolina* (1910), vol. 2, 479–601.

Reports and Resolutions of the General Assembly of the State of South Carolina.

Reports of the South Carolina State Board of Health (in *Reports and Resolutions of the General Assembly of the State of South Carolina*)

Reports of the State Hospital Commission to the General Assembly of South Carolina

Rules and Regulations for the Government of the Lunatic Asylum of South Carolina, Compiled by the Superintendent and Adopted by the Regents, October 8, 1891. Columbia, S.C.: Presbyterian Publishing, 1891.

Testimony Taken Before the Legislative Committee to Investigate the State Hospital for the Insane at Columbia, April 28, May 4, 6, 7, 18, 19, 20, 1909. Columbia, S.C.: Gonzales and Bryan, 1910.

REPORTS AND TRANSACTIONS OF MEETINGS, CONFERENCES, AND COMMISSIONS

Conference on Pellagra Held under the Auspices of the State Board of Health of South Carolina at the State Hospital for the Insane, October 29th, 1908, Columbia, S.C.: State, 1909.

Minutes of the Proceedings [Transactions] of the Fifty-Sixth Annual Meeting of the South Carolina Medical Association held at Darlington, South Carolina, April 20th and 21st, 1904.

Jervey, J. Wilkinson. "The Passing of the Negro: Being Some Further Evidence on the Present Physical Status and Outlook of the Negro Race in America," 183–99.

Minutes of the Third Triennial Meeting of the National Association for the Study of Pellagra, Columbia, S.C., October 21 and 22, 1915 (Babcock papers, box 7, folder 19, SCL).

Pellagra. First Progress Report of the Thompson-McFadden Pellagra Commission of the New York Post-Graduate Medical School and Hospital, by J. F. Siler, P. E. Garrison, and W. J. MacNeal, with the collaboration of A. H. Jennings, W. V. King, V. C. Myers, M. S. Fine, O. S. Hillman, and others [n.p., 1913].

Pellagra II. Second Progress Report of the Thompson-McFadden Pellagra Commission of the New York Post-Graduate Medical School and Hospital, by J. F. Siler, P. E. Garrison, and W. J. MacNeal, with the collaboration of H. Douglas Singer, Paul A. Schule, O. S. Hillman, and others [n.p., 1915].

Pellagra III. Third Report of the Robert M. Thompson Pellagra Commission of the New York Post-Graduate Medical School and Hospital, by J. F. Siler, P. E. Garrison, and W. J. MacNeal, with the collaboration of C. B. Davenport, Elizabeth B. Muncey, and Edward B. Vedder, edited by W. J. MacNeal with the assistance of Lucy Chapin Rich [n.p., 1917].

Proceedings of the Twenty-Seventh Annual Meeting of the Conference of State and Provincial Boards of Health of North America, Washington, D.C., September 20, 21 and 22, 1912. St. Paul, Minn.: Volkszeitung, 1913.

Babcock, J. W. Discussion of Hayne, "Pellagra," 117–18.

Hayne, J. A. "The Communicability of Pellagra" (in "Pellagra" [Report of the Committee on Pellagra, with discussion]), 115–21.

Report of the Pellagra Commission of the State of Illinois, November, 1911. Springfield: Illinois State Journal, 1912.

Forbes, Stephen A. "Black-Flies and Buffalo-Gnats (Simulium) in Illinois," 176–91.

"General Summary," 244–49.

Hirschfelder, Arthur D. "Cutaneous Tests with Corn Extracts in Pellagrins," 165–66.

MacNeal, W. J., and Josephine (Kerr) Allison, "The Intestinal Bacteria of Pellagrins," 55–160.

Rooks, J. T. "Protozoal Infection of Patients at the Kankakee State Hospital," 192–94.

Siler, J. F., and H. J. Nichols, "Report on the Investigation of Pellagra in Illinois for the Illinois Pellagra Commission," 44–52.

Singer, H. Douglas. "Pellagra in Illinois," 9–15.

———. "Meat Used in the State Hospitals," 242–43.

Singer, H. Douglas, W. J. MacNeal, and J. T. Rooks. "Attempts at the Experimental Transmission of Pellagra," 167–75.

Wussow, A. F., and H. S. Grindley, "Dietary Studies and Biochemical Work," 195–241.

"Society Proceedings. National Association for the Study of Pellagra." *Journal of the American Medical Association* 65, no. 23 (1915): 2028–29; 65, no. 24 (1915): 2114–17; and 65, no. 25 (1915): 2195–97.

"Southern Medical Association, Minutes of the Eighth Annual Meeting, Held at Richmond, Va., November 9, 10, 11 and 12, 1914," *Southern Medical Journal* 7, no. 12 (1914): 952–73.

"Symposium on Pellagra" [program], 967.

Transactions of the Forty-Third Annual Session of the Medical Society of Virginia held in Norfolk, October 22–25, 1912. Richmond Press, 1923.

Tucker, Beverley R. "The Nervous and Mental Symptoms of Pellagra," 167–70.

———. Discussion of Thomas W. Merrill, "Skin Symptoms and Treatment of Pellagra," 171–75.

Transactions of the Medical Association of the State of Alabama, Mobile, April 19–22. Montgomery: Brown, 1910.

Cole, Herbert P. Discussion of E. Marvin Mason, "Pellagra," 336–49.

Transactions of the National Conference on Pellagra Held Under Auspices of South Carolina State Board of Health at the State Hospital for the Insane, Columbia, S.C., November 3 and 4, 1909. Columbia, S.C.: State, 1910.

Babcock, J. W. Discussion of Geo. A. Zeller, "Pellagra—Its Recognition in Illinois, and the Measures Taken to Control It," 70–71.

Byrd, Hiram. Discussion of J. H. Taylor, "The Question of the Etiology of Pellagra," 194–95.

Cole, H. P., and Gilman J. Winthrop. "Transfusion in Pellagra," 158–69.

De Jarnet, J. S. "Pellagra, The Corn Curse," 288–93.

Harris, H. F. "Pathology of Pellagra," 86–93.

Jones, J. D. Discussion of J. H. Taylor, "The Question of the Etiology of Pellagra," 195–96.

Kerr, J. W. "Notes on the Hematology of Pellagra" [*sic*; the correct title should be "Pellagra as a National Public Health Problem"], 20–24.

Lavinder, C.M., "Notes on the Hematology of Pellagra," 33–40.

M'Connell, H. E. "Some Facts and Theories of Pellagra," 202–6.

Mobley, J. W. "Pellagra—Its Relation to Insanity and Certain Nervous Diseases," 137–47.

Rohrer, C. W. G. "Pellagra-Its Etiology, Pathology, Diagnosis and Treatment," 94–100.

Sandwith, F. M. "Introductory Remarks," 14–19.

Siler, J. F., and Henry J. Nichols. "Aspects of the Pellagra Problem in Illinois," 53–64.

Taylor, J. H. "The Question of the Etiology of Pellagra," 181–91.

Watson, E. J. "Economic Factors of the Pellagra Problem in South Carolina," 25–32.

Watson, J. J. Discussion of J. H. Taylor, "The Question of the Etiology of Pellagra," 193–94.

Watson, J. J. "Symptomatology of Pellagra and Report of Cases," 207–18.

Zeller, Geo. A., "Pellagra—Its Recognition in Illinois, and the Measures Taken to Control It," 46–52.

Transactions of the National Association for the Study of Pellagra. Second Triennial Meeting at Columbia, South Carolina, October 3 and 4, 1912. Columbia, S.C.: R. L. Bryan, 1914.

Adler, Herman M. "The Experimental Production of Lesions Resembling Pellagra," 261–67.

Alsberg, C. L., and C. F. Black, "Studies of the Metabolism of Moulds Belonging to the Genus Penicillium," 229–33.

Babcock, J. W. "Presidential Address. How Long Has Pellagra Existed in the United States?" 9–22.

———. "Medico-Legal Relations in Pellagra," 391–404.

Babes, Victor. "A Review of Recent Hypotheses upon the Etiology of Pellagra," 113–25.

Beall, K. H. "Pellagra in Texas; Some Suggestions as to Etiology," 177–80.

Blue, Rupert. "The Problem of Pellagra in the United States," 1–7.

Brownston, W. C. "The New Serum Treatment of Pellagra," 387–90.

Cole, H. P. "The Treatment of Pellagra by Direct Transfusion of Blood," 365–68.

Cooper, Ernest. "Intestinal Parasites of Pellagrins and Non-pellagrins—A Comparative Study," 269–73.

Cranston, W. J. "The Use of Salvarsan in Pellagra," 377–85;

Gosio, B., and G. Antonini, "Considerations as to the Etiology of Pellagra," 101–11.

Hunter, S. J. "Pellagra and the Sand-fly," 61–67.

Jennings, Allan H., and W. V. King, "One of the Possible Factors in the Causation of Pellagra," 51–60.

Lavinder, C. H., "The Prevalence and Geographic Distribution of Pellagra in the United States," 23–37. Also in *Public Health Reports* 1912; 27(50): 2076–88.

Martin, E. H. "The Relative Value of Soamin and Salvarsan in the Specific Treatment of Pellagra," 369–75.

Mizell, Geo. C. "Etiologic Factors and Recurrent Attacks of Pellagra," 297–308.

Reed, Howard S. "The Effect of Diplodia Zeae and Some Other Fungi Upon Some Phosphorus Compounds of Maize," 279–85.

Roberts, Stewart R. "The Analogies of Pellagra and the Mosquito," 291–96.

Sandwith, Fleming. "Can Pellagra Be a Disease due to Deficiency in Nutrition?" 97-100.

Saunders, Eleanora B. "The Coexistence of Pellagra and Beri-Beri," 325-31.

Taylor, Julius. "Sambon, the Man, and his Later Investigations on Pellagra," 69-80.

Wood, Edward J. "The Geographical Distribution of Pellagra in North Carolina and its Significance," 173-75.

Secondary Sources

BOOKS, BOOK CHAPTERS, AND PAMPHLETS

Altman, Lawrence K. "Dietary Deprivations." In *Who Goes First? The Story of Self-Experimentation in Medicine*, 240-55. Berkeley: University of California Press, 1998 [1987].

Andrew, Rod. *Wade Hampton: Confederate Warrior to Southern Redeemer.* Chapel Hill: University of North Carolina Press, 2008.

Babcock, J. W. "Public Charity in South Carolina." In *Handbook of South Carolina: Resources, Institutions and Industries of the State*, 2nd ed., 43-65. Columbia, S.C.: State, 1908. Previous versions of this chapter were published as "The Growth of Public Charity in South Carolina," *Reports and Resolutions of the General Assembly of the State of South Carolina*, 1905, volume 2, 933-58; and as "Appendix to Report of State Hospital for the Insane," *Annual Report of the South Carolina State Hospital for the Insane* (1904): 928-58.

————. "State Hospital for the Insane, Columbia, S.C." In *The Institutional Care of the Insane in the United States and Canada*, edited by Henry Mills Hurd, vol. 3, 587-613. Baltimore: Johns Hopkins Press, 1917.

[Babcock, J. H., and Taylor, J. W., eds.] *The State Board of Health and the South Carolina State Hospital for the Insane.* Columbia, S.C.: Gonzales and Bryan, 1909-10.

Baltes, Paul B., and Jacqui Smith, "Toward a Psychology of Wisdom and its Ontogenesis." In *Wisdom: Its Nature, Origins, and Development*, edited by Robert J. Sternberg, 87-120. Cambridge University Press, 1990.

Bass, Jack, and W. Scott Poole. *The Palmetto State: The Making of Modern South Carolina.* Columbia: University of South Carolina Press, 2009.

Beam, Alex. *Gracefully Insane: The Rise and Fall of America's Premier Mental Hospital.* New York: PublicAffairs, 2001.

Beardsley, Edward H. *A History of Neglect: Health Care for Blacks and Mill Workers in the Twentieth-Century South.* Knoxville: University of Tennessee Press, 1987.

Beecher, Henry Knowles, and Mark D. Altschule. *Medicine at Harvard: The First Three Hundred Years.* Hanover, N.H.: University Press of New England, 1977.

Bellamann, Henry. *King's Row.* New York: Simon & Schuster, 1940.

Black, O. F., and C. L. Alsberg. *The Determination of the Deterioration of Maize, with Incidental Reference to Pellagra.* Bulletin 199, Bureau of Plant Industry, U.S. Department of Agriculture. Washington, D.C.: Government Printing Office, 1910.

Blackburn, Laura, and Minier Padgette. *History of Columbia Hospital, 1892–1947.* Columbia, S.C.: R. L. Bryan, 1953.

Blanchard, John A. *The H Book of Harvard Athletics, 1852–1922.* Cambridge: Harvard Varsity Club, 1923.

Bloch, Konrad. "Two Centuries of Pellagra Research." In *Blondes in Venetian Paintings, the Nine-Banded Armadillo, and Other Essays in Biochemistry,* 185–207. New Haven: Yale University Press, 1994.

Bollet, Alfred Jay. "The Pellagra Epidemics: The three M's Produce the Four D's." In *Plagues & Poxes: The Impact of Human History on Epidemic Disease,* 153–72. New York: Demos, 2004.

Bordley, James III, and A. McGehee Harvey. *Two Centuries of American Medicine, 1776–1976.* Philadelphia: W. B. Saunders, 1976.

Broussais, F. J. V. *On Irritation and Insanity,* trans. Thomas Cooper Columbia, S.C.: S. J. M'Morris, 1831.

Brown, E. E. *Life of Oliver Wendell Holmes.* Chicago: E. E. Weeks, 1884.

Brown, Edward M. "Neurology's Influence on American Psychiatry: 1865–1915." In *History of Psychiatry and Medical Psychology, with an Epilogue on Psychiatry and the Mind-Body Reaction,* edited by Edwin R. Wallace and John Gach, 519–31. New York: Springer, 2008.

Bruyn, George W., and Charles M. Poser. "Pellagra." In *The History of Tropical Neurology: Nutritional Disorders,* 109–37. Canton, Mass.: Science History Publications, 2003.

Bryan, Charles S. "Not Like his Father." In *A Most Satisfactory Man: The Story of Theodore Brevard Hayne, Last Martyr of Yellow Fever,* 7–18. Charleston, S.C.: Waring Library Society, 1996.

Bryan, Charles S. "'The Greatest Brahmin.' Overview of a Life." In *Oliver Wendell Holmes: Physician and Man of Letters,* edited by Scott H. Podolsky and Charles S. Bryan, 3–21. Sagamore Beach, Mass.: Boston Medical Library and Science History Publications, 2009.

Bryan, John M. "Robert Mills: Public Architecture in South Carolina, 1820–30." In *Robert Mills: Architect,* 75–104. Washington, D.C.: American Institute of Architects Press, 1989.

Bryan, John M. *Robert Mills: America's First Architect.* New York: Princeton Architectural Press, 2001.

Bryce, James. "Present and Future of the Negro." In *The American Commonwealth*, new ed., vol. 2, 512–39. New York: Macmillan, 1914 [1888].

Burton, Orville Vernon. Introduction to *Pitchfork Ben Tillman, South Carolinian*, Southern Classics ed., by Francis Butler Simkins. Columbia: University of South Carolina Press, 2002 [1944].

Calhoun, Charles W. *Conceiving a New Republic: The Republican Party and the Southern Question, 1869–1900.* Lawrence: University of Kansas Press, 2006.

Campion, Nardi Reeder, and Rosamond Wilfley Stanton. *Look to This Day! The Lively Education of a Great Woman Doctor: Connie Guion, M.D.* Boston: Little, Brown, 1965.

Carpenter, Kenneth J. *Beriberi, White Rice, and Vitamin B: A Disease, a Cause and a Cure.* Berkeley: University of California Press, 2000.

———. *The History of Scurvy and Vitamin C.* Cambridge University Press, 1986.

Censer, Jane Turner. *The Reconstruction of White Southern Womanhood, 1865–1895.* Baton Rouge: Louisiana State University Press, 2003.

Chase, Allan. *The Legacy of Malthus: The Social Costs of the New Scientific Racism.* Urbana: University of Illinois Press, 1980.

Cloyd, Benjamin G. *Haunted by Atrocity: Civil War Prisons in American Memory.* Baton Rouge: Louisiana State University Press, 2010.

Cooper, Ernest. *South Carolina Sanatorium, State Park, S.C.* Columbia, S.C.: R. L. Bryan, n.d.

———. *South Carolina and Palmetto Sanatoria, State Park, S.C.* Columbia, S.C.: McCaw of Columbia, n.d.

Cooper, William J. *The Conservative Regime: South Carolina, 1877–1890.* Baltimore: Johns Hopkins Press, 1968.

Day, Paul L. "The Nutritional Requirements of Primates Other than Man." In *Vitamins and Hormones: Advances in Research and Applications*, edited by Robert S. Harris and Kenneth V. Thimann, vol. 2, 71–105. New York: Academic Press, 1944.

Deaderick, William H., and Loyd Thompson. *The Endemic Diseases of the Southern States.* Philadelphia: W. B. Saunders, 1916.

Doll, Richard. "The Evolution of the Controlled Clinical Trial." In *"Our Lords, the Sick": McGovern Lectures in the History of Medical Humanism*, edited by Lawrence D. Longo, 229–41. Malibar, Fla.: Krieger, 2004.

Donald, David Herbert. *Lincoln.* New York: Simon & Schuster, 1995.

Duffin, Jacalyn. "Wrestling with Demons: History of Psychiatry." In *History of Medicine: A Scandalously Short Introduction*, 276–302. University of Toronto Press, 1999.

Easterlin, Richard A. "State Income Estimates." In *Methodological Considerations and Reference Tables*, edited by Everett S. Lee, Ann Ratner Miller, Carol P. Brainerd, and Richard A. Easterlin, 703–59. Vol. 1 of *Population Redistribution and Economic Growth, United States, 1870–1950*. Philadelphia: American Philosophical Society, 1957.

———. "Interregional Differences in Per Capita Income, Population, and Total Income, 1840–1950." In *Trends in the American Economy in the Nineteenth Century. Studies in Income and Wealth. The Conference on Research in Income and Wealth*, by National Bureau of Economic Research, vol. 24, 73-140. Princeton University Press, 1960.

Edgar, Walter. *South Carolina in the Modern Age*. Columbia: University of South Carolina Press, 1992.

———. *South Carolina: A History*. Columbia: University of South Carolina Press, 1998.

Eliot, Charles W. "The Evils of College Football." In *Charles W. Eliot: The Man and His Beliefs*, edited by William Allan Neilson, vol. 1, 115–20. New York: Harper, 1926.

———. "The Character of a Gentleman." In *Charles W. Eliot: The Man and His Beliefs*, edited by William Allan Neilson, vol. 2, 539–43. New York: Harper, 1926.

Etheridge, Elizabeth W. *The Butterfly Caste: A Social History of Pellagra in the South*. Westport, Conn.: Greenwood, 1972.

———. "Pellagra: An Unappreciated Reminder of Southern Distinctiveness." In *Disease and Distinctiveness in the American South*, edited by Todd L. Savitt and James Harvey Young, 100-19. Knoxville: University of Tennessee Press, 1988.

Faust, Drew Gilpin. "Accounting: 'Our Obligations to the Dead.'" In *This Republic of Suffering: Death and the American Civil War*, 211-49. New York: Vintage, 2008.

Fletcher, Robert, and Fielding H. Garrison, eds. *Index Medicus: A Monthly Classified Record of the Current Medical Literature of the World*. Second series, vol. 9. Washington, D.C.: Carnegie Institution of Washington, 1911.

Forbush, Bliss. *The Sheppard and Enoch Pratt Hospital, 1853-1970: A History*. Philadelphia: J. P. Lippincott, 1971.

Frankenburg, Frances Rachel. *Vitamin Discoveries and Disasters: History, Science, and Controversies*. Santa Barbara, Ca.: Praeger, 2009.

Funk, Casimir. *The Vitamines*, 2nd German ed., translated by Harry E. Dubin. Baltimore: Williams & Wilkins, 1922.

Gibian, Peter. *Oliver Wendell Holmes and the Culture of Conversation*. Cambridge University Press, 2001.

Gladwell, Malcolm. *Outliers: The Story of Success.* New York: Little, Brown: 2008.

———. *The Tipping Point: How Little Things can Make a Big Difference.* New York: Little, Brown, 2000.

Goldberger, Joseph, G. A. Wheeler, Edgar Sydenstricker, and Wilford I. King. *A Study of Endemic Pellagra in Some Cotton-mill Villages of South Carolina.* U.S. Hygienic Laboratory Bulletin no. 153. Washington, D.C.: U.S. Government Printing Office, 1929. Previously published in abbreviated form as "A Study of Endemic Pellagra in Some Cotton-Mill Villages of South Carolina: An Abstract." *Public Health Reports* 43, no. 41 (1928): 2645–47.

Goffman, Erving. *Asylums: Essays on the Social Situation of Mental Patients and Other Inmates.* New York: Anchor, 1961.

Grob, Gerald N. *The Mad Among Us: A History of the Care of America's Mentally Ill.* New York: Free Press, 1994.

———. *Mental Illness and American Society, 1875–1940.* Princeton University Press, 1983.

———. *Mental Institutions in America: Social Policy to 1875.* New York: Free Press, 1973.

———. "The Transformation of American Psychiatry: From Institution to Community, 1800–2000." In *History of Psychiatry and Medical Psychology, with an Epilogue on Psychiatry and the Mind-Body Reaction,* edited by Edwin R. Wallace and John Gach, 533–54. New York: Springer, 2008.

Hale, Nathan G., Jr. *Freud and the Americans: The Beginnings of Psychoanalysis in the United States, 1876–1917.* New York: Oxford University Press, 1971.

Harrington, Thomas Francis, and James Gregory Mumford, *The Harvard Medical School: A History, Narrative, and Documentary, 1782–1905.* Vol. 3. New York: Lewis, 1905.

Harrow, Benjamin. *Casimir Funk: Pioneer in Vitamins and Hormones.* New York: Dodd, Mead, 1955.

Harvard College. *Secretary's Report, Class of 1882: July 1882.* Cambridge, Mass.: Wheeler, 1882.

Harvie, David I. *Limeys: The Conquest of Scurvy.* Phoenix Mill, U.K.: Sutton, 2002.

Hayes, Helen, and Anita Loos. *Twice Over Lightly: New York Then and Now.* New York: Harcourt Brace Jovanovich, 1972.

Helsey, Alexis Jones. *Beaufort: A History.* Charleston, S.C.: History Press, 2005.

Hennig, Helen Kohn. *August Kohn: Versatile South Carolinian.* Columbia, S.C.: Vogue Press, 1949.

Holland, Sir Henry. *Recollections of Past Life.* New York: D. Appleton, 1872.

Hollis, Daniel Walker. *University of South Carolina.* Vol. 2, *College to University.* Columbia: University of South Carolina Press, 1956.

Holmes, Oliver Wendell. "The Young Practitioner." In *Medical Essays: 1842–1882*, 370–95. Boston: Houghton, Mifflin, 1883.

Horsman, Reginald. *Joseph Nott of Mobile: Southerner, Physician, and Racial Theorist.* Baton Rouge: Louisiana State University Press, 1987.

Huisman, Frank, and John Harley Warner, "Medical Histories." In *Locating Medical History: The Stories and Their Meanings*, edited by Frank Huisman and John Harley Warner, 1–30. Baltimore: Johns Hopkins University Press, 2004.

Jarrell, Hampton M. *Wade Hampton and the Negro: The Road Not Taken.* Columbia: University of South Carolina Press, 1950.

Jenerette, Gertrude. *Biographical Sketch of Ernest Cooper, M.D.* Columbia, S.C.: Women's Auxiliary of the Columbia Medical Society, 1940.

Johnson, Steven. *Where Good Ideas Come From: The Natural History of Innovation.* New York: Riverhead, 2010.

Jones, H. Michael. "Pellagra, Progress, and Public Polemics: Joseph Goldberger, E.J. Wood, and the Osler Connection." In *The Persisting Osler—IV: Selected Transactions of the American Osler Society, 2001–2010*, edited by Jeremiah A. Barondess and Charles S. Bryan, 317–27. Sagamore Beach, Mass.: Science History Publications, 2011.

Kantrowitz, Stephen. *Ben Tillman & the Reconstruction of White Supremacy.* Chapel Hill: University of North Carolina Press, 2000.

Kelly, Joseph. *America's Longest Siege: Charleston, Slavery, and the Slow March Toward Civil War.* New York: Overlook, 2013.

Kraut, Alan M. *Goldberger's War: The Life and Work of a Public Health Crusader.* New York: Hill and Wang, 2003.

Kuhn, Thomas S. *The Structure of Scientific Revolutions.* Chicago: University of Chicago Press, 1962.

Lanska, Douglas J. "Historical Aspects of the Major Neurological Vitamin Deficiency Disorders: The Water-Soluble B Vitamins." In *Handbook of Clinical Neurology*, edited by S. Finger, F. Boller, and K. L. Tyler, vol. 95, 445–76. Amsterdam: North Holland, 2010.

Larson, Frances. *An Infinity of Things: How Sir Henry Wellcome Collected the World.* Oxford University Press, 2009.

Lavinder, C. H., A. W. Freeman, and W. H. Frost. *Epidemiologic Studies of Poliomyelitis in New York City and the Northeastern United States During the Year 1916.* Public Health Bulletin 91. Washington, D.C.: Government Printing Office, 1918.

Link, William A. *The Paradox of Southern Progressivism, 1880–1930.* Chapel Hill: University of North Carolina Press, 1992.

Lisman, Gary L., and Arlene Parr. *Bittersweet Memories: A History of the Peoria State Hospital*. Bartonville, Ill.: Namsil, 2005.

Little, Nina Fletcher. *Early Years of the McLean Hospital*. Boston: Francis A. Countway Library of Medicine, 1972.

Logan, Rayford W. *The Betrayal of the Negro, from Rutherford B. Hayes to Woodrow Wilson*. New York: Da Capo, 1997 [1965].

——. *The Negro in American Life and Thought: The Nadir, 1877–1901*. New York: Dial, 1954.

——. Ludmerer, Kenneth M. *Learning to Heal: The Development of American Medical Education*. New York: Basic Books, 1885.

McCandless, Peter. "James Woods Babcock." In *American National Biography*, edited by John A. Garraty and Mark C. Carnes, vol. 1, 810–11. New York: Oxford University Press, 1999.

——. *Moonlight, Magnolias, & Madness: Insanity in South Carolina from the Colonial Period to the Progressive Era*. Chapel Hill: University of North Carolina Press, 1996.

——. *Slavery, Disease, and Suffering in the Southern Lowcountry*. New York: Cambridge University Press, 2011.

McCollum, Elmer V. *A History of Nutrition: The Sequence of Ideas in Nutrition Investigations*. Boston: Houghton Mifflin, 1957.

McPherson, James M. *Battle Cry of Freedom: The Civil War Era*. New York: Oxford University Press, 2003 [1988].

Major, Ralph H., and Mahlon H. Delp. *Physical Diagnosis*, 6th ed. Philadelphia: W. B. Saunders, 1962.

Manson-Bahr, Sir Philip. *History of the School of Tropical Medicine in London (1899–1949)*. London: H. K. Lewis, 1956.

Marie, A. *Pellagra*, translated by C. H. Lavinder and J. W. Babcock. Columbia, S.C.: State, 1910.

Marscher, Bill and Fran. *The Great Sea Island Storm of 1893*. Macon, Ga.: Mercer University Press, 2003.

Moran, Michael E., and Sakti Das. "William Beaumont, M.D. and the Ethics of Research." In *The Persisting Osler—IV: Selected Transactions of the American Osler Society, 2001–2010*, edited by Jeremiah A. Barondess and Charles S. Bryan, 229–37. Sagamore Beach, Mass.: Science History Publications, 2011.

Moore, John Hammond. *Carnival of Blood: Dueling, Lynching, and Murder in South Carolina, 1880–1920*. Columbia: University of South Carolina Press, 2006.

——. *Columbia and Richland County: A South Carolina Community, 1740–1990*. Columbia: University of South Carolina Press, 1993.

Morens, David M., Victoria A. Harden, Joseph Kinyoun Houts Jr., and Anthony S. Fauci. "Plague in San Francisco: 1900, the Year of the Rat." In *The Indispensible Man: Joseph Kinyoun and the Founding of the National Institutes of Health*, 26–35. Bethesda, Md.: U.S. Department of Health and Human Services, National Institutes of Health, National Institute of Allergy and Infectious Diseases, 2012.

Niles, George M. *Pellagra: An American Problem*. Philadelphia: W. B. Saunders, 1912.

One Hundredth Annual Catalog of the Medical School (Boston) of Harvard University, 1882–1883. Cambridge, Mass.: Charles W. Sever, 1882.

Osler, William. "Books and Men." In *Aequanimitas, With other Addresses to Medical Students, Nurses and Practitioners of Medicine*, 3rd ed., 207–15. Philadelphia: P. Blakiston's Son, 1932

———. *The Growth of Truth as Illustrated in the Discovery of the Circulation of the Blood*. London: Henry Frowde, 1906.

———. *The Principles and Practice of Medicine*, 6th ed. New York: D. Appleton Company, 1907.

———. *The Principles and Practice of Medicine*, 7th ed. New York: D. Appleton, 1910.

Osler, William, and Thomas McCrae. *The Principles and Practice of Medicine*, 8th ed. New York: D. Appleton, 1918.

Parsons, Robert P. *Trail to Light: A Biography of Joseph Goldberger*. Indianapolis: Bobbs-Merrill, 1943.

Payne, Christopher. *Asylum: Inside the Closed World of State Mental Institutions*. Cambridge, Mass.: MIT Press, 2009.

Porter, Roy. *Madness: A Brief History*. Oxford University Press, 2002.

Postlethwait, John H., and Janet L. Hopson. *Modern Biology*. Orlando, Fl.: Holt, Rinehart and Winston, 2009.

Reiss, Benjamin. *Theaters of Madness: Insane Asylums and Nineteenth-century American Culture*. University of Chicago Press, 2008.

Rice, John Andrew. *I Came out of the Eighteenth Century*. New York: Harper, 1942.

Roberts, Stewart R. *Pellagra: History, Distribution, Diagnosis, Prognosis, Treatment, Etiology*. St. Louis: C. V. Mosby, 1913.

Roe, Daphne A. *A Plague of Corn: The Social History of Pellagra*. Ithaca: Cornell University Press, 1973.

Rose, Willie Lee Nichols. *Rehearsal for Reconstruction: The Port Royal Experiment*. Athens: University of Georgia Press, 1999 [1964].

Rosen, George. *A History of Public Health*. New York: MD Publications, 1958.

Rosenberg, Charles E. *The Cholera Years: The United States in 1832, 1849, and 1866*. University of Chicago Press, 1987 [1962].

————. "Explaining Epidemics." In *Explaining Epidemics and other Studies in the History of Medicine*, 293–303. Cambridge University Press, 1992.

Roussel, Théophile. *Traité de la Pellagra et des Pseudo-Pellagres*. Paris: J. B. Ballière, 1966.

Rubillo, Tom. *Hurricane Destruction in South Carolina: Hell and High Water*. Charleston, S.C.: History Press, 2006.

Sandwith, F. M. *Egypt as a Winter Resort*. London: Kegan Paul, Trench, 1889.

————. *Medical Diseases of Egypt*. London: H. Kimpton, 1905.

Scull, Andrew. *Madhouse: A Tragic Tale of Megalomania and Modern Medicine*. New Haven: Yale University Press, 2005.

Shorter, Edward. *A History of Psychiatry: From the Era of the Asylum to the Age of Prozac*. New York: John Wiley & Sons, 1997.

Simkins, Francis Butler. *Pitchfork Ben Tillman, South Carolinian*, Southern Classics ed. Columbia: University of South Carolina Press, 2002 [1944].

Smith, Mark M. *Mastered by the Clock: Time, Slavery, and Freedom in the American South*. Chapel Hill: University of North Carolina Press, 1997.

Snowden, Yates. *Old Books and Their Lovers*, vol. 2. Columbia, S.C.: privately printed, 1908.

Stephens, Lester D. *Science, Race, and Religion in the American South: John Bachman and the Charleston Circle of Naturalists, 1815–1895*. Chapel Hill: University of North Carolina Press, 2000.

Still, Charles N. "Nicotinic Acid and Nicotinamide Deficiency: Pellagra and Related Disorders of the Nervous System." In *Handbook of Clinical Neurology*, edited by P. J. Vinkin and G. W. Bruyn, vol. 28, part 2: 59–104. Amsterdam: North Holland, 1976.

Stokes, Allen H. "The Kohn-Hennig Library." In *The Kohn-Hennig Library: A Catalog*, edited by Stephen G. Hoffius, vii–xv. Columbia: South Caroliniana Library, University of South Carolina, 2011.

Strauss, Maurice B., ed. *Familiar Medical Quotations*. Boston: Little, Brown, 1968.

Sutton, S.B. *Crossroads in Psychiatry: A History of the McLean Hospital*. Washington, D.C.: American Psychiatric Press, 1986.

Taylor, Isaac M. *An Appeal for State Care for All the Insane from an Economic Standpoint: The Report of the Chairman of the Section on State Medicine and Medical Jurisprudence Made to the Medical Society of the State of North Carolina, May 28th, 1891*. Wilmington, N.C.: James & Bell, Steam Power Presses, 1891.

Taylor, J. H. *Dr. James Woods Babcock: An Appreciation*. Greenville, S.C.: Peace Printing, 1922.

Terris, Milton. *Goldberger on Pellagra*. Baton Rouge: Louisiana State University Press, 1964.

Tetzlaff, Monica Maria. *Cultivating a New South: Abbie Holmes Christensen and the Politics of Race and Gender, 1852–1938*. Columbia: University of South Carolina Press, 2002.

Thielman, Samuel B. "Southern Madness: The Shape of Mental Health Care in the Old South." In Ronald L. Numbers and Todd L. Savitt, eds. *Science and Medicine in the Old South*, 256–75. Baton Route: Louisiana State University Press, 1989.

Thompson, Frances E., and Amy F. Subar. "Dietary Assessment Methodology." In *Nutrition in the Prevention and Treatment of Disease*, edited by Ann M. Coulston, Carol J. Boushey, and Mario G. Ferruzzi, 3rd ed., 5–46. London: Academic Press, 2013.

Thompson, James Lawrence. *Of Shattered Minds: Fifty Years at the South Carolina State Hospital for the Insane*, edited by Anita Wyric Ruth. Columbia, S.C.: South Carolina Department of Mental Health, [ca. 1989].

Tillman, B.R. *A Farewell to Public Life. Address of Senator Tillman to his Constituents before the Primary Election in South Carolina, August 15, 1914*. Washington, D.C.: Government Printing Office, 1915.

———. *The Negro Problem and Immigration, delivered by invitation before the South Carolina House of Representatives, January 24, 1908*. Columbia, S.C.: Gonzales and Bryan, 1908.

Tindall, George Brown. *South Carolina Negroes, 1877–1900*. Columbia: University of South Carolina Press, 1952.

Townsend, Joseph. *A Journey through Spain in the Years 1786 and 1787*, vol. 2. London: C. Dilly, 1792.

Tuttle, George T. "McLean Hospital, Waverley, Mass." In *The Institutional Care of the Insane in the United States and Canada*, edited by Henry Mills Hurd, vol. 2, 599–615. Baltimore: Johns Hopkins Press, 1917.

Vaillant, George E. *Adaptation to Life*. Boston: Little, Brown, 1977.

Vedder, Edward B. *Beriberi*. New York: William Wood, 1913.

Wallace, Edwin R., and John Gach, eds., *History of Psychiatry and Medical Psychology, with an Epilogue on Psychiatry and the Mind-Body Reaction*. New York: Springer, 2008.

Ward, James Sheridan, and Arlene Parr. *Asylum Light: Stories from the George A. Zeller Era and Beyond*. Springfield, Ill.: Phillips, 2004.

Waring, Joseph Ioor. *A History of Medicine in South Carolina, 1825–1900*. Columbia, SC: South Carolina Medical Association, 1967.

Waring, Joseph Ioor. *A History of Medicine in South Carolina, 1900–1970*. Columbia: South Carolina Medical Association, 1971.

Warman, Arturo. *Corn & Capitalism: How a Botanical Bastard Grew to Global Dominance*, trans. Nancy L. Westrate. Chapel Hill: University of North Carolina Press, 2003.

Washington-Williams, Essie Mae, and William Stadiem. *Dear Senator: A Memoir by the Daughter of Strom Thurmond*. New York: Regan, 2005.

Weiner, Dora B. "The Madman in the Light of Reason: Enlightenment Psychiatry. Part II: Alienists, Treatises, and the Psychologic Approach in the Era of Pinel." In *History of Psychiatry and Medical Psychology, with an Epilogue on Psychiatry and the Mind-Body Reaction*, edited by Edwin R. Wallace and John Gach, 281–303. New York: Springer, 2008.

Weinstein, Michael A. "Oliver Wendell Holmes's Depth Psychology." In *Oliver Wendell Holmes: Physician and Man of Letters*, edited by Scott H. Podolsky and Charles S. Bryan, 93–103. Sagamore Beach, Mass.: Boston Medical Library and Science History Publications, 2009.

Wilkinson, Lise, and Anne Hardy. *Prevention and Cure: The London School of Hygiene & Tropical Medicine; A 20th Century Quest for Global Health*. London: Kegan Paul, 2001.

Wood, Edward Jenner. *A Treatise on Pellagra for the General Practitioner*. New York: D. Appleton, 1912.

Zuczek, Richard. *State of Rebellion: Reconstruction in South Carolina*. Columbia: University of South Carolina Press, 1996.

JOURNAL ARTICLES

Alsberg, C.L. "Agricultural Aspects of the Pellagra Problem in the United States." *New York Medical Journal* 90 (July 10, 1909): 50–54.

Anderson, John F., and Joseph Goldberger, "An Attempt to Infect the Rhesus Monkey with Blood and Spinal Fluid from Pellagrins." *Public Health Reports* 26, no. 26 (1911): 1003–4.

Anderson, Uta P. "Eleanora Bennette Saunders: A Pioneering Psychiatrist." *Journal of the South Carolina Medical Association* 93, no. 6 (1997): 223–26.

"Attempts to Produce Experimental Pellagra." *Scientific American* 105 (December 2, 1911): 490.

Babcock, J.W. "The Colored Insane." *Alienist and Neurologist* 16, no. 4 (1895): 423–47. Also in *Proceedings of the American Medico-Psychological Association. Sixty-Fifth Annual Meeting, Atlantic City, N.J., June 1–4, 1909*. Baltimore: American Medico-Psychological Association, 1909.

———. "Communicated Insanity and Negro Witchcraft." *American Journal of Insanity* 51, no. 4 (1895) 518–23.

————."The Diagnosis and Treatment of Pellagra." *Journal of the South Carolina Medical Association* 4, no. 11 (1908): 563–67.

————. "A History of Columbia's Trees." *State* (Columbia, S.C.), November 13, 1904.

————. "How Long has Pellagra Existed in S.C." *Journal of the South Carolina Medical Association* 8, no. 7 (1912): 200-10. Previous version in *Proceedings of the American Medico-Psychological Association. Sixty-Seventh Annual Meeting, Denver, Colorado, June 19–22, 1911*. Baltimore: American Medico-Psychological Association, 1911. Slightly revised reversions as "How Long has Pellagra Existed in South Carolina? A Study of Local Medical History," in *American Journal of Insanity* 69, no. 1 (1912): 185–200; and as "Presidential Address: How Long Has Pellagra Existed in the United States?" in *Transactions of the National Association for the Study of Pellagra. Second Triennial Meeting at Columbia, South Carolina, October 3 and 4, 1912*. Columbia, S.C.: R. L. Bryan, 1914.

————. "Medico-legal Relations of Pellagra." *Southern Medical Journal* 7, no. 10 (1914): 771–78. An earlier version was published as "Medico-Legal Relations in Pellagra," *Transactions of the National Association for the Study of Pellagra. Second Triennial Meeting at Columbia, South Carolina, October 3 and 4, 1912*. Columbia, S.C.: R. L. Bryan, 1914, 391–404.

————. "Pellagra in Egyptian Asylums, 1913." *Southern Medical Journal* 8, no. 8 (1915): 688–90.

————. "The Prevalence of Pellagra." *Journal of the South Carolina Medical Association* 6, no. 9 (1910): 445–49. Also published as *Prevalence of Pellagra: Article Reprinted from the Journal of the South Carolina Medical Association by J. W. Babcock, M.D., and Consular Report on the Prevalence of Pellagra in Italy and Southern Europe by Vice Consul W. Bayard Cutting, Jr.; Presented by Mr. Tillman*. Document no. 706, Washington, D.C.: Government Printing Office, 1911.

————. "The Prevalence and Psychology of Pellagra." *American Journal of Insanity* 67, no. 3 (1911) 517–40.

————. "The Prevention of Tuberculosis in Hospitals for the Insane." *American Journal of Insanity* 51, no. 2 (1894): 182–95. Also in *Proceedings of the American Medico-Psychological Association at the Fiftieth Annual Meeting held in Philadelphia, May 15–18, 1894* (Utica, NY: American Medico-Psychological Association, 1895).

————. "The Proud Record of South Carolina in the Care of the Insane." *News and Courier* (Charleston, S.C.), April 20, 1904, Centennial Edition supplement.

————. "The Psychology of Pellagra." *Journal of the South Carolina Medical Association* 6, no. 11 (1910): 563–89.

[Babcock, J. W., and C. H. Lavinder.] "Pellagra." *South Carolina State Board of Health Monthly Bulletin* 1, no. 10 (December 1910).

Baker, Robert B., Harriet A. Washington, Ololade Olakanmi, Todd L. Savitt, Elizabeth A. Jacobs, Eddie Hoover, and Matthew K. Wynia. "Creating a Segregated

Medical Profession: African American Physicians and Organized Medicine, 1846–1910." *Journal of the National Medical Association* 101, no. 6 (2009): 501–12.

"Baughn's Pellagra Remedy: A Worthless Nostrum Sold Under Fraudulent Claims." *Journal of the American Medical Association* 61, no. 20 (1913): 1828–30.

Bean, Robert Bennett. "Some Racial Peculiarities of the Negro Brain." *American Journal of Anatomy* 5, no. 4 (1906): 353–432.

Beardsley, Edward H. "Making Separate, Equal: Black Physicians and the Problems of Medical Segregation in the Pre-World War II South." *Bulletin of the History of Medicine* 57, no. 3 (1983): 382–96.

Benedek, Thomas G., and Jonathon Erlen, "The Scientific Environment of the Tuskegee Study of Syphilis, 1920–1960." *Perspectives in Biology and Medicine* 43, no. 1 (1999): 1–30.

"Beverley Randolph Tucker 1874–1945." *American Journal of Psychiatry* 102, no. 11 (1945): 431–32.

Blue, Rupert. "Pellagra in California." *California State Journal of Medicine* 8, no. 3 (1910): 101–2.

Bollet, Alfred Jay. "Politics and Pellagra: The Epidemic of Pellagra in the U.S. in the Early Twentieth Century." *Yale Journal of Biology and Medicine* 65, no. 3 (1992): 211–21.

Bryan, Charles S. "Are We a Profession or a Business? A Brief History of the Columbia Medical Society (Part II)." *Recorder of the Columbia Medical Society of Richland County, S.C., Inc.*, 48, no. 2 (1992): 10–16.

Bryan, Charles S., Sandra W. Moss, and Richard J. Kahn. "Yellow Fever in the Americas." *Infectious Disease Clinics of North America* 18, no. 2 (2004): 275–92.

Bryan, John M., and Julie M. Johnson. "Robert Mills' Sources for the South Carolina Lunatic Asylum, 1822." *Journal of the South Carolina Medical Association* 75, no. 6 (1979): 264–68.

Caccini, A. "Pellagra as We See it in Italy: Old and New Theories; with Report of Cases Seen in New York City." *Medical Record* 79, no. 10 (1911): 421–30.

"Carl Voegtlin, 1879–1960." *Journal of the National Cancer Institute* 25, no. 4 (1960): iii–xv.

Carpenter, K. J. "Effects of Different Methods of Processing Maize on its Pellagra-genic Activity." *Federation Proceedings* 40, no. 5 (1981); 1531–35.

Carter, K. Codell. "The Germ Theory, Beriberi, and the Deficiency Theory of Disease." *Medical History* 21, no. 2 (1977): 119–36.

"Cesare Lombroso." *Journal of the American Medical Association* 53, no. 20 (1909): 1644–45.

Chacko, Elizabeth. "Understanding the Geography of Pellagra in the United States: The Role of Social and Place-Based Identities." *Gender, Place and Culture* 12, no. 2 (2005): 197–212.

Chick, Harriette, and Eleanor Margaret Hume. "The Production in Monkeys of Symptoms Closely Resembling Those of Pellagra, by Prolonged Feeding on a Diet of Low Protein Content." *Biochemical Journal* 14, no. 2 (1920): 135–46.

Chittenden, Russell H., and Frank P. Underhill. "The Production in Dogs of a Pathological Condition which Closely Resembles Human Pellagra." *American Journal of Physiology* 44, no. 1 (1917): 13–16. Also in *Proceedings of the National Academy of Sciences of the United States of America* 3, no. 3 (1917): 195–97.

Christensen, Niels Jr. "The State Dispensaries in South Carolina." *Annals of the American Academy of Political and Social Science* 32, no. 3 (1908): 545–55.

Clarke, F. B., et al. "Studies on Pellagra Based on its Occurrence in 1910 in the Cook County Institutions at Dunning, Illinois." *Journal of Infectious Diseases* 10, no. 2 (1912): 186–90.

Concato, John, Nirav Shah, and Ralph I. Horwitz. "Randomized, Controlled Trials, Observational Studies, and the Hierarchy of Research Designs." *New England Journal of Medicine* 342, no. 25 (2000): 1887–92.

"Conference on Pellagra." *Journal of the South Carolina Medical Association* 4, no. 10 (1908): 523.

"The Conference on Pellagra." *Journal of the American Medical Association* 53, no. 20 (1909): 1645–46.

Cook, G. C. "Patrick Manson (1844–1922) FRS: *Filaria (Mansonella) perstans* and Sleeping Sickness (African Trypanosomiasis)." *Journal of Medical Biography* 20, no. 2 (2012): 69–70.

Cooper, E. A., and Casimir Funk, "Experiments on the Causation of Beriberi." *Lancet* 178 (November 4, 1911): 1266–67.

Cowles, Edward. "The Advancement of Psychiatry in America." *American Journal of Insanity* 52, no. 3 (1896): 364–86.

———. "Advanced Professional Work in Hospitals for the Insane." *American Journal of Insanity* 55, no. 1 (1898): 21–29.

Crabb, Mary Katherine. "An Epidemic of Pride: Pellagra and the Culture of the American South." *Anthropologica* 34, no. 1 (1992): 89–103.

Davenport, C. B. "The Hereditary Factor in Pellagra." *Archives of Internal Medicine* 18, no. 1 (1916): 4–31. Also in *Pellagra III. Third Report of the Robert M. Thompson Pellagra Commission of the New York Post-Graduate Medical School and Hospital*, 417–44.

Davis, John Martin Jr. "Coosaw Rock Alchemy: A Short History of River-Phosphate Mining in Beaufort County." *South Carolina Historical Magazine* 109, no. 4 (2008): 269–94.

Dean, Charles E. "The Death of Specificity in Psychiatry: Cheers or Tears?" *Perspectives in Biology and Medicine* 55, no. 3 (2012): 443–60.

Dick, George F. "Inoculation of Monkeys with Pellagrous Blood and Serum, and the Occurrence of B. maydis in Pellagra." *Journal of Infectious Diseases* 10, no. 2 (1912): 196–99.

"Dr. Edward Cowles." *Journal of Nervous and Mental Diseases* 50, no. 5 (1919): 504–10.

"Dr. J. W. Babcock." *Boston Medical and Surgical Journal* 186, no. 24 (1922): 828.

Donald, Alexander G. "James Higgins McIntosh, M.D.: An Archetype for the Family Practitioner?" *Journal of the South Carolina Medical Association* 76, no. 5 (1980): 245–48.

Eliot, Charles W. "The Defect in Football." *Baseball Magazine* 2, no. 2 (1908): 17–19.

Elmore, Joann G., and Alvan R. Feinstein, "Joseph Goldberger: An Unsung Hero of American Clinical Epidemiology." *Annals of Internal Medicine* 121, no. 5 (1994): 372–75.

Elvehjem, C. A., R. J. Madden, F. M. Strong, and D. W. Wooley. "Relation of Nicotinic Acid and Nicotinic Acid Amide to Canine Blacktongue." *Journal of the American Chemical Society* 59, no. 9 (1937): 1767–68

Elvehjem, C. A., Robert J. Madden, F. M. Strong, and D. W. Wooley. "The Isolation and Identification of the Anti-Black-Tongue Factor." *Journal of Biological Chemistry* 123, no. 1 (1938): 137–49.

"F. M. Sandwith, C.M.G., M.D., F.R.C.P." *British Medical Journal* 1 (March 2, 1918): 273.

Flannery, Michael A. "Fighting Pellagra in Alabama: Carl A. Grote's Forgotten Contribution to Conquering a Southern Scourge." http://contentdm.mh.sl. uab.edu/u?/PELLAGRA,13 (accessed May 23, 2013).

"Fleming Mant Sandwith, M.D. DURH., F.R.C.P. LOND., C.M.G." *Lancet* 1 (March 2, 1918): 347–48.

Funk, Casimir. "The Etiology of the Deficiency Diseases, Beri-Beri, Polyneuritis in Birds, Epidemic Dropsy, Scurvy, Experimental Scurvy in Animals, Infantile Scurvy, Ship Beri-Beri, Pellagra." *Journal of State Medicine* 20 (1912): 341–68.

———. "Nicotinic Acid and Vitamin B." *Journal of the American Medical Association* 109, no. 25 (1937): 2086.

———. "Studies on Beri-beri VII: Chemistry of the Vitamine-fraction from Yeast and Rice Polishings." *Journal of Physiology* 46, no. 3 (1913): 173–79.

———. "Studies on Pellagra I: The Influence of the Milling of Maize on the Chemical Composition and the Nutritive Value of Maize-Meal." *Journal of Physiology* 47, no. 4–5 (1913): 389–92.

Garrison, P. E. "The Recent Pellagra Clinic at Columbia, S.C." *United States Naval Bulletin for the Information of the Medical Department of the Service* 6, no. 1 (1912): 152–57.

Gibbes, James H. "Fifty Years of Medicine: Retrospect and Prospect." *Journal of the South Carolina Medical Association* 51, no. 6 (1955): 192–93.

Goldberger, Joseph. "The Cause and Prevention of Pellagra." *Public Health Reports* 29, no. 37 (1914): 2354-57.

———. "The Etiology of Pellagra. The Significance of Certain Epidemiological Observations with Respect Thereto." *Public Health Reports* 29, no. 26 (1914): 1683–86.

Goldberger, Joseph, C. H. Waring, and David G. Willets. "The Prevention of Pellagra: A Test of Diet Among Institutional Inmates." *Public Health Reports* 30, no. 43 (1915): 3117-31.

Goldberger, Joseph, and W. F. Tanner. "A Study of the Pellagra-Preventive Action of Dried Beans, Casein, Dried Milk, and Brewers' Yeast, with a Consideration of the Essential Preventive Factors Involved." *Public Health Reports* 40, no. 2 (1925): 54-80.

Goldberger, Joseph, and G. A. Wheeler. "Experimental Pellagra in the Human Subject Brought About by a Restricted Diet." *Public Health Reports* 30, no. 46 (1915): 3336-39.

Goldberger, Joseph, G. A. Wheeler, Edgar Sydenstricker, and R. E. Tarbetto. "A Study of the Relation of Factors of a Sanitary Character to Pellagra Incidence in Seven Cotton-Mill Villages of South Carolina in 1916." *Public Health Reports* 35, no. 29 (1920): 1701-14.

Goldberger, Joseph, G. A. Wheeler, and Edgar Sydenstricker. "A Study of the Relation of Family Income and Other Economic Factors to Pellagra Incidence in Seven Cotton-Mill Villages of South Carolina in 1916." *Public Health Reports* 35, no. 46 (1920): 2673-714.

Goldberger, Joseph, G. A. Wheeler, and W. F. Tanner, "Yeast in the Treatment of Pellagra and Black Tongue. A Note on Dosage and Mode of Administration." *Public Health Reports* 40, no. 19 (1925): 927-28.

Goldsmith, Grace A., Herbert P. Sarett, U.D. Register, and Janis Gibbins. "Studies of Niacin Requirement in Man I: Experimental Pellagra in Subjects on Corn Diets Low in Niacin and Tryptophan." *Journal of Clinical Investigation* 31, no. 6 (1952): 533-42.

Green, H. M. "Report for the National Pellagra Commission." *Journal of the National Medical Association* 6, no. 1 (1914): 1-9.

Griminger, Paul. "Casimir Funk: A Biographical Sketch (1884-1967)." *Journal of Nutrition* 102, no. 9 (1972): 1105-13.

Grimm, R. M. "Pellagra: A Report of an Epidemiologic Study." *Public Health Reports* 27, no. 8 (1912): 255–64.

Gross, Dominik, and Gereon Schäfer. "100th Anniversary of the Death of Ricketts: Howard Taylor Ricketts (1871–1910); The Namesake of the Rickettsiaceae Family." *Microbes & Infection* 13, no. 1 (2011): 10–13.

Hall, William S. "Psychiatrist, Humanitarian, and Scholar: James Woods Babcock, M.D." *Journal of the South Carolina Medical Association* 66, no. 10 (1970): 366–71.

Haller, John S. Jr. "Race, Mortality, and Life Insurance: Negro Vital Statistics in the Late Nineteenth Century." *Journal of the History of Medicine and Allied Sciences* 25, no. 3 (1970): 247–61.

Halstead, Scott B. "Etiologies of the Experimental Dengues of Siler and Simmons." *American Journal of Tropical Medicine and Hygiene* 23, no. 5 (1974): 974–82.

Harden, Victoria A. "Koch's Postulates and the Etiology of Rickettsial Diseases." *Journal of the History of Medicine and Allied Sciences* 42, no. 3 (1987): 277–95.

Harkness, Jon M. "Prisoners and Pellagra." *Public Health Reports* 111, no. 5 (1986): 463–67.

Harris, S. J. "Pellagra." *Kentucky Medical Journal* 16, no. 3 (1918): 106–8.

Harris, William H. "The Experimental Production of Pellagra in the Monkey by a Berkefeld Filtrate Derived from Human Lesions: A Preliminary Note." *Journal of the American Medical Association* 60, no. 25 (1913): 1948–50.

Hayne, James A. "The History of Pellagra in South Carolina." *Journal of the South Carolina Medical Association* 28, no. 8 (1932): 205–9.

"Historical Perspectives. Notifiable Disease Surveillance and Notifiable Disease Statistics: United States June 1946 and June 1996." *Morbidity and Mortality Weekly Report* 45, no. 25 (1996): 530–36.

Holland, Henry. "On the Pellagra, a Disease Prevailing in Lombardy." *Medico-Chirurgical Transactions of London* 8 (1817): 315–46.

Horwitt, Max K., Alfred E. Harper, and LaVell M. Henderson. "Niacin-tryptophan relationships for evaluating niacin equivalents." *American Journal of Clinical Nutrition* 34, no. 3 (1981): 423–27.

Horwitz, Allan V., and Gerald N. Grob. "The Checkered History of American Psychiatric Epidemiology." *Milbank Quarterly* 89, no. 4 (2011): 628–57.

"The Hospital and the Doctors." *Journal of the South Carolina Medical Association* 5, no. 5 (1909): 238–39.

Howard, Herbert B. "James Woods Babcock, A.B., M.D., L.L.D." *American Journal of Psychiatry* 78 [1, n.s.], no. 4 (1922): 709–11.

Humphreys, Margaret. "How Four Once Common Diseases were Eliminated from the American South." *Health Affairs* 28, no. 6 (2009): 1734–44.

Hurd, Henry M. "Three-Quarters of a Century of Institutional Care of the Insane in the United States." *American Journal of Insanity* 69, no. 3 (1913): 469–81.

Hyde, James Nevins. "Pellagra and Some of its Problems." *American Journal of the Medical Sciences* 139, no. 1 (1910): 1–26.

Ihde, Aaron J., and Stanley L. Backer, "Conflict of Concepts in Early Vitamin Studies." *Journal of the History of Biology* 41, no. 1 (1971): 1–33.

"The Importance of Rational Inductive Methods in Advancing Knowledge." *Journal of Tropical Medicine and Hygiene* 11, no. 3 (1908): 41–42.

"In Memoriam: H. Douglas Singer, 1875–1940." *American Journal of Psychiatry* 97, no. 4 (1941): 1002–4.

"The Increasing Prevalence of Pellagra." *Journal of the American Medical Association* 96, no. 8 (1931): 614.

Jennings, Allan H. "Summary of Two Years' Study of Insects in Relation to Pellagra." *Journal of Parasitology* 1, no. 1 (1914): 10–21. Also published in abbreviated form as "Summary of Two Years' Study of Insects in Relation to Pellagra." *Science* 39, n.s., no. 1013 (1914): 794–95.

Jennings, Allan H., and W. V. King. "An Intensive Study of Insects as a Possible Etiologic Factor in Pellagra." *American Journal of the Medical Sciences* 146, no. 3 (1913): 411–40. Also in *Pellagra. First Progress Report of the Thompson-McFadden Pellagra Commission of the New York Post-Graduate Medical School and Hospital*, 81–110.

Jukes, Thomas H. "The Prevention and Conquest of Scurvy, Beri-Beri, and Pellagra." *Preventive Medicine* 18, no. 6 (1989): 877–83.

Kamminga, Harmke. "Credit and Resistance: Eijkman and the Transformation of Beri-beri into a Vitamin Deficiency Disease." *Clio Medica* 48 (1998): 232–54.

Kerr, W. J. W. "The Cause of Pellagra, as Seen by a Veteran." *American Journal of Clinical Medicine* 23, no. 9 (1916), 785–86.

King, Barrington. "The Conquest of Pellagra." *The State Magazine* (Columbia, S.C.; supplement to *The State*), August 23, 1953, 6–7.

King, Howard D. "The Etiologic Controversy Regarding Pellagra." *Journal of the American Medical Association* 54, no. 11 (1910): 859–66.

Kirkland, Larry R., and Charles S. Bryan. "Osler's Service: A View of the Charts." *Journal of Medical Biography* 15 (2007, supplement 1): 50–54.

Klein, Alexander. "Personal Income of U.S. States: Estimates for the Period 1880–1910." http://www2.warwick.ac.uk/fac/soc/economics/research/papers_2009/twerp_916.pdf (accessed July 16, 2013).

Koo, Denise, and Stephen B. Thacker. "In Snow's Footsteps: Commentary on Shoe-Leather and Applied Epidemiology." *American Journal of Epidemiology* 172, no. 6 (2010): 737–39.

Kushner, Howard I. "The Art of Medicine: Medical Historians and the History of Medicine." *Lancet* 372 (August 30, 2008): 710–11.

———. "Cesare Lombroso and the Pathology of Left-Handedness." *Lancet* 377 (January 8, 2011): 118–19.

Lanska, Douglas J. "Stages in the Recognition of Epidemic Pellagra in the United States, 1865–1960." *Neurology* 47, no. 3 (1996): 829–34.

"The Late Colonel F. M. Sandwith." *Lancet* 1 (May 25, 1918): 754.

Lavinder, C. H. "The Association for the Study of Pellagra: A Report of the Second Triennial Meeting Held at Columbia, S.C., October 3–4, 1912." *Public Health Reports* 27, no. 44 (1912): 1776–79.

———. "The National Congress on Pellagra, Held at Columbia, S.C., November 3 and 4, 1909." *Public Health Reports* 24, no. 46 (1909): 1697–1702.

———. "A Note on the Inoculation of the Rhesus Monkey with Blood, Spinal Fluid, and Nervous Tissue from Pellagrins." *Public Health Reports* 26, no. 26 (1911): 1005–6.

———. "The Prevalence and Geographic Distribution of Pellagra in the United States." *Public Health Reports* 27, no. 50 (1912): 2076–88.

———. "The Prophylaxis of Pellagra." *Public Health Reports* 24, no. 44 (1909): 1617–24.

———. "The Theory of the Parasitic Origin of Pellagra." *Public Health Reports* 25, no. 21 (1910): 735–37.

Lavinder, C. H., C. F. Williams, and J. W. Babcock. "The Prevalence of Pellagra in the United States—A Statistical and Geographical Note, with Bibliography." *Public Health Reports* 24, no. 25 (1909): 849–52. Revised versions in *Journal of the South Carolina Medical Association* 5, no. 8 (1909): 351–54; in *Proceedings of the American Medico-Psychological Association. Sixty-Fifth Annual Meeting, Atlantic City, N.J., June 1–4, 1909.* Baltimore: American Medico-Psychological Association, 1909; and as *The Prevalence of Pellagra in the United States: A Statistical and Geographical Note, with Bibliography.* Washington, D.C.: Government Printing Office, 1909.

Lavinder, C. H., Edward Francis, R. M. Grimm, and W. F. Lorenz. "Attempts to Transmit Pellagra to Monkeys." *Journal of the American Medical Association* 63, no. 13 (1914): 1093–94.

Lewinsohn, Rachel. "Prophet in his Own Country: Carlos Chagas and the Nobel Prize." *Perspectives in Biology and Medicine* 46, no. 4 (2003) 532–49.

Little, Y. A. "The Dietetic Treatment of Pellagra, with Report of Eleven Cases." *Southern Medical Journal* 8, no. 8 (1915): 659–62.

Livingstone, David N. "Tropical Climate and Moral Hygiene: The Anatomy of a Victorian Debate." *British Journal of the History of Science* 32, no. 1 (1999): 93–110.

"Louis Sambon, M.D." *British Medical Journal* 2 (September 12, 1931): 514-15.

"Louis Sambon, M.D. Naples." *Lancet* 2 (September 12, 1931): 613.

MacNeal, W. J. "The Infectious Etiology of Pellagra." *Southern Medical Journal* 15, no. 11 (1922): 899-902.

"Mandatory Reporting of Infectious Diseases by Clinicians." *Morbidity and Mortality Weekly Reports* 33, no. RR-9 (1990): 1-11, 16-17.

Manson, Patrick, E. R. Rost, L. W. Sambon, Ronald Ross, C. W. Daniels, James Cantlie, W. T. Prout, P. A. Nightingale, and Wm. Kynsney. "A Discussion on Beri-Beri." *British Medical Journal* 2 (September 20, 1902): 830-39.

Mariani-Costantini, Renato, and Aldo Mariani-Costantini. "An Outline of the History of Pellagra in Italy." *Journal of Anthropological Sciences* 85 (2007): 163-71.

Marks, Harry M. "Epidemiologists Explain Pellagra: Gender, Race, and Political Economy in the Work of Edgar Sydenstricker." *Journal of the History of Medicine and Allied Sciences* 58, no. 1 (2003): 34-55.

Mazzarello, Paolo. "Cesare Lombroso: An Anthropologist between Evolution and Degeneration." *Functional Neurology* 26, no. 2 (2011): 97-101.

McCandless, Peter. "A Female Malady? Women at the South Carolina Lunatic Asylum, 1828-1915." *Journal of the History of Medicine and Allied Sciences* 54, no. 4 (1999): 543-71.

McConnell, H. E. "Clinical Observations of Pellagra." *Journal of the South Carolina Medical Association* 4, no. 11 (1908): 569-71.

McKie, Thomas J. "A Brief History of Insanity and Tuberculosis in the Southern Negro." *Journal of the American Medical Association* 28, no. 12 (1897): 537-38.

Miller, Donald F. "Pellagra Deaths in the United States." *American Journal of Clinical Nutrition* 31, no. 4 (1978): 558-59.

Miller, Henry W. "Report of a Case of Pellagra in Maine with Remarks upon Recent Work on the Etiology of the Disease." *American Journal of Insanity* 69, no. 3 (1913); 551-57.

Milling, C. J. "Pellagra and the New Deal." *Journal of the South Carolina Medical Association* 32, no. 9 (1936): 209-13.

Mitchener, Kris James, and Ian W. McLean, "U.S. Regional Growth and Convergence, 1880-1980." *Journal of Economic History* 59, no. 4 (1999): 1016-42.

Monaco, Francesco, and Marco Mula, "Cesare Lombroso and Epilepsy 100 Years Later: An Unabridged Report of his Original Transactions." *Epilepsia* 52, no. 4 (2011): 679-88.

Moore, Noel M. "Etiology of Pellagra." *Journal of the South Carolina Medical Association* 4, no. 11 (1908): 558-60.

Muncey, Elizabeth B. "A Study of the Heredity of Pellagra in Spartanburg County, South Carolina." *Archives of Internal Medicine* 18, no. 1 (1916): 32-75. Also in

Pellagra III. Third Report of the Robert M. Thompson Pellagra Commission of the New York Post-Graduate Medical School and Hospital, 373–416.

Munyon, Paul Glenn, "A Critical Review of Estimates of Net Income from Agriculture for 1880 and 1900: New Hampshire, a Case Study." *Journal of Economic History* 37, no. 3 (1977): 634–54.

Nakagawa, Itsiro, Tetsuzo Takahashi, Atsuko Sasaki, Masatoshi Kajimoto, and Taeko Suzuki, "Efficiency of Conversion of Tryptophan to Niacin in Humans," *Journal of Nutrition* 103, no. 8 (1973): 1195–99.

"National Conference on Pellagra." *Southern Medical Journal* 5, no. 5 (1912): 361–62.

"News from the Classes." *Harvard Graduates' Magazine* 30, no. 120 (June 1922): 563.

Nichols, Henry J., and William H. Hough. "Demonstration of *Spirochaeta Pallida* in the Cerebrospinal Fluid from a Patient with Nervous Relapse Following the Use of Salvarsan." *Journal of the American Medical Association* 60, no. 2 (1913): 108–10.

"Notes and Comment." *American Journal of Insanity* 65, no. 2 (1908–1909): 377–84.

"Notes and Comment: South Carolina and Her State Hospital." *American Journal of Insanity* 71, no. 4 (1915): 799–805.

Novy, Frederick G., and Ward J. MacNeal. "On the Trypanosomes of Birds." *Journal of Infectious Diseases* 2, no. 2 (1905): 256–308.

"Obituary Notice of James Woods Babcock, M.D., L.L.D." *Bulletin of the Phillips Exeter Academy,* April 1922: 25.

Paneth, Nigel, Ezra Susser, and Mervyn Susser. "Origins and Early Development of the Case-Control Study: Part 1, Early Evolution." *Arbeitsmed Soz Praventivmed* 47, no. 5 (2002): 282–88.

Park, Youngmee K., Christopher T. Sempos, Curtis N. Barton, John E. Vanderveen, and Elizabeth A. Yetley. "Effectiveness of Food Fortification in the United States: The Case of Pellagra." *American Journal of Public Health* 90, no. 5 (2000): 727–38.

"The Pellagra Conference." *Journal of the South Carolina Medical Association* 8, no. 10 (1912): 262–66.

"Pellagra Conference." *Southern Medical Journal* 6, no. 10 (1913): 690–91.

"Pellagra in this Country." *Journal of the South Carolina Medical Association* 4, no. 2 (1908): 60–61.

"Pellagra Symposium, Report of Committee on Prevention and Treatment of Pellagra." *Journal of the American Medical Association* 65, no. 23 (1915): 2029–31.

"Pellagracide and Ez-X-Ba: Fraudulent Nostrums Sold as Cures of Pellagra." *Journal of the American Medical Association* 58, no. 9 (1912): 648–49.

Peloquin, Suzanne M. "Occupational Therapy Service: Individual and Collective Understandings of the Founders, Part 1." *American Journal of Occupational Therapy* 45, no. 4 (1991): 352–60.

"Personal." *Journal of the South Carolina Medical Association* 5, no. 5 (1909): 237.

Piro, Anna, Giuseppe Tagarelli, Paolo Lagonia, Antonio Tagarelli, and Aldo Quattrone. "Casimir Funk: His Discovery of the Vitamins and their Deficiency Disorders." *Annals of Nutrition and Metabolism* 57, no. 2 (2010): 85–88.

Powell, Theophilus O. "The Increase of Insanity and Tuberculosis in the Southern Negro since 1860, and its Alliance, and Some of the Supposed Causes." *Journal of the American Medical Association* 27, no. 23 (1896): 1185–88.

Powers, Bernard E. Jr. "'The Worst of all Barbarism': Racial Anxiety and the Approach of Secession in the Palmetto State." *South Carolina Historical Magazine* 112, nos. 3–4 (2011): 139–56.

Preskill, Stephen. "Educating for Democracy: Charles W. Eliot and the Differentiated Curriculum." *Educational Theory* 39, no. 4 (1989): 351–58.

Rajakumar, Kumaravel. "Pellagra in the United States: A Historical Perspective." *Southern Medical Journal* 93, no. 3 (2000): 272–77.

Randolph, James H. "Notes on Pellagra and Pellagrins, with Report of Cases." *Archives of Internal Medicine* 2, no. 6 (1908–1909): 553–68.

Ray, W. W., J. H. Taylor, J. W. Babcock, J. L., J. L. Thompson, H. H. Griffin, and Eleanora B. Saunders. "What are Pellagra and Pellagrous Insanity? Does Such a Disease Exist in South Carolina, and What are its Causes? An Inquiry and a Preliminary Report to the South Carolina State Board of Health." *Journal of the South Carolina Medical Association* 4, no. 2 (1908): 64–76. Also in *American Journal of Insanity* 64, no. 4 (1907–1908), 703–25.

"Recent Investigations on Pellagra." *Nature* 84 (October 27, 1910): 538–39.

"Reconciled." *New Yorker*, May 18, 1963, 30–32.

"Requiem for a Gracious Gentlewoman." *Journal of the South Carolina Medical Association* 64, no. 5 (1968): 205–7.

Johnson, Steven. Review of *Where Good Ideas Come From*. *New Yorker*, November 8, 2010, 84.

Rice, H. W. "The Etiology of Pellagra in Children: A Study of Two Hundred Cases in Orphanages." *Southern Medical Journal* 9, no. 9 (1916): 778–85.

———. "Pellagra in Children, with Observations on Eighty-Five Cases in Two Orphanages." *Journal of the South Carolina Medical Association* 9, no. 6 (1913): 146–52.

Roberts, Stewart R. "Sambon's New Theory of Pellagra and its Application to Conditions in Georgia." *Journal of the American Medical Association* 56, no. 23 (1911): 1713–15.

Russell, William L. "The Medical Service of State Hospitals for the Insane." *American Journal of Insanity* 66, no. 3 (1910): 365–82.

Sambon, Louis W. "The Elucidation of Sleeping Sickness." *Journal of Tropical Medicine* 7, no. 4 (1904): 61-63; 7, no. 5 (1904): 68-74; 7, no. 6 (1904): 87–91. Also in *Transactions of the Epidemiological Society of London* 23 n.s. (1904): 16–78.

———. "Progress Report on the Investigation of Pellagra." *Journal of Tropical Medicine and Hygiene* [London] 13, no. 18 (1910): 271–82; 13, no. 19 (1910): 287–300; 13, no. 20 (1910): 306–15; 13, no. 21 (1910): 319–21.

———. "Remarks on the Geographical Distribution and Etiology of Pellagra." *British Medical Journal* 2 (November 11, 1905): 1272–75. Also in *Journal of the South Carolina Medical Association* 5, no. 2 (1909): 68–73; and in "Proceedings of the Section on Tropical Diseases, Seventy-Third Annual Meeting of the British Medical Association, held at Leicester, July 24th, 25th, 26th, 27th, and 28th, 1905." *British Medical Journal* 2 (November 11, 1905): 1272-75.

"Sand-fly Transmission of Pellagra." *Journal of the American Medical Association* 55, no. 22 (1910): 1898.

Sandwith, F. M. "Is Pellagra a Disease due to Deficiency of Nutrition?" *Transactions of the Society of Tropical Medicine and Hygiene* 6, no. 5 (1913): 143–48.

———. "Pellagra in the Thirty-Five States of America." *Transactions of the Society of Tropical Medicine and Hygiene* 5, no. 3 (1912): 120–24.

Sandifer, S. Hope. "Pellagra in South Carolina." *Journal of the South Carolina Medical Association* 77, no. 12 (1981): 602-4.

Saunders, Eleanora B. "The Gynecological, Obstetrical, and Surgical Aspects of Pellagra. *American Journal of Insanity* 67, no. 3 (1911): 541–51. Also in *Transactions of the National Conference on Pellagra Held Under Auspices of South Carolina State Board of Health at the State Hospital for the Insane, Columbia, S.C., November 3 and 4, 1909.* Columbia, S.C.: State, 1910; and in expanded form as "The Gynecological, Obstetrical, and Surgical Aspects of Pellagra: A Second Report," in *Proceedings of the American Medico-Psychological Association. Sixty-Seventh Annual Meeting, Denver, Colorado, June 19–22, 1911.* Baltimore: American Medico-Psychological Association, 1911.

———. "A Study of Depressions in Late Life with Special Reference to Content." *American Journal of Insanity* 88, no. 5 (1932): 925–48.

Savitt, Todd L. "Entering a White Profession: Black Physicians in the New South, 1880-1920." *Bulletin of the History of Medicine* 61, no. 4 (1987): 507-40.

———. "Walking the Color Line: Alonzo McClennan, the *Hospital Herald*, and Segregated Medicine in Turn-of-the-Twentieth Century Charleston, South Carolina." *South Carolina Historical Magazine* 104, no. 4 (2003): 228–57.

Schultz, Myron G. "Joseph Goldberger and Pellagra." *American Journal of Tropical Medicine and Hygiene* 26, no. 5, pt. 2 suppl. (1977): 1088–92.

Searcy, George H. "An Epidemic of Acute Pellagra." *Transactions of the Medical Association of the State of Alabama*, April 1907, 387–92. Also in abbreviated form as "An Epidemic of Acute Pellagra," *Journal of the American Medical Association* 49, no. 1 (1907): 37–38.

Seidell, Atherton. "A Stable Form of Vitamine, Efficient in the Prevention and Cure of Certain Nutritional Deficiency Diseases." *Public Health Reports* 31, no. 7 (1916): 364–70.

Semba, Richard D. "Thèophile Roussel and the Elimination of Pellagra from 19th Century France." *Nutrition* 16, no. 3 (2000): 231–33.

Siler, Joseph F., and Philip E. Garrison. "An Intensive Study of the Epidemiology of Pellagra. Report of Progress." *American Journal of the Medical Sciences* 146, no. 1 (1913): 42–66, 238–77. Also in *Pellagra. First Progress Report of the Thompson-McFadden Pellagra Commission of the New York Post-Graduate Medical School and Hospital*, 17–80.

Siler, J. F., P. E. Garrison, and W. J. MacNeal. "Pellagra: A Summary of the First Progress Report of the Thompson-McFadden Commission." *Journal of the American Medical Association* 62, no. 1 (1914): 8–12. Also in *Pellagra: First Progress Report of the Thompson-McFadden Pellagra Commission of the New York Post-Graduate Medical School and Hospital*, 3–14.

———. "Further Studies of the Thompson-McFadden Commission: A Summary of the Second Progress Report." *Journal of the American Medical Association* 63, no. 13 (1914): 1090–93. Also in *Pellagra II: Second Progress Report of the Thompson-McFadden Pellagra Commission of the New York Post-Graduate Medical School and Hospital*, 1–10.

———. "Introduction to the Third Report of the Robert M. Thompson Pellagra Commission of the New York Post-Graduate Medical School and Hospital." *Archives of Internal Medicine* 18, no. 1 (1916): 1–3. Also in *Pellagra III: Third Report of the Robert M. Thompson Pellagra Commission of the New York Post-Graduate Medical School and Hospital*, 1–3.

Smith, David T., and Julian M. Ruffin. "Effect of Sunlight on the Clinical Manifestations of Pellagra." *Archives of Internal Medicine* 59, no. 4 (1937): 631–45.

"South Carolina and Her State Hospital." *American Journal of Insanity* 71, no. 4 (1915): 799–805.

Spencer, T. N. "Is 'Black Tongue' in Dogs Pellagra?" *American Journal of Veterinary Medicine* 11 (1916): 325.

Spies, Tom Douglas, William Bennett Bean, and Robert E. Stone. "The Treatment of Subclinical and Classical Pellagra: Use of Nicotinic Acid, Nicotinic Acid Amide and Sodium Nicotinate, with Special Reference to the Vasodilator Action and the Effect on Mental Symptoms." *Journal of the American Medical Association* 111, no. 7 (1938): 584–92.

"State Health Officer." *Journal of the South Carolina Medical Association* 4, no. 2 (1908): 61.

Stone, Clarence N. "Bleaseism and the 1912 Election in South Carolina." *North Carolina Historical Review* 40 (January 1963): 54–74.

Streeter, Carrie. "Theatrical Entertainments and Kind Words: Nursing the Insane in Western North Carolina, 1882–1907." *Journal of Psychiatric and Mental Health Nursing* 18, no. 10 (2011): 904–13.

"Studies of Pellagra." *Journal of the American Medical Association* 65, no. 21 (1915): 1818–19.

Summers, Martin. "'Suitable Care of the African When Afflicted With Insanity': Race, Madness, and Social Order in Comparative Perspective." *Bulletin of the History of Medicine* 84, no. 1 (2010): 58–91.

Sydenstricker, V. P. "The History of Pellagra, Its Recognition as a Disorder of Nutrition and its Conquest." *American Journal of Clinical Nutrition* 6, no. 4 (1958): 409–14.

———. "The Impact of Vitamin Research upon Medical Practice." *Proceedings of the Nutrition Society* 12, no. 3 (1953): 256–69.

Taylor, Isaac M. "Personal Experience with Some Cases of Nervous and Mental Diseases Showing the Pellagra Syndrome." *Journal of the South Carolina Medical Association* 4, no. 11 (1908): 573–75.

Taylor, J. H. "The Protozoan Theory of Pellagra." *Journal of the South Carolina Medical Association* 4, no. 11 (1908): 552–56.

Thompson, J. L. "The Roumanian Theory as to the Cause of Pellagra." *Journal of the South Carolina Medical Association* 4, no. 11 (1908): 560–62.

Tillman, Benjamin R. "How I Restored my Health and Vigor." *Physical Culture* 37, no. 4 (1917): 7–15.

Tomes, Nancy J., and John Harley Warner, "Introduction to Special Issue on Rethinking the Reception of the Germ Theory of Disease: Comparative Perspectives," *Journal of the History of Medicine and Allied Sciences* 52, no. 1 (1997): 7–16.

Vedder, Edward B. "Dietary Deficiency as the Etiological Factor in Pellagra." *Archives of Internal Medicine* 18, no. 2 (1916): 137–72. Also in *Pellagra III: Third Report of the Robert M. Thompson Pellagra Commission of the New York Post-Graduate Medical School and Hospital,* 337–73.

———. "Some Further Remarks on Beri-beri." *American Journal of Tropical Diseases and Preventive Medicine* 1, no. 12 (1914): 826–47.

Voegtlin, Carl. "Recent Work on Pellagra." *Public Health Reports* 35, no. 25 (1920): 1435–52.

————."The Treatment of Pellagra." *Journal of the American Medical Association* 63, no. 13 (1914): 1094–98.

Wan, P., S. Moat, and A. Antsley. "Pellagra: A Review with Emphasis on Photosensitivity." *British Journal of Dermatology* 164, no. 6 (2011): 1188–200.

Watson, J. J. "Etiology of Pellagra: The Italian Maize Theory, or the Theory of Lombroso." *Journal of the South Carolina Medical Association* 4, no. 11 (1908): 549–52.

"Waverley Sanitarium, Inc." (advertisement). *Journal of the South Carolina Medical Association* 31, no. 1 (1935): 19.

"What is the Cause of Pellagra?" *Journal of the American Medical Association* 76, no. 23 (1921): 1577.

Wheeler, G. A., Joseph Goldberger, and M. R. Blackstock. "On the Probable Identity of the Chittenden-Underhill Pellagralike Syndrome in Dogs and 'Blacktongue.'" *Public Health Reports* 37, no. 18 (1922): 1063–69.

White, William A. "Presidential Address." *American Journal of Psychiatry* 5, [82], no. 1 (1925): 1–20.

"Why Blease Won." *Literary Digest* 45, no. 11 (14 September 1912): 410.

Wilkinson, J. G. "Pellagra: Symptoms, Diagnosis, and Treatment." *Southern Medical Journal* 4, no. 8 (1911): 607–9.

Wilkinson, Lise. "AJE Terzi and LW Sambon: Early Italian Influences on Patrick Manson's 'Tropical Medicine,' Entomology, and the Art of Entomological Illustration in London." *Medical History* 46, no. 4 (2002): 569–79.

Willcock, Edith G., and F. Gowland Hopkins, "The Importance of Individual Amino-acids in Metabolism," *Journal of Physiology* 35, nos. 1–2 (1906): 88–102.

Williams, Adrian C., and David B. Ramsden, "Pellagra: A Clue as to why Energy Failure Causes Diseases?" *Medical Hypotheses* 69, no. 3 (2007): 618–28.

Williams, Robert R. "Edward Bright Vedder: A Biographical Sketch (June 28, 1878–1952)." *Journal of Nutrition* 77 (May 1962): 3–6.

Wilson, Robert Jr. Discussion of James A. Hayne, "The History of Pellagra in South Carolina," *Journal of the South Carolina Medical Association* 28, no. 8 (1932): 205–9.

Wolff. "Are the Jews Immune to Pellagra?" *Southern Medical Journal* 5, no. 2 (1912): 116–24.

Wood, Edward Jenner. "The Appearance of Pellagra in the United States." *Journal of the American Medical Association* 53, no. 4 (1909): 274–82.

————. "The Etiology of Pellagra: A Consideration of Vitamin Deficiency." *American Journal of the Medical Sciences* 152, no. 6 (1916): 813–22.

————."'Pellagra sine Pellagra' with a Differential Diagnosis from Sprue." *Transactions of the Tri-State Medical Association* 11 (1909): 446–50.

————."Pellagra: Some Problems in the Study of its Etiology." *Journal of the South Carolina Medical Association* 4, no. 11 (1908): 556–58.

Wood, Edward Jenner, and R. Harlee Bellamy. "Pellagra." *Bulletin of the North Carolina Board of Health* 24, no. 7 (1909): 83–91.

Worthington, W. Curtis Jr., "Psychiatrist and Humanitarian Sarah Campbell Allan (1861–1954): South Carolina's First Licensed Woman Physician." *Journal of the South Carolina Medical Association* 89, no. 1 (1993): 9–14.

————."A Study in Post-Flexner Survival: The Medical College of the State of South Carolina, 1913." *Journal of the American Medical Association* 266, no. 7 (1991): 981–84.

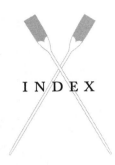

INDEX

Page numbers in italics denote illustrations.

Medical College of the State of South
Carolina, 32, 33, 34, 53, 124, 198,
201, 223, 224
medical history, usefulness of, 149–52,
321n36
mental illness: diseases and their
classifications (nosology), 69–71,
299n159, 334n19; history of, 17. *See
also* drug therapy, for mental illness;
hydrotherapy, for mental illness;
mechanotherapy, for mental illness;
moral therapy, for mental illness;
psychiatry; restraint of patients,
mechanical
metabolism, role of niacin in, 78–79
Metchnikoff, Eli, 305n41
Meyer, Adolf, 250
Milady, John, 296n105
Miller, George N., 164
Miller, Stephen D., 28
Mills, Robert, 28, 289n5
Minot, Charles S., 13
Minot, Francis, 14
Mississippi State Penitentiary (Rankin
Farm), 233, 240, 244, 248, 273,
347n64
Mitchell, J. M., 123–24
Mitchell, Silas Weir, 110, 310n112
Mizell, George C., 178, 320n34
molds (fungi). *See* Pellagra, causal
explanations of,
Moore, Noel M., 98
Mt. Vernon Hospital for the Colored
Insane (Ala.), 104
moral therapy, for mental illness, 17, 26
Muncey, Elizabeth B., 348n77
Murphy, Patrick Livingston, 66, 67, 141
Murray, Patrick J., 226

NAD+/NADH, 77–79, 301n3, 302n4
National Association for the Study of
Pellagra, xxvi, 77, 102, 111, 173, 176,
185, 233, 240, 246–47, 261, 271,

285n10. *See also*, Columbia, South
Carolina, pellagra, conferences in
National Hygienic Laboratory
(Washington, D.C.), 158, 167–69,
226, 245, 308n79
National Medical Association, 236,
323n58
National Pure Food and Drug Act,
157, 158
Native Americans, 75. *See also* Catawba
Indians, Cherokee Nation, Pre-
Columbian Indians
neurology, as medical specialty, 14, 26,
110, 289n2
New Jersey State Hospital, 134
New York Hospital, 254
niacin, xxiii, 77–81, 79, 111, 173,
199, 242, 248, 267, 274, 275, 276,
301n3, 302n7. *See also* nicotinamide,
nicotinic acid
Nichols, Henry J., 110, 111, 163
Nicolaidi, Jean, 177, 178
nicotinamide, 78–79, 79, 271, 274, 275,
302n4, 302n7
nicotinic acid, 78–79, 79, 173, 188, 191,
248, 272, 274, 275, 302n4, 302n7
Niles, George M., 149
Noguchi, Hideyo, 334n21
Nott, Josiah Clark, 50
Novy, Frederick G., 164
Nurses. *See* South Carolina State
Hospital for the Insane, nurses at
nursing schools, 18–19, 73–74, 224,
299n168
nutrition. *See* diet

occupational therapy, at asylums, 30,
135, 290n15, 314n54
Odoardi, Jacopo, 83
Olmsted, Frederick Law, 18
orphanages, pellagra in, 100. *See also*
Epworth Orphanage; Jackson
(Miss.) orphanages

U.S. Public Health and Marine
   Hospital Service, 77, 96, 101,
   107–8, 143, 160, 162, 164–65, 176,
   309n81
U.S. Public Health Service, 101,
   166–71, 186, 225, 229–30, 236, 255,
   309n81

Vedder, Edward B., 174, *243*, 244, 256,
   348n76
Vienna (Austria) Asylum, 46
vitamin A deficiency, xxiii, 285n1
vitamin C deficiency, 285n1
vitamin D deficiency, 285n1
vitamin P-P, 78, 274
"vitamine" hypothesis, 173–76, 179–82,
   268, 272
vitamins, 77–81; definitions of, 78, 173;
   history of discovery of, 173–76,
   328n1. *See also* niacin, riboflavin,
   thiamine, vitamin C
Voegtlin, Carl, 230, 237, 249

War of 1812, 1
Waring, C. H., 238
Warren, Frederic, 286n14
Warren, John Collins, 14
Wassermann, August Paul von, 334n21
Wassermann test, 198, 199, 203–6,
   334n21
Watkins, Rachel, 163
Watson, Ebbie J., 108
Watson, Joseph Jenkins, 75, 96, 98,
   100, 108, 262, 263, 271, 306n54,
   306n55, 320n22
Waverley Sanitarium, 23, 224, 258
Weidel, Hugo, 80, 270
Wellcome, Henry, 249
Western State Hospital (Virginia), 108
Weston, Francis Hopkins, 138–39, 263
Whaley, E. M., 317n4
"What are Pellagra and Pellagrous
   Insanity?" (Ray et al.), 89–92

Wheeler, George A., 240, *241*, 348n79
white supremacy, 42, 51, 292n45
Wilkinson, J. G., 148
Willcock, Edith G., 328n2
Willets, David G., 238
Williams, Charles Frederick, 97, *101*,
   102, 104, 111, 234, 239–40, 262,
   305n39, 344n36
Williams, Robert R., 174
Williams, Robert Runnels, 268
Wilson, Robert Jr., xxiii, 97, 102, 111,
   188, 194–95, *195*, 201
Wines, Frederick Howard, 128–29
Winthrop College, 40, 198
Winthrop, Gilman J., 111
"wisdom" criteria, 287n26
Withers, John S., 22
Wofford College, 96, 187
womanhood, white southern, 53, 207
women's issues: in medicine, 53–54;
   pellagra in, 246. *See also* Allan,
   Sarah Campbell; race and gender
   disparities; womanhood, white
   southern
Women's Medical College of the New
   York Infirmary, 53
Wood, Edward Jenner, 98, 143, 149,
   179
Worcester (Massachusetts) State
   Asylum, 18
World War I, 245, 247, 251, 255
Wyman, Walter, 144, 160
Wyman, Rufus, 18

Yale College, 1, 7, 9
yellow fever, 17, 50, 160, 226, 308n80,
   327n120
Youndin, William, 81

zeist and anti-zeist hypotheses, 87. *See
   also* pellagra, causal explanations of
Zeller, George A., *109*, 110–11, 158,
   162, 271, 310n110